Myelopathy

Benjamin Greenberg
Editor

Myelopathy

A Guide to Diagnosis and Treatment

Springer

Editor
Benjamin Greenberg
Department of Neurology
University of Texas Southwestern
Dallas, TX, USA

ISBN 978-3-030-99905-6 ISBN 978-3-030-99906-3 (eBook)
https://doi.org/10.1007/978-3-030-99906-3

This Springer imprint is published by the registered company Springer Nature Switzerland AG
The registered company address is: Gewerbestrasse 11, 6330 Cham, Switzerland

Contents

Contributors

A. Karim Ahmed, BS, MD Candidate Department of Neurosurgery, The Johns Hopkins Hospital, Baltimore, MD, USA

Matthew N. Andersen, MD Department of Neurosurgery, Warren Alpert School of Medicine, Brown University, Rhode Island Hospital, Providence, RI, USA

Carlos Antonio Bagley, MD, MBA Department of Neurological Surgery, University of Texas Southwestern Medical Center, Dallas, TX, USA

Tarek Y. El Ahmadieh, MD Department of Neurological Surgery, University of Texas Southwestern Medical Center, Dallas, TX, USA

John K. Fink, MD Department of Neurology, University of Michigan, Ann Arbor, MI, USA

Matthew J. Fogarty, BVSc, PhD Department of Physiology and Biomedical Engineering, Mayo Clinic, Rochester, MN, USA

School of Biomedical Sciences, The University of Queensland, Brisbane, QLD, Australia

Jared S. Fridley, MD Department of Neurosurgery, Warren Alpert School of Medicine, Brown University, Rhode Island Hospital, Providence, RI, USA

Philippe Gailloud, MD Division of Interventional Neuroradiology, The Johns Hopkins Hospital, Baltimore, MD, USA

Ziya L. Gokaslan, MD Department of Neurosurgery, Warren Alpert School of Medicine, Brown University, Rhode Island Hospital, Providence, RI, USA

C. Rory Goodwin, MD, PhD Department of Neurosurgery, Duke University Medical Center, Durham, NC, USA

Benjamin Greenberg, MD, MHS, FANA, FAAN, CRND Department of Neurology, University of Texas Southwestern, Dallas, TX, USA

Manraj K. S. Heran, MD, FRCPC Department of Radiology, The University of British Columbia, Vancouver, BC, Canada

Benjamin Kafka, MD Department of Neurological Surgery, University of Texas Southwestern Medical Center, Dallas, TX, USA

Thomas Kosztowski, MD Department of Neurosurgery, Warren Alpert School of Medicine, Brown University, Rhode Island Hospital, Providence, RI, USA

Cornelia Laule, PhD Department of Radiology, The University of British Columbia, Vancouver, BC, Canada

Department of Pathology & Laboratory Medicine, Department of Physics & Astronomy, International Collaboration on Repair Discoveries (ICORD), The University of British Columbia, Vancouver, BC, Canada

Camilo Molina, MD Department of Neurosurgery, Washington University in St Louis, St Louis, MO, USA

Olwen C. Murphy, MBBCh, MRCPI Division of Neuroimmunology and Neuroinfectious Diseases, Department of Neurology, Johns Hopkins University School of Medicine, Baltimore, MD, USA

Ram N. Narayan, MD, MHS Barrow Neurological Institute, Phoenix, AZ, USA

Om James Neeley, MD Department of Neurological Surgery, University of Texas Southwestern Medical Center, Dallas, TX, USA

Adetokunbo A. Oyelese, MD, PhD Department of Neurosurgery, Warren Alpert School of Medicine, Brown University, Rhode Island Hospital, Providence, RI, USA

Zach Pennington, BS, MD Candidate Department of Neurosurgery, The Johns Hopkins Hospital, Baltimore, MD, USA

Department of Neurosurgery, Mayo Clinic, Rochester, MN, USA

Cristina L. Sadowsky, MD Kennedy Krieger Institute, International Center for Spinal Cord Injury, Baltimore, MD, USA

Daniel M. Sciubba, MD Department of Neurosurgery, The Johns Hopkins Hospital, Baltimore, MD, USA

Department of Neurosurgery, Northwell Health/Donald and Barbara Zucker School of Medicine, Manhasset, NY, USA

Jason R. Shewchuk, MD, FRCPC Department of Radiology, The University of British Columbia, Vancouver, BC, Canada

Gary C. Sieck, PhD Department of Physiology and Biomedical Engineering, Mayo Clinic, Rochester, MN, USA

Owen D. M. Stechishin, MD, PhD Department of Radiology, The University of British Columbia, Vancouver, BC, Canada

Sohail Syed, MD, BS Department of Neurosurgery, Warren Alpert School of Medicine, Brown University, Rhode Island Hospital, Providence, RI, USA

Arun Venkatesan, MD, PhD Division of Neuroimmunology and Neuroinfectious Diseases, Department of Neurology, Johns Hopkins University School of Medicine, Baltimore, MD, USA

A. Talia Vertinsky, MD, FRCPC Department of Radiology, The University of British Columbia, Vancouver, BC, Canada

Anatomy of the Spinal Cord

1

Vascular Anatomy of Spinal Cord

Om James Neeley, Tarek Y. El Ahmadieh, Benjamin Kafka, and Carlos Antonio Bagley

Contents

Introduction

A precise understanding of the vascular anatomy of the spinal cord has been an elusive target prior to angiographic elucidation. The inaccessibility of the intramedullary regions of the cord prohibits in vivo studies, combined with the complex and variable blood supply, has limited our knowledge of the anatomy and physiology of the entire cord. In many published texts as late as 1958, vascular anatomy discussions had to be introduced by a reminder of the normal blood supply [1]. Vascular pathologies including infarctions, intermittent spinal claudication, and vascular myelopathies remain largely unexplained in their etiology and pathogenesis. An improved understanding of spinal cord vascular anatomy helps form a base from which we can investigate and explain these complex pathologies. The use of new imaging techniques, including selective spinal angiography, myelography, and magnetic resonance imaging with angiography focus have expanded our

O. J. Neeley · T. Y. El Ahmadieh · B. Kafka · C. A. Bagley (✉)
Department of Neurological Surgery, University of Texas Southwestern Medical Center, Dallas, TX, USA
e-mail: Carlos.bagley@utsouthwestern.edu

B. Greenberg (ed.), *Myelopathy*, https://doi.org/10.1007/978-3-030-99906-3_1

understanding of spinal cord vascular anatomy and enabled researchers to unlock these mysteries [2].

Knowledge of vascular anatomy of the spinal cord is essential for clinicians when diagnosing and treating pathologies affecting the cord. As with all of the neuro-axis, embryologic development dictates the evolution of vascular anatomy in the spinal cord. Therefore, a thorough understanding of this embryology is helpful in understanding both normal vascular anatomy and pathologies that may impact it. In this chapter, we intend to describe – in a simple fashion – the common arteries and veins that are part of spinal cord vascular anatomy as well as some of the more common vascular pathologies that are relevant to the spinal cord. In order to do so, we will begin with a discussion of the embryologic development of the cord, then discuss the arterial and venous anatomy by region of the vertebral column, and finally the pathologies affecting each of these vessels along with common clinical presentations.

Embryology

The spinal cord begins to develop during the third week of gestation [3]. Following the gastrulation phase, the 'notochord' is formed and serves as a foundation for the axial skeleton [3]. Early in the fourth gestational week, the ectodermal tissue overlying the notochord and the adjacent mesoderm differentiates into the neural plate [4] The margins of the neural plate subsequently form neural folds that continue to elevate and ultimately fuse along the dorsal midline creating the neural tube [5, 6] The neural tube and the caudal one-third of the neural plate constitute the future spinal cord, whereas the paraxial mesodermal somites form the axial skeleton [4].

While the embryologic development of the brain vasculature is well-established [7, 8], reports on the development of the spinal cord vasculature are limited [9, 10]. In 1987, Thron et al. studied the spinal cord vascular anatomy of 13 bovine embryos after injecting their umbilical arteries with a dye and gelatin [9]. They noted the first evidence of a primitive vertebral arch surrounding the neural tube in the fifth gestational week as well as a preliminary intramedullary capillary network within the cervical spine [9]. At the seventh gestational week, immature blood vessels with branching segments were noted to invade the dorsolateral aspect of the spinal cord. This occurred in association with the cellular maturation and metabolic demand of the spinal grey matter [9]. By the tenth and eleventh gestational weeks, the spinal cords were found to receive blood supply from a well-formed anterior spinal artery [9]. This anterior spinal artery is formed from longitudinal anastomoses between segmental arteries arising from the dorsal aorta. The majority of these segmental arteries eventually regress as the longitudinal arterial supply matures. Only a few segmental arteries remain until adulthood and form the radiculomedullary arteries. In 2001, Zawilinski et al. studied the developing vasculature of the spinal cords of 50 human fetuses between the tenth and twenty-eighth weeks of gestation [10]. The anterior spinal artery was found to already exist at tenth week of gestation, which is consistent with findings from the previous bovine study. The two posterior spinal arteries were found to mature at a later stage between the fifteenth and the twentieth gestational weeks [10].

The venous system of the spinal cord has shown high variability as compared to the arterial system [10, 11]. Zawilinski et al. found that only the anterior spinal artery and central arteries of the spinal cord were consistently accompanied by venous counterparts [10]. Other veins did not follow the regular arterial distribution. The spinal venous system has been reported to develop as early as the fourth gestational week and begins with the development of the anterior and posterior cardinal veins [11]. Segmental veins later arise from cardinal veins and drain the developing spinal elements into the azygous, renal, and iliac venous systems [11].

Arterial Anatomy

The arterial supply to the spinal cord depends on the level of the cord that is being evaluated and is divided into anterior and posterior networks. At the most rostral end of the spinal cord, the anterior network is supplied by the anterior spinal artery, which arises from the distal vertebral artery. The anterior spinal artery most commonly originates from the medial surface of each vertebral artery and travels medially to converge on the midline near the cervicomedullary junction. This artery then travels caudally along the entire length of the spinal cord in the anterior median fissure, which is the midline cleft that divides the spinal cord into left and right hemicords. This artery sends small perforators into the parenchyma of the spinal cord called the sulcocommisural branches, which supply most of the white and grey matter of the anterior spinal cord [1]. At regular intervals, circumferential pial arteries will take off the anterior spinal artery at 90° angles and travel radially around to the lateral surface of the spinal cord. The anterior spinal artery and its circumferential pial branches perfuse the anterior two-thirds of the spinal cord including the cortical spinal tracts, the anterior horns, and the spinothalamic tracts [12].

The posterior one-third of the cervical spinal cord, including the posterior columns and a small portion of the corticospinal tracts, is supplied by an arterial network formed by two posterior spinal arteries. These posterior spinal arteries can arise from the posterior inferior cerebellar artery or the distal vertebral artery and then travel caudally on the posterior surface of the spinal cord [13]. These arteries give rise to smaller branches that form a network or arcade of arterioles along the posterior surface of the spinal cord. The anterior and posterior spinal arteries form a plexiform network of collaterals between the circumferential pial arteries of the anterior spinal artery and the posterior spinal network on the surface of the spinal cord.

At multiple levels, usually 6–10 in adults [14], along the entire length of the spinal cord there are also arteries known as medullary arteries which anastomose with the anterior and posterior spinal arteries to supply the cord. In the cervical spine, these medullary arteries arise from the vertebral arteries rostrally and the thyrocervical trunk in the caudal cervical spine. The thoracic and lumbar spinal cord is supplied by bilateral segmental arteries, which arise from the aorta rostrally and the iliac arteries at the most caudal levels. Each of these posterior segmental arteries originates from intercostal arteries in the thoracic spine and segmental or radicular arteries in the lumbar spine. They then travel posteriorly from the aorta around the vertebral body and send off a spinal ramus that enters into the nerve root sleeve dura within the vertebral foramen. This artery then divides, sending radicular arteries supplying both the anterior and posterior nerve rootlets arising from the spinal cord, the nerve root sleeve, as well as contributing to the vascular supply of the spinal dura at that level. The spinal ramus will also give off medullary arteries that travel through the dura along the dorsal root ganglion and ascend along the spinal cord to contribute to the anterior and posterior spinal arteries. The anterior and posterior spinal arteries both travel caudally and anastomose at the conus medullaris. The anterior spinal artery continues with the filum terminale after it anastomoses with the posterior spinal artery.

The middle thoracic and lumbar segments of the spinal cord are supplied by the largest medullary artery, the artery of Adamkiewicz or arteria radicularis magna. This most commonly arises from the left segmental artery between T8-L2, but can be seen anywhere from T3-L4. It also can rarely originate from the right segmental artery [15].

The watershed zone of the spinal cord vascular supply lies in the region of T2-4 – between the well-collateralized cervical region and the uppermost region supplied by the artery of Adamkiewicz. The anterior spinal artery is the smallest in this region, which makes this region susceptible to ischemia or infarction during periods of profound hypotension [16]. A lesser watershed zone exits on the anterolateral surface of the spinal cord between the circumferential pial branches of the anterior spinal artery and the posterior spinal arterial arcade [17].

Figure 1.1 shows the arterial anatomy of spinal cord.

Venous Anatomy

The venous drainage of the spinal cord and spinal column can be divided into three systems or plexuses: the intrinsic, extrinsic, and extradural. The intrinsic system is further divided into axial and longitudinal components, both of which drain radially outward and are symmetrically arranged [18]. The arterial supply from the medial portion of both sides of the spinal cord drain to axially oriented ventral and dorsal sulcal. The ventral sulcal vein drains the anterior horns, anterior commissure, and the white matter of the anterior funniculus [19]. The number of ventral sulcal veins varies depending of the segment of spinal cord with increasing number of veins in the lumbosacral when compared to the cervical [20]. The dorsal sulcal veins are smaller and fewer in number, and drain the posterior columns and posterior grey matter [19]. The peripheral grey and white matter not drained by either the dorsal or ventral sulcal veins are drained to the pial surface by small radial veins, which anastomose with the extrinsic network at the pial surface [20]. There is also a intricate anastomotic system of smaller veins connecting the sulcal and radial veins [18].

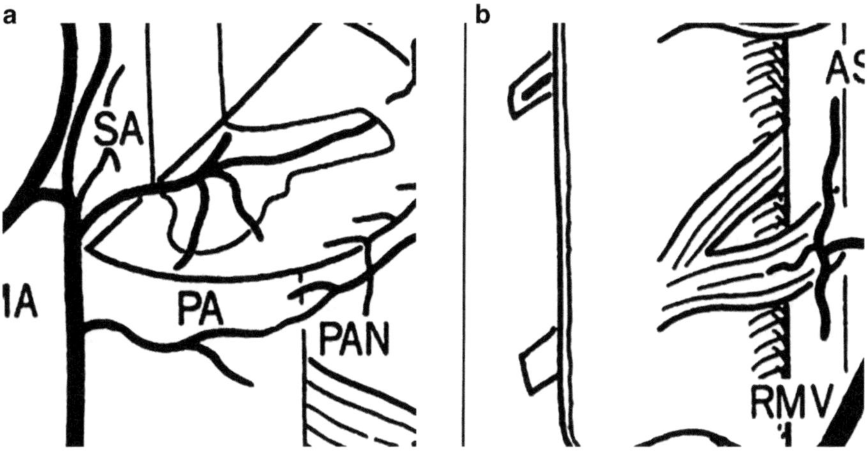

Fig. 1.1 Arterial Anatomy of Spinal Cord. (**a**) Schematic drawing of the arterial supply to the spinal cord. *ASA* anterior spinal artery, *PA* pial artery, *PAN* pial arterial network, *PSA* posterior spinal artery, *RA* radicular artery, *RPA* radiculopial artery, *RMA* radiculomedullary artery, *SA* sulcul artery. (**b**) Schematic drawing of the venous drainage of the spinal cord. *ASV* anterior spinal vein, *SV* sulcul vein, *PSV* posterior spinal vein, *PV* pial vein, *PVN* pial venous network, *RPV* radial perforating vein, *TA* transmedullary anastomosis, *RV* radicular vein, *RMV* radiculomedullary vein. (Credit: Ref. [13])

The longitudinal veins of the intrinsic system are fewer in number, and ascend or descend the spinal cord obliquely connecting the axial venous networks [20, 21].

The extrinsic system is made up of the intradural extramedullary veins. Whereas the intrinsic venous system is mostly axially oriented, the extrinsic system tends to follow a coronal orientation. Pial veins located laterally on the spinal cord drain into the ventral and dorsal median pial veins which are usually large and solitary, midline longitudinal veins located on the ventral and dorsal surfaces of the spinal cord, however up to three may be present. These make up the major drainage of the extrinsic system [20]. The sulcal veins drain directly into the ventral and dorsal median pial veins [21]. The ventral median pial vein continues at the end of the spinal cord onto the filum terminale to the end of the dural sac [19]. The extrinsic system is connected to the extradural system via radiculomedullary veins, analogous to the previously described medullary arteries. These radiculomedullary veins receive blood from both the dorsal and ventral median pial veins and exit the dura through the nerve root sleeve or less frequently between two nerve roots and empty into the extradural system [19]. It had long been assumed that these radicular veins had valves within them as an anti-reflux mechanism, but recent studies have found no such valves. Instead, the radicular veins have intravenous dural folds, very tortuous oblique paths through the dura, a smaller lumen, and smooth muscle fibers in the vascular walls all of which may help regulate reflux in an environment of venous hypertension [22, 23].

The extradural system not only drains the spinal cord but also drains the spinal column, including vertebra and intervertebral discs, and is also to a lesser degree is involved with CSF reabsorption by draining small amounts of arachnoid granulations within the spinal nerve roots [20]. The radiculomedullary veins exit the dura and drain into the vertebral venous plexus or Batson's plexus [20]. This plexus is located extradurally within the spinal canal circumferentially around the spinal dura and continues superiorly where it is continuous with the suboccipital venous system [24]. The vertebral venous plexus is larger anteriorly and increases in caliber as it travels caudally [22]. The extradural system is drained to the systemic circulation through intervertebral veins. The cervical level drains into the vertebral veins, the deep cervical and jugular veins; the thoracic and lumbar levels drain to the azygous or hemiazygous system and ascending lumbar veins; the lumbosacral levels drain to ascending lumbar veins or sacral veins which empty into the inferior vena cava [20].

Pathologies

Spinal cord vascular pathologies can be generally divided into three categories: (1) Spinal vascular malformations (SVM); (2) Cavernomas; and (3) Infarctions. Each of these topics is explored below with a discussion of hallmark clinical and radiologic findings.

Spinal vascular malformations are a heterogeneous group of pathologies which are among the most difficult to diagnose and understand of all spinal cord pathology. This group comprises about 3–4% of all intradural spinal lesions [18]. Though they are similar to the analogous cranial conditions, they often go unrecognized leading to dramatic clinical deficits. Their first clinical observation was published in 1890; however, the initial treatment of these lesions was not attempted until 1914.

Imaging of SVMs is fundamental to their diagnosis and to understanding their pathophysiology. The development of spinal angiography in the 1960s is the foremost modern event in the diagnosis and treatment of these lesions. Before the advent of this technique, most descriptions were from post-mortem pathology. Among the modern modalities to discuss for diagnosis of these lesions are: (1) MRI and MRA, (2) Angiography and (3) CT.

MRI is the first study typically ordered in the workup of SVMs. MRI findings typically include: hyperintense T2 cord signal indicating edema of the cord, which may enhance on post-gadolinium sequences; dilated, serpinginous peri-medullary vessels lining the dorsal or ventral surface of the spinal cord on T2 weighted MRIs which will be visualized as flow voids; cord atrophy can also be seen in advanced stages of disease. If hemorrhage is present, varying cord signal and enhancement patterns can elucidate the age of the hemorrhage [20]. Although MRI can show signs of SVMs, the findings seen on MRI are not predictive of the vessel of origin or location of the lesion. MRA, especially with recent advances, new sequences, and protocols, better elucidate SVMs and, frequently, have the detail and clarity to localize the lesion to a spinal level. Currently spinal MRA does not have the detail or resolution to make treatment decisions. However, this technology does make spinal angiograms safer by requiring less radiation exposure, contrast load, and fewer levels needing to be accessed.

CT angiography (CTA) as well as CT myelography can also be used to diagnosis SVMs. CT myelography will reveal dilated serpentine filling defects representative of vascular pathology. Studies have shown comparable detection rates compared to MRA, CTA however may not have as good of resolution in obese patients [21].

The gold standard for diagnosis and characterization of spinal vascular lesions of SVMs is spinal angiography. Spinal angiography allows for determination of the exact vessels and levels involved in the malformation and, in some instances, identify the exact location of the fistulous connection. It is also very useful in defining the surrounding vascular anatomy. The addition of 3D rotational spinal angiography has further improved the imaging quality of SVMs. Another benefit of spinal angiography is the extent of anatomy investigated. If no lesion is seen by injecting the segmental or radicular arteries, arteries such as the internal iliacs, the lateral sacrals or the arterial supply to the posterior fossa of the cranium can all be injected to further investigate the source of the lesion.

Spinal vascular malformations can be split into two subcategories: spinal dural arterio-venous fistulas (AVF) and arterio-venous malformations (AVM). Spinal AVFs are the result of a direct connection between an artery with a vein or venous plexus that drains intrathecally. They can occur extradurally and drain intrathecally through an incompetent valve in the spinal dura, but most occur intradurally. Spinal AVMs are defined as higher flow lesions when compared to AVFs that flow through a nidus or tangle of multiple abnormal vessels to a dilated venous system. There have been multiple classification schemes proposed as SVMs have been investigated. The most commonly used classification scheme is known as the American/British/French connection classification (ABF) (Table 1.1) [22].

SVMs present to clinical attention in two different categories: acute or protracted. Acute neurologic deterioration is seen in patients with hemorrhage into the spinal cord, hematomyelia, or subarachnoid hemorrhage in the spinal column. This can be due to intradural or intramedullary AVMs or aneurysms associated with AVMs or AVFs, although AVFs present acutely much less frequently than AVMs [18]. Acute presentation is often sudden onset of excruciating back pain or meningismus. This can be with or without the sudden onset of a neurologic deficit such as paresis/paralysis, paresthesias, pain, bowel/bladder dysfunction. There is also a

Table 1.1 ABF classification of spinal vascular malformations

Type I	Spinal dural arteriovenous fistula (previous angioma racemosum venosum): located at the dural sleeve of a spinal root, associated with a single-coiled vessel on the dorsal pial surface of the spinal cord
Type II	Glomus AVM (previous angioma racemosum arteriovenosum): Characterized by a true intramedullary nidus and with the arteriovenous shunting occurring deep into the pia
Type III	Metameric or juvenile AVM (previous cobb syndrome): Involvement of one or more metameres (and consequently of portions of the neural tissue, dura, bone, muscle, and skin)
Type IV	Direct or perimedullary AVF: Direct arteriovenous fistula, usually supplied by anterior spinal artery with venous drainage through pial venous network, resulting in aneurysmal dilation of the draining veins

small subset of the AVFs that will present suddenly with acute neurologic deterioration from extreme venous hypertension and possible subsequent venous thrombosis. This was first described in 1926 by Foix and Alajouanine and has since been described as Foix-Alajouanine syndrome [23]. Pathologically, the spinal cord will show extensive necrosis and hypertrophy of the pial and intramedullary veins and venous thrombosis. Acute presentation with hemorrhage is less likely than protracted clinical course, with subarachnoid or intramedullary hemorrhage being the first imaging finding in 35% of SVM patients [23]. Children appear to be more prone to hemorrhage and acute presentation with 84% of children diagnosed with SVMs presenting with sudden onset of symptoms and hemorrhage on imaging [25].

Protracted or chronic presentations are secondary to venous hypertension, cord ischemia or mass effect. This often presents as signs of progressive myelopathy such as upper or lower extremity weakness, loss of pain and temperature sensation, bowel or bladder incontinence, and increased muscular tone [24]. Patients with SVMs, especially AVFs, can also present with neurogenic claudication with symptoms of back and thigh pain exacerbated by physical exertion and relieved by sitting. In one study of 110 patients with SVM, the most common presentation was paresis or paralysis (75.5%), paresthesias (60%), pain (51.8%), and bowel or bladder dysfunction (41.8%) [19]. Arterial venous fistulas more commonly present with a protracted clinical course. These lesions also have a strong male predilection (>80%), 80% occur after the age of 40, and the majority are located in the thoracolumbar region [26].

Venous hypertension seen in patients with an SVM presenting with a protracted or chronic clinical course is due to the arterialization of the coronal venous plexus caused by the fistulous connection of an artery with a vein. This produces the dilated serpiginous veins seen on the surface of the spinal cord on imaging and during surgery. The arterialization of these veins transmits the high pressure of the valveless veins on the substance of the cord in a retrograde fashion to the veins within the spinal cord leading to venous congestion, venous hypertension, diminished arterial perfusion, ischemia, and then myelopathy [23]. Mass effect on the spinal cord can occur with large AVFs or AVMs with massively dilated venous structures, which form as a result of venous hypertension and venous congestion, or feeding vessel aneurysms [18]. Massively dilated epidural veins caused by AVFs can also cause mass effect on the spinal cord resulting in neurologic deficits. Vascular steal is another mechanism through which SVMs may cause symptoms. SVMs cause steal phenomenon by increasing the blood flow through their high flow low resistance vascular beds diverting flow away from the spinal cord causing regional ischemia [27].

As there are no large randomized studies regarding the treatment of SVMs, there is no data to support a standardized treatment algorithm. Depending on the vascular architecture, presenting symptoms, and location, SVM can be treated with open microsurgery, endovascular therapies, radiosurgery or a combination of therapies. The goal of treatment is to halt, and potentially reverse, progressive neurologic deficit by eliminating flow through the abnormal vascular connection in an effort to restore normal perfusion pressure and circulation patterns to the spinal cord. The outcome of any treatment strongly correlates with the degree of preoperative neurologic function, with those with lesser degree of neurologic impairment doing better overall [28]. Motor symptoms tend to respond better to treatment while sensory symptoms (numbness, dysethesias, burning pain) tend to respond less frequently. Bowel and bladder symptoms also have poor recovery after treatment with persistence of symptoms in up to 73% of patients [29]. Clinical recovery is possible in patients with severe deficits including paraplegia, so treatment should not be withheld; even slight increases in function can have large impacts in quality of life [30].

Spinal Cavernomas (also known as cavernous malformations or cavernous hemangiomas) are angiographically occult vascular malformations of the central nervous system. Cavernomas in the spinal cord are histologically identical to those found in the brain. Histologically, they consist of dilated sinusoidal venous channels lacking a complete vascular wall without intervening normal nervous tissue [31]. They account for 5%–12% of all spinal vascular abnormalities [32]. These lesions are most commonly intramedullary, but can also rarely present in the epidural space [33]. Most spinal cavernomas occur sporadically (80%) but some do present in a familial form (20%), especially within the Hispanic community. The familial form will also present more commonly with multiple lesions [34]. Cavernoma formation has also been associated with exposure to spinal irradiation [35].

Spinal cavernomas are angiographically occult but can be evaluated with CT and MRI imaging modalities. CT scans will show focal hyperdense lesions with indistinct margins containing areas of hemorrhage or speckles of calcific density [36]. These findings are non-specific and could represent lesions such granulomas or as hemorrhage from other causes such as other SVMs or neoplasms. MRI is the imaging modality of choice for diagnosing spinal cavernous malformations. An MRI of a spinal cavernous malformation will exhibit characteristic appearance of a well-defined circumscribed nodular lesion displaying reticulated heterogeneous intensity within the core resembling a mulberry or popcorn kernel on both T1 and T2 weighted sequences [37]. This mixed signal core is caused but areas of thrombosis, fibrosis, calcification and various blood breakdown products within the lesion [38]. There is also a characteristic peripheral ring of hypointensity, which corresponds to hemosiderin and iron deposition [38]. Post gadolinium MRIs do not usually add any findings to aid in diagnosis of spinal cavernomas, but do sometimes detect associated nearby developmental venous anomalies [39]. The imaging appearance of cavernomas will vary and will change with time as their appearance depends on the size and stage of evolution of the blood products within them. The blood products within the lesion and their representation on different MRI sequences can help determine the chronicity of any hemorrhage. MRI sequences such as T2-weighted, GRE, or SWI are very sensitive in detecting hemosiderin containing blood products and calcium. Their signal characteristics will also appear larger due to the blooming effect, which makes them even more sensitive for detecting small cavernomas that have not recently hemorrhaged [40].

Symptomatic spinal cavernomas can clinically present with discrete acute episodic progression over time, slowly and gradual progressive decline in function over time, acute onset with rapidly progression of deficit, or a slow progression after an acute development of a neurologic deficit [41]. The progressive presentation of some patients is likely due to the irritation and disruption of neural pathways within the spinal cord, which has a very high density of eloquent structures. The irritation and disruption is thought to result from slow enlargement of the lesion, which may be caused by micro-hemorrhages, hyalinization of vascular channels, intraluminal thrombosis, microcirculatory changes, gliosis of the surrounding tissue, or capillary proliferation [42]. Acute presentation is most likely caused by lesional hemorrhage into the spinal cord parenchyma causing mass effect and irritation of the surrounding neural tissue. Reported rates of symptomatic spinal cavernoma hemorrhage in the literature range from 1.4–6.8% per year [43]. One meta-analysis showed 45% of patients present with an acute or stepwise clinical course while 55% present with progressive neurologic decline [43]. The distribution of symptoms on presentation where 60% motor, 58% sensory, 34% pain, and 24% with bowel or bladder disfuction [43]. These symptoms can also be seen in the setting of myelopathy. Spinal cord cavernomas most frequently occur in the thoracic (57%) and cervical (38%) spinal cord [44].

Spinal cord cavernomas are managed with either surgical resection or observation. The decision making process to take a patient to surgery must include location of lesion, the presence of pial presentation, the duration of symptoms, the acuity of the neurologic decline, and the patient's ability to tolerate surgery. When taken to surgery the goal is complete resection because residual cavernoma left behind will often result in symptomatic hemorrhage [45]. In patients presenting with severe neurologic deterioration or progrèssive symptoms, surgical resection must be considered. In asymptomatic cases or patients with only mild symptoms, the indications for surgery are less clear. As with any surgery, the risk of further deterioration or hemorrhage must be weighed against the morbidity associated with surgical resection. Postsurgical outcomes are mostly dependent on preoperative neurologic status, with patients with lesser deficits having better outcomes [46]. Duration of symptoms greater than 3 years also has been shown to be a predictor of a poorer outcome [43]. Postoperatively 15–25% of patients will experience a worsening of their neurologic deficit immediately after surgery but most of these deficits will resolve, and after the acute post-surgical period the neurologic outcomes have been reported in a meta-analysis as 51% improved, 38% unchanged and 11% worse [43, 47].

Infarctions

Spinal cord infarction is a rare and devastating disorder that may be recognized quickly due to the unique clinical presentation. In discussing infarction syndromes, it is imperative to first discuss factors that modulate blood flow, spinal cord autoregulation, and discuss the common diseases that present with infarction.

The factors that modulate blood flow in the spinal cord are similar to those that regulate cerebral perfusion. Both hypoxia and hypercapnia increase blood flow via autoregulation [48]. Gray matter has a higher metabolic demand and, therefore, requires higher perfusion pressures. The cervical and lumbar levels have the largest amount of gray matter due to their motor control of upper and lower extremities, making these levels the most sensitive to perfusion pressure changes [48].

Perfusion pressure is paramount to maintaining metabolic function in the spinal cord. Through autoregulatory mechanisms, the spinal blood flow is maintained at a near constant level despite mean arterial pressure differences. As with the brain, there are limits to this regulation [49]. Failure to regulate pressure may precipitate vascular injury and subsequent cord edema. Because the spinal cord exists in a fixed space, resultant cord edema may cause further vascular compression and irreversible injury. This constraint is analogous to the Kelli-Monro doctrine of the cerebrum.

Spinal cord infarction is secondary to a number of pathologies. These pathologies are outlined in Table 1.2. Broadly, these pathologies include: (1) Diseases and Intervention of the thoraco-abdominal aorta, (2) Hypoperfusion, (3) Arterial Occlusion, and (4) Venous Infarction.

The thoraco-abdominal aorta plays an important role in cord perfusion, as discussed in the arterial anatomy section. Disease or intervention on this vessel are predominant causes of spinal cord ischemia. First, surgery to repair thoracic aortic aneurysms is the most common cause of spinal cord infarction [51]. Reported rates vary but typically average between 10 and 11% in most retrospective studies. As endovascular techniques have improved, there are early indications that the risk may be lower with endovascular methods. However, there is clear selection bias of patients and pathology for these procedures [52]. The onset of clinical symptoms

Table 1.2 Causes of spinal cord infarction

Aorta Diseases, Procedures	**Infection**
Aortic surgery	Bacterial meningitis
Thoracic endovascular aorta repair (TEVAR)	Syphillis
Traumatic rupture of the aorta	Mucormycosis
Aortic thrombosis	**Hematologic Diseases**
Aortic aneurysm	Hypercoagulable conditions
Coarctation of the aorta	Sickle cell anemia
Aortography	**Non-Aortic Surgeries**
Systemic Hypoperfusion	**Spine Disease**
Cardiac arrest	Spine surgery
Systemic bleeding	Cervical spondylosis
Cardiogenic Embolism	Fibrocartilagenous embolism
Atrial Myxoma	Epidural steroid injection
Mitral valve disease	**Miscellaneous**
Patent foramen Ovale	Cocaine abuse
Bacterial endocarditis	Vertebral artery dissection
Cardiac catheterization	Spinal vascular malformation
Vasculitis	Decompression sickness
Systemic lupus erythematosus	
Polyarteritis Nodosa	
Behcet syndrome	
Giant cell arteritis	

Credit: Ref. [50]

ranges from immediate to delayed with reports of ischemia induced injury 27 days after surgical repair [53]. There are a number of factors that play a role in the pathogenesis – systemic hypotension before, during, or after procedure; aortic cross clamping with decreased perfusion pressure; occlusion of important feeding arteries such as Adamkiewicz or intercostal arteries by ligation, resection, or embolization. Systemic hypotension appears to be the most strongly correlated with delayed ischemia [54]. Of note, many interventions are anecdotally employed to reduce risk of ischemia including the placement of lumbar drains, reimplantation of intercostal arteries, intraoperative neurophysiologic monitoring, epidural cooling, use of distal aortic perfusion, and blood pressure augmentation. However, these interventions have not been studied in randomized fashion with sufficient follow up necessary to reach definitive conclusions regarding efficacy. Second, aortic dissection of the descending aorta has a number of complications, including occlusion of the radicular arteries. Due to the high immediate mortality, the incidence of spinal cord ischemia is not well elucidated but has been estimated at 4% [55]. Spinal cord ischemia has also been reported with non-aortic interventions, though these cases are likely due to either radicular artery injury or systemic hypoperfusion, particularly in the setting of known aortic disease.

Arterial occlusion is the second important mechanism of spinal cord ischemia. Vessel-to-vessel embolus is the most frequent example of this pathology. A rare phenomenon, fibrocartilagenous embolism develops from herniated intervertebral discs and may result in arterial occlusion. The history occasionally reveals antecedent heavy lifting and most frequently the injury involves the cervical cord. Given its proximity to the brainstem, this injury has a high morality rate. Although the exact pathogenesis is unclear, the hypothesis is that axial loading causes pressurized ejection of nucleus pulposus with retrograde occlusion of local arteries and veins [56]. Others have postulated that dynamic instability in the spine could transiently compress vasculature, though this has not been substantiated. Improvements in dynamic imaging will confirm or refute this hypothesis in due time.

Other etiologies of spinal cord infarction include venous infarction (emboli, hypertension secondary to SVM), vasculitis, and autoimmune or toxic arteriopathy. Venous infarction has a divergent clinical presentation – hemorrhagic infarction precipitates a flaccid paraparesis while non-hemorrhagic infarction produces a progressive decline in function.

Infarction syndromes can be divided into two main categories: (1) radicular artery infarcts (anterior and posterior spinal artery); and (2) hypoperfusion infarcts (central and transverse infarcts) [57]. Radicular artery infarcts include unilateral and bilateral anterior and posterior spinal artery infarcts.

Anterior spinal artery syndrome is the most common form of spinal cord infarction. Clinically, it presents with a loss of motor function and pain/temperature sensation and sparing of proprioception and vibration below the level of the lesion. The above deficits are explained by the anatomic sparing of the dorsal columns, which are perfused by posterior spinal arteries. Acutely, the patient typically presents with flaccid paresis and reflexes with possible hypotension. It is important to recognize hypotension as a cause and result of spinal cord ischemia. Unilateral forms are explained by an incomplete connection between the posterior systems or duplication of the anterior system [58]. Posterior spinal artery syndrome results in loss of vibration and proprioception and total anesthesia below the level of the injury. Weakness on the other hand may be transient or partial.

Hypoerfusion infarcts include a less well-defined group of stroke presentations including Brown-Sequard syndrome, transverse lesions, and central cord distributed lesions. These lesions likely represent different points on a continuum depending on the degree of collateralization and duration of hypoperfusion. Clinical presentations vary among these infarct patterns.

The final consideration in spinal cord infarction is the diagnostic imaging modalities. T2 changes on MRI are the most widely recognized finding but this change is significantly delayed from ictus. MRI-DWI is significantly more sensitive but also shows delay. However, the findings of diffusion restriction and T2 hyperintensity are not specific to infarct and can be seen in transverse myelitis and other intrinsic pathologies. The presence of vertebral body infarction adjacent to cord signal can serve to reinforce the suspicion of infarct but it is only present in 4–35% of patients [59]. Further testing is not necessary, particularly if there is a compelling clinical history (eg: aortic surgery); however, in the absence of a recognized clinical precedent, other tests should be ordered. These tests include: (1) vascular imaging to investigate for intrinsic cord lesion or aortic injury; (2) cranial imaging to investigate for neuromyelitis optica or multiple sclerosis; (3) lumbar puncture to investigate for acute inflammatory demyelinating polyneuropathy and infectious etiologies; (4) blood tests to investigate for auto-immune markers [60].

References

1. Gilbilan LA. The arterial blood supply of the human spinal cord. J Comp Neurol. 1958;110(1):75–103.
2. Thron AK. Vascular anatomy of the spinal cord: neuroradiological investigations and clinical syndromes. Springer; 1988.
3. Macdonald RL, Schwartz ML, Lewis AJ. Neurenteric cyst located dorsal to the cervical spine: case report. Neurosurgery. 1991;28:583–7. discussion 7-8
4. Saker E, Henry BM, Tomaszewski KA, Loukas M, Iwanaga J, Oskouian RJ, et al. The human central canal of the spinal cord: a comprehensive review of its anatomy, embryology, molecular development, variants, and pathology. Cureus. 2016;8:e927.
5. Gupta P, Kumar A, Goel S. Congenital spinal cord anomalies: a pictorial review. Curr Probl Diagn Radiol. 2013;42:57–66.
6. Nikolopoulou E, Galea GL, Rolo A, Greene ND, Copp AJ. Neural tube closure: cellular, molecular and biomechanical mechanisms. Development. 2017;144:552–66.
7. Schmidt-Lademann S, Stoeter P, Voigt K. Embryonal and fetal development of capillaries: microangiographic investigations. II. The telencephalon. Diagn Imaging. 1980;49:177–87.
8. Stoeter P, Schmidt-Lademann S, Voigt K. Embryonal and fetal development of capillaries: microangiographic investigations. I. The brain stem. Diagn Imaging. 1980;49:131–40.
9. Thron A, Stoeter P, Hauss C, Dietz R, Drews U, Sonntag W. Embryonal and fetal vascularisation of the spinal cord: microangiographic examinations. In: Nadjmi M, editor. Imaging of brain metabolism spine and cord interventional neuroradiology free communications. Berlin Heidelberg: Springer; 1989. p. 239–40.

10. Zawilinski J, Litwin JA, Nowogrodzka-Zagorska M, Gorczyca J, Miodonski AJ. Vascular system of the human spinal cord in the prenatal period: a dye injection and corrosion casting study. Ann Anat Off Organ Anat Ges. 2001;183:331–40.
11. Griessenauer CJ, Raborn J, Foreman P, Shoja MM, Loukas M, Tubbs RS. Venous drainage of the spine and spinal cord: a comprehensive review of its history, embryology, anatomy, physiology, and pathology. Clin Anat. 2015;28:75–87.
12. Nelson PK, Decske T. The vascular anatomy of the vertebro-spinal axis. Neurosurg Clin N Am. 2009;20:259–64.
13. Miyasaka K, Asano T, Ushikoshi S, Kida K, Koyangi I. Vascular anatomy of the spinal cord and classification of spinal ateriovenous malformations. Interv Neuroradiol. 2000;6(Suppl1):195–8.
14. Kendall BE, Logue V. Spinal epidural angiomatous malformations draining into intrathecal veins. Neuroradiology. 1977;13:181–9.
15. Hurst RW. Spinal vascular disorders. In: Atlas SW, editor. Resonance imaging of the brain and spine. 2nd ed. Philadelphia: Lippincott; 2006. p. 1387.
16. Mohr JP, Benavente O, Barnett HJ. Spinal cord ischemia. In: Barnett HJ, Mohr JP, Stein BM, Yatsu FM, editors. Stroke pathophysiology, diagnosis, and management. Philadelphia: Churchill Livingstone; 1998. p. 423.
17. Gailloud P, Gregg L, Galan P, Becker D, Pardo C. Periconal arterial anastomotic circle and posterior lumbosacral watershed zone of the spinal cord. J NeuroIntervent Surg. 2015;7:848–53.
18. Griessenauer CJ, Raborn J, Foreman P, Shoja MM, Loukas M, Tubbs RS. Venous drainage of the spin and spinal cord: a comprehensive review of its history, embryology, Amatomy, physiology, and pathology. Clin Anat. 2015;28:75–87.
19. Santillan A, Nacarino V, Greenberg E, Riina H, Gobin Y, Patsalides A. Vascular anatomy of the spinal cord. J NeuroIntervent Surg. 2012;4:67–74.
20. Lasjaunias P, Berenstein A. Spinal and spinal cord arteries and veins. In: Surgical neuroangiography: functional vascular anatomy of brain, spinal cord, and spine. New York: Springer; 1990.
21. Thron A, Rossberg C. Vascular anatomy of the spinal cord: Neuroradiological investigations and clinical syndromes. New York: Springer; 1988.
22. Groen R, Groenewegen H, van Alphen H, Hoogland P. Morphology of the human internal vertebral venous plexus: a cadaver study after intravenous Araldite CY 221 injection. Anat Rec. 1997;249:285–94.
23. van der Kuip M, Hoogland P, Groen R. Human radicular veins: regulation of venous reflux in the absence of valves. Anat Rec. 1999;254:173–80.
24. Tubbs RS, Hansasuta A, Loukas M, Louis RG Jr, Shoja MM, Salter EG, Oakes WJ. The basilar venous plexus. Clin Anat. 2007;20:755–9.
25. Rangel-Castilla L, Russin J, Zaidi HA, Martinez-del-Campo E, Park MS, Albuquerque FC, McDougall CG, Nakaji P, Spetzler RF. Contemporary management of spinal AVFs and AVMs: lessons learned from 110 cases. Neurosurg Focus. 2014;37:E14.
26. Morris JM. Imaging of dural arteriovenous fistula. Radiol Clin N Am. 2012;50:823–39.
27. Flores BC, Klinger DR, White JA, Hunt Batjer H. Spinal vascular malformations: treatment strategies and outcome. Neurosurg Rev. 2017;40(1):15–28.
28. Si-jia G, Meng-wei Z, Xi-ping L, Yu-shen Z, Jing-hong L, Zhong-hui W, Pei-zhuo Z, Qiang S, Qiang W, Chuan-sheng L, Ke X. The clinical application studies of CT spinal angiography with 64- detector row spiral CT in diagnosing spinal vascular malformations. Eur J Radiol. 2009;71:22–8.
29. Black P. Spinal vascular malformations: an historical per- spective. Neurosurg Focus. 2006;21:1–7.
30. Rosenblum B, Oldfield EH, Doppman JL, et al. Spinal arteriovenous malformations: a comparison of dural arteriovenous fistulas and intradural AVM's in 81 patients. J Neurosurg. 1987;67:795–802.
31. Aminoff MJ, Logue V. Clinical features of spinal vascular malformations. Brain. 1974;97:197–210.
32. Taylor CL, Selman WR, Ratcheson RA. Steal affecting the central nervous system. Neurosurgery. 2002 Apr;50(4):679–88.

33. Riché MC, Modenesi-Freitas J, Djindjian M, et al. Arteriovenous malformations (AVM) of the spinal cord in children. A review of 38 cases. Neuroradiology. 1982;22:171–80.
34. Oldfield E. Surgical treatment of spinal dural arteriovenous fistulas. Semin Cerebrovasc Dis Stroke. 2002;2:209–26.
35. Watson JC, Oldfield E. The surgical management of spinal dural vascular malformations. Neurosurg Clin N Am. 1999;10:73–87.
36. Fugate JE, Lanzino G, Rabinstein AA. Clinical presentation and prognostic factors of spinal dural arteriovenous fistulas: an overview. Neurosurg Focus. 2012;32:E17.
37. Narvid J, Hett SW, Larsen D, Neuhaus J, Singh TP, McSwain H, Lawton MT, Dowd CF. Spinal dural arteriovenous fistulae: clinical features and long-term results. Neurosurgery. 2008;62:159–67.
38. Clatterbuck RE, Eberhart CG, Crain BJ, Rigamonti D. Ultrastructural and immunocytochemical evidence that an incompetent blood-brain barrier is related to the pathophysiology of cavernous malformations. J Neurol Neurosurg Psychiatry. 2001;71:188–92.
39. Jellinger K. Pathology of spinal vascular malformations and vascular tremors. In: Pia HW, Djindjian R, editors. Spinal Angiomas: advances in diagnosis and therapy. New York: Springer; 1978.
40. Hemalatha AL, Ravikumar T, Chamarthy NP. A pure epidural spinal cavernous hemangioma—with an innocuous face but a perilous behaviour! J Clin Diagn Res. 2013;7:1434–5.
41. Rigamonti D, Hadley MN, Drayer BP, et al. Cerebral cavernous malformations. Incidence and familial occurrence. N Engl J Med. 1988;319:343–7.
42. Maraire JN, Abdulrauf SI, Berger S, et al. De novo development of a cavernous malformation of the spinal cord following spinal axis radiation. Case report J Neurosurg. 1999;90(suppl):234–8.
43. Robinson J, Awad IA, Masaryk TJ, et al. Pathological heterogeneity of angiographically occult vascular malformations of the brain. Neurosurgery. 1993;33:547–54.
44. Kivelev J, Niemela M, Hernesniemi J. Outcome after microsurgery in 14 patients with spinal cavernomas and review of the literature. J Neurosurg Spine. 2010;13:524–34.
45. Rivera PP, Willinsky RA, Porter PJ. Intracranial cavernous malformations. Neuroimaging Clin N Am. 2003;13:27–40.
46. Abe T, Singer RJ, Marks MP, et al. Coexistence of occult vascular mal- formations and developmental venous anomalies in the central nervous system: MR evaluation. AJNR Am J Neuroradiol. 1998;19:51–7.
47. Atlas SW, Mark AS, Grossman RI, et al. Intracranial hemorrhage: gradient-echo MR imaging at 1.5 T. Comparison with spin-echo imaging and clinical applications. Radiology. 1988;168:803–7.
48. Ogilvy CS, Louis DN, Ojemann RG. Intramedullary cavernous angiomas of the spinal cord: clinical presentation, pathological features, and surgical management. Neurosurgery. 1992;31:219–29.
49. Badhiwala JH, Farrokhyar F, Alhazzani W, Yarascavitch B, Aref M, Algird A, Murth N, Kachur E, Cenic A, Reddy K, Almenawer SA. Surgical outcomes and natural history of intramedullary spinal cord cavernous malformations: a single center series and meta-analysis of individual patient data. J Neurosurg Spine. 2014;21:662–7.
50. Mullen MT. Spinal cord infarction: clinical presentation and diagnosis; 2017. UpToDate. Retrieved October 1, 2017.
51. Gross BA, Du R, Popp AJ, et al. Intramedullary spinal cord cavernous malformations. Neurosurg Focus. 2010;29:E14.
52. Maslehaty H, Barth H, Petridis AK, et al. Symptomatic spinal cavernous malformations: indication for microsurgical treatment and outcome. Eur Spine J. 2011;10:1765–70.
53. Oldfield EH. Spinal vascular malformations. In: Swash M, editor. Outcomes in neurological disorders. Cambridge, UD: Cambridge University Press; 1998.
54. Amenta PS, Medel R, Singh MK, Dumont AS, Oldfield EH. Microsurgical treatment of spinal vascular malformations. In: Winn HR, editor. Youmans and Winn neurological surgery. 7th ed. Elsevier; 2017.

55. Cheshire WP, Santos CC, Massey EW, Howard JF. Spinal cord infarction etiology and outcome. Neurology. 1996;47(2):321–30.
56. Marcus ML, Heistad DD, Ehrhardt JC, Abboud FM. Regulation of total and regional spinal cord blood flow. Circ Res. 1977;41(1):128–34.
57. Hickey R, Albin MS, Bunegin L, Gelineau J. Autoregulation of spinal cord blood flow: is the cord a microcosm of the brain? Stroke. 1986;17(6):1183–9.
58. Sandson TA, Friedman JH. Spinal cord infarction: report of 8 cases and review of the literature. Medicine. 1989;68(5):282–92.
59. Messé SR, Bavaria JE, Mullen M, Cheung AT, Davis R, Augoustides JG, Gutsche J, et al. Neurologic outcomes from high risk descending thoracic and thoracoabdominal aortic operations in the era of endovascular repair. Neurocrit Care. 2008;9(3):344–51.
60. Maniar HS, Sundt TM, Prasad SM, Chu CM, Camillo CJ, Moon MR, Rubin BG, Sicard GA. Delayed paraplegia after thoracic and thoracoabdominal aneurysm repair: a continuing risk. Ann Thorac Surg. 2003;75(1):113–20.

Spinal Cord Physiology: Neuromotor Control of Diaphragm Muscle

2

Matthew J. Fogarty and Gary C. Sieck

Contents

Introduction

Spinal cord physiology can be broadly categorized into motor and sensory systems, which are integrated to accomplish motor behaviors. This chapter will focus primarily on sensorimotor control of the diaphragm muscle, which displays a range of fairly simple to complex motor behaviors. In neuromotor control of any skeletal muscle, the motor unit is the final common output. Sherrington first defined the motor unit as comprising a motor neuron and all the muscle fibers it innervates via axonal projections and synapses termed neuromuscular junctions [1]. Subsequently, it was discovered that all muscle fibers comprising a motor unit are homogeneous in their mechanical, fatigue and biochemical properties, which match contractile protein expression and define muscle fiber types [2–7]. Accordingly, slow-twitch, fatigue resistant (type S) motor units comprise type I muscle fibers. Fast-twitch, fatigue resistant (type FR) motor units comprise type IIa muscle fibers. Fast-twitch, fatigue intermediate (type FInt) motor units comprise type IIx muscle fibers, and

M. J. Fogarty
Department of Physiology and Biomedical Engineering, Mayo Clinic, Rochester, MN, USA

School of Biomedical Sciences, The University of Queensland, Brisbane, QLD, Australia

G. C. Sieck (✉)
Department of Physiology and Biomedical Engineering, Mayo Clinic, Rochester, MN, USA
e-mail: sieck.gary@mayo.edu

B. Greenberg (ed.), *Myelopathy*, https://doi.org/10.1007/978-3-030-99906-3_2

fast-twitch fatigable (type FF) motor units comprise type IIx and/or IIb muscle fibers co-expressed in varying proportions.

Phrenic motor neurons innervating diaphragm muscle fibers are located in the cervical spinal cord, and all four motor unit types are typically present – at least in lab animals (rodents and cats). Innervation of the diaphragm is segmentally organized in a dorsal-ventral direction based on phrenic motor neurons located in the C_3 to C_6 segments depending on species [8–15]. Phrenic motor neurons display a wide range of sizes (somal and total surface areas), reflecting systematic size dependent recruitment of diaphragm motor units [11, 16, 17].

Motor units are recruited systematically according to the size motor neurons (Henneman size principle [18]) and motor unit type [19–21]. Henneman showed that those motor units recruited first had slower axonal conduction velocities compared to motor units recruited later. Axonal conduction velocity is directly related to axonal diameter, which in turn reflects motor neuron somal volume and surface area (i.e., motor neuron size). Biophysically, the surface area of motor neurons determines electrical membrane capacitance (Cm), and depolarization of a motor neuron (i.e., the change in membrane potential – dVm/dt) for a given amount of synaptic current (Ic) is inversely related to Cm (dVm/dt = Ic/Cm). The size principle for motor unit recruitment in the diaphragm muscle has been confirmed [19, 20, 22–29] and underlies neuromotor control of force generation across a range of motor behaviors.

Motor units are also recruited systematically depending on motor unit type to develop a range of forces required to accomplish different motor behaviors [19, 20, 24, 27, 28, 30–33]. Accordingly, type S and FR motor units, which develop lower forces but are fatigue resistant, are recruited first, especially during sustained motor behaviors [24, 25, 34, 35]. Higher force, shorter duration motor behaviors are achieved by the additional recruitment of type FInt and FF motor units.

The diaphragm muscle is the major inspiratory pump muscle and contributes to inspiratory airflow via the generation of a pressure gradient (transdiaphragmatic pressure [P_{di}]) across the diaphragm reflected as the difference between abdominal pressure (P_{abd}) and pleural pressure (P_{pl}), which is the. During diaphragm contraction, P_{abd} increases and P_{pl} decreases resulting in an increase in P_{di}. In addition to inspiration, the diaphragm muscle also functions to generate force required for deep sighs that protect against lung atelectasis, and even greater forces required for expulsive behaviors, such as expectoration (coughing) and sternutation (sneezing), which are essential for expelling phlegm, clearing the airways and maintaining airway patency [19, 25, 26, 29, 30, 33, 36, 37]. Further, the diaphragm muscle contributes to non-respiratory related activities, such as swallowing and vocalization [38–40]. Accordingly, diaphragm motor units display a range of contractile and fatigue properties and this repertoire is available for neuromotor control to accomplish these different motor behaviors. Following the Henneman Size Principle, smaller phrenic motor neurons innervating type S and FR motor units are recruited first to accomplish low force sustained ventilatory pump behaviors. By contrast, larger phrenic motor neurons innervating type FInt and FF motor units are recruited later to accomplish deep sighs and higher force, airway clearance behaviors [6, 19, 20, 22–30, 36].

Motor units display a wide degree of adaptability. Phrenic motor units are particularly plastic, and all components of the motor unit undergo alterations in a wide range of conditions, including during development, injury, infection, drug effects and nutritional status. Denervation and aging show similar characteristics of reduced muscle specific force (force per cross-sectional area) generation, and selective atrophy of type IIx and/or IIb muscle fibers that comprise type FInt and FF motor units. Based on converging indirect evidence, it appears that with aging, there is a decrease in the number of type FInt and FF motor units due to the specific loss of these motor neurons [41–44]. This chapter will focus on the diaphragm muscle and present a coherent outline regarding neuromotor control of ventilator (inspiratory pump) and non-ventilatory (airway clearance) behaviors within the context of motor unit specificity, and explore the plasticity of motor unit properties, with a particular emphasis on changes associated with the aging spectrum – from birth to old age.

Diaphragm Motor Unit Physiology

Phrenic Motor Neurons

Diaphragm motor units are innervated by phrenic motor neurons located within the ventral horn (lamina IX) of the cervical spinal cord, segments C_3-C_5 in rats [8, 10, 11, 13, 14], C_{3}-$_{6}$ in mice [12], C_{4}-$_{6}$ in cats [15] and C_{3}-$_{5}$ in humans [9]. In the rat, there are ~230 phrenic motor neurons on each side of the cervical spinal cord [8, 10, 11, 13], bilaterally innervating the diaphragm muscle (providing a total of ~460 motor units). Innervation of the diaphragm muscle displays a somatotopic organization with more rostral cervical segments of the phrenic motor neuron pool innervating more ventral regions of the costal and crural regions of the diaphragm muscle, whereas more caudal segments innervate more dorsal portions of both the costal and crural regions [45].

During late embryonic and early postnatal development, ~50% of motor neurons within the mammalian spinal cord undergo pruning or programmed cell death [46]. Within the phrenic motor pool of the rat, this motor neuron loss occurs days before birth and numbers remain stable during late embryogenesis and early postnatal life within the mammalian spinal cord [47, 48]. In older animals, an age-related loss of spinal cord motor neurons has been observed in locomotor muscles [49], and ongoing investigations within our lab suggest that there is an age-related loss of phrenic motor neurons – primarily larger motor neurons.

Adult phrenic motor neurons display a wide range of sizes, matching the range of diaphragm motor unit types. In the rat, the somal surface areas of phrenic motor neurons range from 1000 to 8000 μm^2 with a median of 4500 μm^2 [10, 11, 13, 50]. In ~80% of cases, somal surface areas of phrenic motor neurons display a significant biomodal distribution, perhaps reflecting differences between phrenic motor neurons innervating type S and FR motor units (possibly including some more fatigue resistant FInt units) and larger phrenic motor neurons innervating type FInt and FF motor units. Other than size, it is difficult to identify phrenic motor neurons innervating different motor unit types. It has been reported that larger motor neurons (FInt and FF motor units) do not express the synaptic vesicle protein SV2A [51], and we have recent evidence to support the absence of SV2A mRNA in larger phrenic motor neurons.

Importantly, phrenic motor neurons during embryogenesis and early postnatal development are smaller and relatively homogeneous in size [11]. The full gamut of size-based heterogeneity of phrenic motor neurons is established only after weaning, a period of rapid growth of phrenic motor neurons and diaphragm muscle fibers [11, 52, 53]. This growth appears to be exclusively of the larger phrenic motor neurons that innervate type IIx and/or IIb muscle fibers [11]. By contrast to postnatal development, we found an age-related loss of larger phrenic motor and for surviving motor neurons a striking reduction in size.

Synaptic Inputs to Phrenic Motor Neurons

There are five main components of the neuronal circuitry of the phrenic/diaphragm motor system: (1) a central pattern generator (for ventilation or other motor behaviors); (2) premotor neurons responsible for transmitting the output of the central pattern generator; (3) interneurons responsible for modulating or coordinating premotor neuron and/or phrenic motor neuron excitability – these interneurons also serve to integrate sensory feedback (e.g., chemoreceptive, lung stretch, propriospinal or other afferent inputs); (4) direct cortical premotor input to motor neurons via the corticospinal pathway, and (5) phrenic motor neurons as the final common output for generating the forces necessary for the desired motor behaviors.

It is likely that several distinct central pattern generators affect activation of the diaphragm muscle to accomplish motor behaviors, e.g., ventilation, sneeezing, coughing, swallowing, vocalization, etc. Of these, the neuronal circuitry responsible for generating the rhythmic behavior of breathing (ventilation) is the best characterized central pattern generator affecting phrenic motor neurons and diaphragm muscle activation. For ventilatory behaviors, this central pattern generator plays an indispensable role in determining the timing and duration of the different phases of the respiratory pattern. Other central pattern generators affecting diaphragm muscle neuromotor control may also exist in the brainstem and spinal cord, e.g., for swallowing [54], coughing and sneezing. The output of these other pattern generators must be integrated with that of the pattern generator for respiration. For example, the central pattern generator for respiration is interrupted during swallowing.

Respiration consists of three main phases, inspiration, post inspiration and expiration [55, 56]. The precise mechanisms underlying the central pattern generator for respiration are still debated, but it is now generally agreed that the Pre-Bötzinger Complex (PreBötC) in the medulla provides the spontaneously active 'kernel' of neurons for the metronomic drive for the inspiratory phase, via interactions of various membrane channels [57]. It now appears that the PreBötC is essential for inspiration [58], and is the prime source of inspiratory excitatory drive to respiratory premotor neurons [59] via a core subpopulation of glutamatergic (Glu) pacemaker cells that project bilaterally [60]. Inhibitory neurotransmission at premotor neurons also plays an important role in modulating respiratory pattern generator outputs [61, 62].

The Bötzinger Complex located rostral to the PreBötC provides for switching from inspiration to expiration [55, 56] possibly via inhibitory inputs to the PreBötC [63]. Normally, expiration is passive; however, active expiration appears to have a distinct central pattern generator located in the region of the retrotrapezoid nucleus (RTN) [64].

Premotor neurons providing monosynaptic drive to phrenic motor neurons during inspiration (ventilatory behavior) are located primarily in the ventrolateral medulla (ventral respiratory group – VRG), although there is some contribution from a dorsal respiratory group (DRG) in the dorsomedial medulla [65, 66]. These descending excitatory (Glu) premotor inputs are predominantly ipsilateral [67–70], transmitted via bulbospinal pathways located in the ventrolateral and ventromedial funiculi [59, 69, 71], and generally thought to be widely distributed [72, 73].

It remains unclear whether the other central pattern generators that affect diaphragm neuromotor control share common or distinct premotor neurons. It is likely that the central pattern generator involved in breathing compared to expulsive motor behaviors of the diaphragm muscle will have a certain degree of overlap in premotor components of neuromotor control [59, 74]. For ventilatory behaviors, it is generally thought that phrenic motor neurons receive distributed descending premotor input that is predominantly ipsilateral. However, retrograde tracing studies that examine the connectivity of phrenic motor neurons have indicated a variety of premotor inputs both from the brainstem and spinal cord [22, 23, 68, 75–78]. Perhaps these connections reflect premotor inputs mediating the output of central pattern generators other than that involved in rhythmic breathing behavior.

Premotor neurons that relay the output from central pattern generator for respiration are also a major site of integration of sensory (e.g., chemoreceptor and pulmonary stretch receptor) and behavioral (e.g., sleep-wake state) modulations within the context of respiratory neuromotor control. Modulation of the respiratory pattern and/or of phrenic motor neuron activity may occur directly or indirectly in response to afferent inputs to phrenic motor neurons, from signaling initiated by mechanoreceptors in the lung and airway, peripheral and central chemoreceptors, to behavioral state influence mediated by serotonergic projections emanating from the raphe. Mechanoreceptors in the lung respond to lung inflation, are sensitive to the mechanical loading of breathing and prevent airway over-inflation by increasing their afferent activity – peaking at the end of inspiration [79, 80]. These afferent inputs exert effects on ventilatory phrenic motor neuron discharge indirectly, via vagal nerve inputs in the nucleus tractus solitarius (NTS) [81, 82]. Laryngeal mechanoreceptors also exert an indirect effect on phrenic motor neurons, decreasing inspiratory drive during upper airway collapse [83]. Peripheral chemoreceptors, primarily in the carotid bodies, respond to hypoxia and hypercapnea by increasing ventilation [84–87] indirectly effect via signaling to brainstem respiratory centres indirectly via the carotid sinus nerve [88]. Central chemoreceptors are found in many brainstem areas [89] and are exquisitely sensitive [90] and increase ventilation in response to hypercapnea [91]. The interactivity of peripheral and central chemoreceptors is subject to intense study and debate in the field. Regardless, chemoreceptors act in an indirect modulatory fashion on the overall drive to phrenic motor neurons. Serotinergic neurons located in the caudal raphe project to brainstem respiratory regions and the phrenic motor pool [92], and thus may have effects on rhythmic central pattern generator and premotor outputs [93, 94] as well as on phrenic motor neuron excitation [95, 96]. Catecholamine modulation of respiration also occurs via activation of the α_1 or α_2 adrenoreceptors, enhancing or inhibiting, respectively respiratory rhythmic central pattern generation [97–100].

Phrenic motor neuron also receive input from spinal cord interneurons, including those involved in proprioception. However, in stark contrast to muscles involved in locomotor behaviors [101], the diaphragm muscle has few muscle spindles [102]. Thus, direct muscle spindle proprioceptive feedback from the diaphragm does not contribute substantially to modulation of phrenic motor neuron excitability [103, 104]. However, phrenic motor neurons do receive feedback from muscle spindles in intercostal muscles, and this input has primarily inhibitory effects on phrenic motor neuron excitability [105, 106]. In particular, the intercostal to phrenic reflex suppresses phrenic nerve activity following strain on the chest wall [107, 108], an effect that appears to involve both disfacilitation of VRG premotor input [108–110] and interneuronal inhibition of phrenic motor neurons [111]. Additional, local inhibition provided to phrenic motor neurons from interneurons within the spinal cord have been characterized [111–115]. Local interneurons within the spinal cord may provide some of the substrate (increased respiratory drive) for recovery of ventilatory and non ventilatory behaviors following spinal cord injury [116, 117].

In humans, direct corticospinal inputs onto phrenic motor neurons allow for voluntary control of breathing [118, 119] and the interplay between ventilation and behaviors such as speech [120]. Phrenic motor neuron integration of rhythmic pattern inputs, modulatory inputs and cortical inputs is illustrated in the difference in drive to breathe during the waking state [121], whereby the awake state provides a resilience to apnea in hypercapnic conditions [121, 122]. In contrast, sleep predisposes to episodes of apnea in the hypercapnic condition [122, 123], yet it remains unknown how influential cortical arousal states are in the maintenance of eupnea.

Although much is still to be defined in regard to phrenic motor neuron inputs and the central pattern generation of ventilatory and other motor behaviors of the diaphragm muscle, the individual phrenic motor neuron is the final integrator of these signals. The diaphragm motor unit remains the final executor of neuromotor control and produces motor force output across a range of ventilatory and higher force, non-ventilatory behaviors. It remains unclear whether phrenic motor neurons innervating different types of diaphragm motor units receive different premotor inputs. Regardless, neuromotor control of the diaphragm muscle during different motor behaviors requires production of different levels of force generation, a property dependent on recruitment and rate coding of motor units themselves.

Classification of Diaphragm Motor Units

Diaphragm muscle force generation is dependent on the interplay between phrenic motor neurons and the muscle fibers they innervate. Motor units are commonly classified into four types (type S, FR, FInt and FF – see Fig. 2.1), according to the mechanical and fatigue properties of their constituent muscle fibers [6, 26, 37,

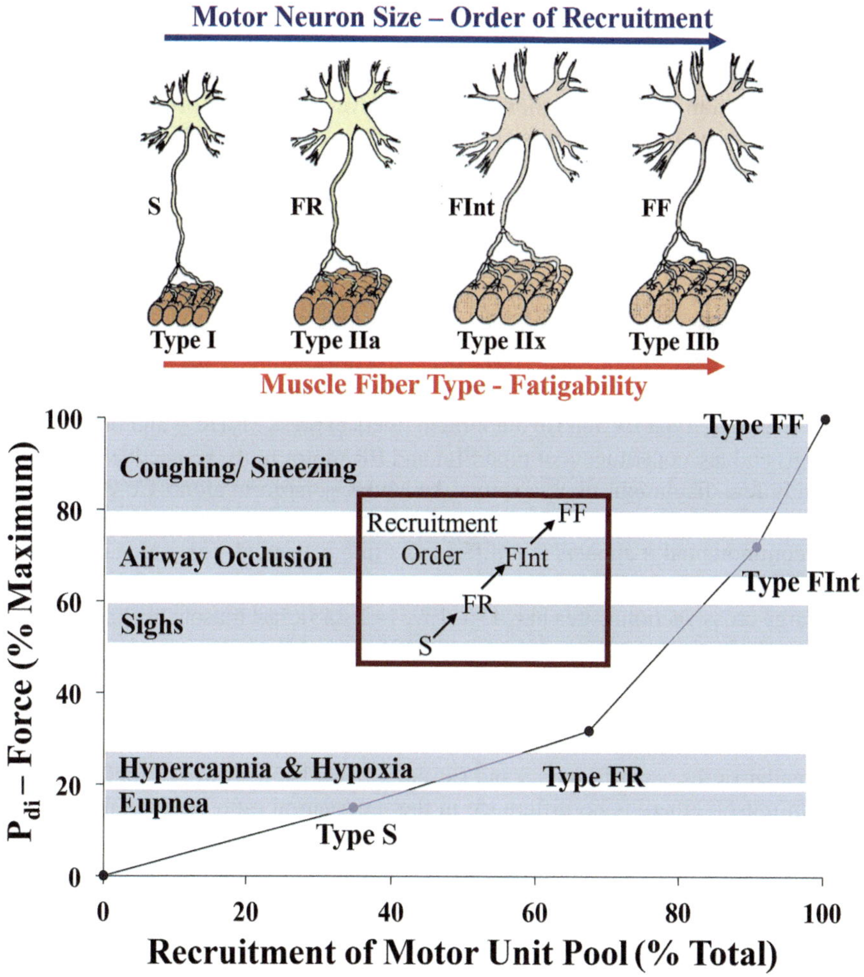

Fig. 2.1 Different DIAm motor unit types are recruited based on PhMN size to accomplish a range of motor behaviors. Ventilation (eupnea and hypercapnia & hypoxia) is accomplished by recruitment of smaller PhMNs comprising type S and FR motor units, whereas higher force, airway clearance behaviors require recruitment of larger PhMNs comprising more fatigable DIAm motor units. Diaphragm motor units are classified into four types, type S motor units have smaller motor neurons and muscle fibers and exhibit slower contraction times than other motor unit types, produce lower forces and are particularly resistant to fatigue

124–130]. Importantly, within an individual motor unit, all of the muscle fibers display homogeneous contractile protein expression and biochemical properties that define a specific muscle fiber type [124, 131–133]. This homogeneity of muscle fiber type within motor units has been confirmed in the adult cat diaphragm [5, 6, 134, 135].

In modern classification schemes, different muscle fiber types are identified by the expression of different MyHC isoforms. Type I muscle fibers in type S motor units express $MyHC_{Slow}$ and have a high mitochondrial volume density and oxidative capacity [130, 134], have smaller cross-sectional areas [11, 136–139], generate less force per cross-sectional area (specific force) [125, 126, 140, 141] and display slower maximum velocity of shortening and have lower rates of ATP hydrolysis compared to type II muscle fibers [125, 126, 140, 141]. Type IIa diaphragm muscle fibers that express $MyHC_{2A}$ and constitute type FR motor units, have mitochondrial volume densities and oxidative capacities comparable to type I fibers, which may account for their greater fatigue resistance. The cross-sectional areas of type IIa fibers is generally small similar to type I fibers, but the specific force they generate is comparable to other type II muscle fibers [125, 126, 140, 141]. The maximum velocity of shortening of type IIa fibers is faster than type I fibers but slower than other type II fibers [125, 126, 140, 141]. Correspondingly, the maximum ATP hydrolysis rate of type IIa fibers is lower than other type II fibers but higher than type I fibers [7]. Type IIx and IIb diaphragm fibers express $MyHC_{2X}$ and/or $MyHC_{2B}$ isoforms and are constituents of type FInt and FR motor units, respectively. In fact, relatively few diaphragm fibers express the $MyHC_{2B}$ isoform alone. Co-expression of expression of $MyHC_{2X}$ and $MyHC_{2B}$ isoforms in diaphragm muscle fibers is fairly common, and it appears that differences in mechanical, energetic and fatigue properties depend on the extent of co-expression [130]. These muscle fibers that have large cross-sectional area [11, 136–139, 142, 143], fast muscle fiber shortening velocity and higher muscle specific forces [125, 126, 140, 141].

An important factor in the force generated by a motor unit is the innervation ratio, defined as the number of muscle fibers innervated by a single motor neuron. In limb muscles, the largest innervation ratios occur in type FInt and FF motor units and smaller ratios occur in type S and FR units [144, 145]. However, in the cat diaphragm muscle, there is no difference in the innervation ratio between motor unit types [27, 33, 146]. Taken together, the larger muscle fiber cross-sectional areas and the greater specific forces of type FInt and FF diaphragm motor units result in markedly greater levels of force contributed by these motor units compared to type S and FR units [24, 26, 30, 124, 129, 147].

Diaphragm Motor Unit Recruitment

Motor units are recruited in an orderly fashion based on the intrinsic size-dependent electrophysiological properties of motor neurons [26, 148, 149]. For a given magnitude of synaptic input, smaller more excitable motor neurons are recruited before larger motor neurons. Henneman first observed that motor units recruited first had slower conduction velocities than motor units recruited later and concluded that the slower conduction velocities corresponded to smaller axon diameters and smaller more excitable motor neurons-the "size principle" [18, 150]. Two key observations provide evidence for the size principle concept of neuromotor control. First, recordings from ventral root nerve filaments have shown that the action potentials of motor units recruited first have smaller amplitudes and slower conduction velocities than those units recruited later [18, 151–153]. Second, nerve action potential amplitude and conduction velocity correspond with axon diameter and motor neuron size [154, 155].

Recruitment of motor units also generally matches their mechanical and fatigue properties, with type S and FR motor units recruited first followed by type FInt and FF motor units (Fig. 2.1). Thus, motor unit type also appears to be an important determinant of motor unit recruitment order [156–158]. In agreement, it has been shown that the force developed by a motor unit is highly indicative of its recruitment order [159]. In the diaphragm muscle, it is very likely that type S and FR motor units are recruited first, especially to accomplish the lower force, high duty cycle (active vs. inactive) behavior of breathing. During rhythmic breathing, inspiration typically has a duty cycle of 30–40%, which would cause fatigue if type FInt and FF motor units were recruited. Higher force, expulsive sneezing and coughing behaviors of the diaphragm muscle have very short durations allowing sufficient time for recovery from any fatigue that might occur.

Based on these observations, a model of diaphragm motor unit recruitment was formulated based on an orderly recruitment of type S, FR, FInt and FF motor units [24–28, 30, 33, 124]. In the initial model in the cat diaphragm, the force contribution of each motor unit type was based on direct measurements of motor unit mechanical properties [26, 27, 37, 124, 147, 160]. Subsequently, in the rat diaphragm muscle the force contributed by different motor unit types was estimated based on measurements of specific force generated by single muscle fibers of different types [125, 126, 140, 141], the cross-sectional area of different muscle fiber types [11, 136–139], the proportion of different fiber types in the diaphragm muscle [6, 37, 124, 130, 134] and the assumption of comparable innervation ratios across motor unit types [27, 33, 146]. In these models, ventilatory behaviors (i.e., eupnea and response to hypoxia/hypercapnea) can be accomplished by the recruitment of type S and FR motor units [19, 20, 24, 26, 27, 30, 33]. In this model, the number of phrenic motor neurons recruited during inspiration in cats is ~23% of the total pool [23], which corresponds with the proportion of type S and FR motor units in the diaphragm muscle [6, 26, 124]. To perform higher force, expulsive behaviors (i.e., coughing and sneezing), the recruitment of additional FInt and FF motor units is required [19, 20, 24, 26, 27, 30, 33]. The gradations in force generated by diaphragm motor units (type FF > FInt > FR > S) [26, 124–126, 140, 141, 147] results in various slopes of force development during the sequential recruitment of motor units (Fig. 2.1).

Diaphragm Muscle Force

Transdiaphragmatic pressure (P_{di}) measurements have been used to measure diaphragm muscle force generated during different ventilatory and non-ventilatory behaviors in a variety of species [20, 24, 26, 28, 30, 33, 161–165]. While ventilatory behaviors are accomplished by activating only ~10–25% of diaphragm total force-generating capacity [19, 20, 24, 26–28, 30, 33, 166, 167] a greater amount of activation is required to achieve higher force, expulsive behaviors (Fig. 2.1). For normalization purposes and to determine maximal force generation, bilateral phrenic nerve stimulation was used to obtain the maximum P_{di} (P_{di}max) in anesthetized animals. In cats, Pdi generated during eupnea was ~10% of P_{di}max, and ~20% of P_{di}max in the rat. In humans, estimates of the P_{di} generated by the diaphragm muscle during eupnea is approximately 10% of P_{di}max [165]. When ventilation was stimulated by exposing animals to hypoxic (10% O_2) and hypercapnic (5% CO_2) gas mixtures, the forces generated increased to ~30% P_{di}max in cats and rats [19, 20, 24, 26–28, 30, 33, 166, 167]. Although exposure to hypoxia-hypercapnia represents a robust ventilatory stimulus, it does not even approach the maximal force generation of the diaphragm muscle, so there is considerable reserve capacity (Fig. 2.1). Indeed, even during sustained airway occlusion the forces generated by the diaphragm muscle were only ~50% of P_{di}max in cats, ~45% of P_{di}max in hamsters and ~65% of P_{di}max in rats [19, 20, 24, 26–28, 30, 33, 166, 167]. Only during high force, expulsive behaviors (e.g., coughing, sneezing) were maximal diaphragm muscle forces generated in both cats and rats [19, 20, 24, 26–28, 30, 33, 166, 167]. It is important to note that sneezing and coughing behaviors constitute physiological patterns of motor activation that can be elicited in anesthetized animals [19, 20, 24, 26–28, 30, 33, 166, 167], and thus do not depend on voluntary control of respiratory muscle activity. These results indicate that measures of diaphragm muscle activity during a variety of motor behaviors is necessary in assessing muscle weakness or diminished functional reserve [165, 168–170].

Ventilatory behaviors of the diaphragm muscle can be accomplished by the recruitment of fatigue resistant type S and FR motor units, even during hypoxic/hypercapnic conditions. However, during ventilatory challenges such as sustained airway occlusion, the additional recruitment of type FInt motor units would be required. The P_{di} generated during sneezing and coughing was near the maximal generated by bilateral phrenic nerve stimulation, and would require full recruitment of more fatigable type FInt and FF diaphragm motor units [20, 24, 26, 28, 30, 33, 161–165]. Although considerable force reserve exists for the diaphragm muscle to generate higher forces surpassing those necessary for sustaining ventilation, this comes at the expense of fatigue. Adaptations of motor unit properties during early postnatal development or with advanced aging (e.g., sarcopenia), as well as following injury or disease (e.g., cachexia) may impact this force reserve and differentially impair ventilatory and non-ventilatory behaviors, potentially placing patients at increased risk of respiratory failure [171].

Diaphragm Motor Unit Plasticity

Motor unit plasticity can occur at each of its components, namely, the motor neuron, neuromuscular junctions and/or muscle fibers. Altered use of the diaphragm muscle, whether it is an increase or decrease in activity, or non-activity/loading dependent hypertrophy/atrophy or strengthening/weakening will impact motor unit properties and thus, cause adaptations in neuromotor control. At the muscle fiber level, there may be hypertrophy or atrophy of muscle fibers, altered expression of contractile proteins and/or changes in fiber mechanical properties. At neuromuscular junctions, there may be remodeling of pre- and postsynaptic elements and altered synaptic efficacy. At phrenic motor neuron, there may be changes in somal surface area or dendritic branching. These adaptations may affect orderly motor neuron recruitment, synaptic transmission, and/or the ability of the diaphragm muscle to generate sufficient force for different motor behaviors. It is important to recognize that neuromotor control of the diaphragm muscle may be altered in differing ways depending on how different motor unit types are affected.

A myriad of past investigations have demonstrated that the biochemical and mechanical properties of skeletal muscles are altered in response to changes in their innervation [172–176]. Denervation elicits a profound effect on diaphragm muscle fibers, with specific atrophy and weakening (reduced specific force) of type IIx and/or IIb muscle fibers, thereby markedly affecting the force contribution of type FInt and FF motor units and higher force, expulsive motor behaviors [138, 139, 165, 177–187]. In contrast, diaphragm muscle paralysis induced by motor neuron inactivity causes remarkably few changes in the mechanical and biomechanical properties of muscle fibers from any of the motor unit types [138]. These results indicate that muscle inactivity *per se* is not the major determinant of diaphragm motor unit plasticity. Indeed, it appears that mismatched activity of nerve and muscle, and disrupted trophic support are likely players in the adaptation of muscle fibers within diaphragm motor units.

The consequence of a mismatch in nerve and muscle activity was explored in previous studies, where the effects of diaphragm paralysis induced by C_2 spinal cord hemisection (inactivating phrenic motor neurons) were compared to the effects of tetrodotoxin (TTX)-induced nerve blockade (phrenic motor neurons remained active) [138, 184, 188]. After two weeks of TTX-induced phrenic nerve blockade, there were dramatic effects at neuromuscular junctions (synaptic vesicle depletion) and neuromuscular transmission failure at diaphragm muscle fibers. In contrast after two weeks of diaphragm muscle paralysis induced by C2 hemisection neuromuscular transmission was actually enhanced. These results are consistent with a Hebbian plasticity at the neuromuscular junction where it is important to match the activity of motor neurons with the activity of the muscle fiber target cell.

Type IIx and/or IIb muscle fibres are almost exclusively affected in a wide variety of conditions perturbing diaphragm muscle function including postnatal development, denervation, TTX nerve blockade, hypothyroidism, corticosteroid treatment, undernutrition, obesity, chronic obstructive pulmonary disease, emphysema and aging [135, 138, 140, 141, 143, 163, 178–180, 189–209]. The fact that atrophy and weakness induced by these conditions are limited to type IIx and/or IIb muscle fibers indicates that type FInt and FF motor units are more vulnerable to mal-adaptations [208, 210–212]. If motor unit specific differences in neurotrophic support underlie neuroplasticity of phrenic motor neurons and diaphragm motor units, then neurotrophins would make an ideal target for therapeutic interventions to improve diaphragm muscle function.

Aging of Diaphragm Motor Units

Sarcopenia is an age-related loss of muscle mass (atrophy of type IIx and/or IIb muscle fibers) and a decrease in specific force (weakness) [36, 213, 214]. In rodents, sarcopenia has profound effects on the diaphragm muscle with a selective atrophy of type IIx and/or IIb muscle fibers that constitute type FInt and FF motor units and a reduction in maximum specific force [143, 163, 190, 194, 215]. Functionally, diaphragm muscle sarcopenia impairs the high force, expulsive motor behaviors necessary to clear the airways [143, 163, 190, 194, 215]. This inability to perform high force, expulsive motor behaviors may underlie respiratory complications that are particularly common in older humans [216–218].

A plethora of human and rodent studies have identified other age-related impairments of motor units including neuromuscular junction withdrawal and motor neuron loss [163, 215, 219–232], and converging evidence suggests that type FInt and FF motor units are specifically involved [125]. This raises the important questions of why and how are type S and FR motor units spared [143, 190, 233]. In the diaphragm muscle, the why is readily apparent since breathing must be unimpaired during aging for life to continue [163]. The how question is more difficult to answer but most likely relates to differences in trophic and/or metabolic support of type S and FR motor units.

Previous reports have established aging-related motor neuron loss in spinal cords of humans [234, 235] and rodent models [42–44, 236, 237], including in the cervical segments supplying the phrenic nerve [238]. Impairments in neuromuscular transmission, cholinergic receptor density and nerve terminal fragmentation occur during aging [239–247]. However, there is a surprising paucity of motor unit type-specific neuromuscular junction studies. One rare report illustrates that fragmentation of the neuromuscular junction occurs selectively in those of type FInt and FF motor units, with type S and FR motor units showing little adaption to age [231]. A concentration of efforts upon motor unit adaptations at the neuronal, neuromuscular junction and muscle fiber level are required if we are to untangle the specific mechanisms of sarcopenia. Our current conceptual framework (Fig. 2.2) underlining the specific vulnerability of type FInt and FF motor units and the sparing of type S and FR motor units during aging is based on complimentary observations of loss of larger phrenic motor neurons, fragmentation of neuromuscular junctions at type IIx

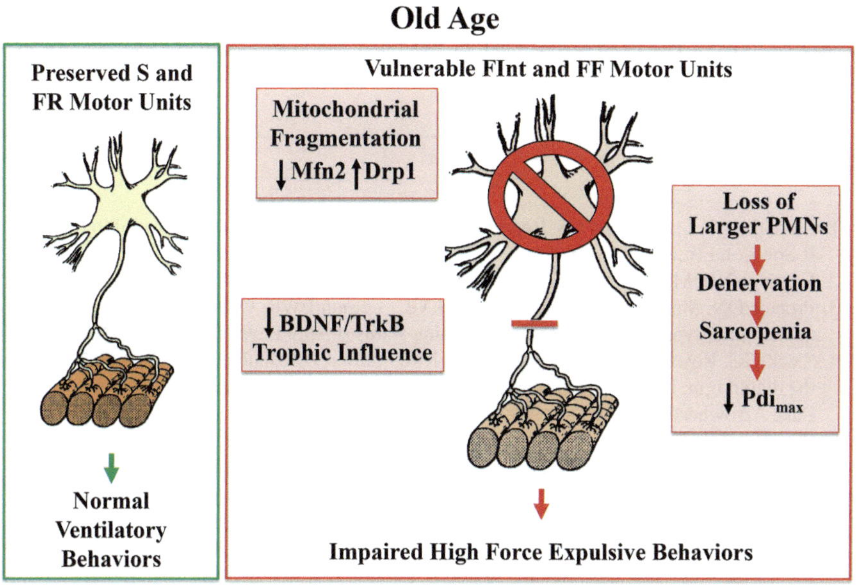

Fig. 2.2 We hypothesize that impaired high force behaviors in old age are underpinned by mitochondrial fragmentation, resulting from decreased Mfn2 and increased Drp1 expression and a decrease in BDNF/TrkB signaling. The resulting denervation of type IIx and/or IIb fibers leads to selective atrophy and weakness (sarcopenia) of the DIAm and selective vulnerability of larger phrenic motor neurons

and IIb muscle fibers and selective atrophy of type IIx and/or IIb muscle fibers. Preliminary results also suggest that mitochondrial fragmentation and reduced neurotrophic support may be essential to this process.

Conclusions

Diaphragm motor units and phrenic motor neurons are not a passive amorphous relay of premotor signals, they integrate the myriad of synaptic messages they receive and according to the discrete biochemical and contractile properties of constituent muscle fibers, they accomplish the wide range of force generations required to accomplish different motor behaviors. These motor behaviors include ventilatory pump actions that require low levels of force generation, deep inspirations (sighs) that require higher force to mitigate lung airway atelectasis, and expulsive airway clearance behaviors, such as coughing and sneezing, that require the generation of near maximal forces of the diaphragm. Curiously, conditions that impair motor unit function such as aging, seem to affect type FInt and FF motor units and thus the generation of larger forces while sparing type S and FR motor units and the generation of lower force ventilatory behaviors essential for life.

Acknowledgements Supported by a National Institutes of Health grants R01-AG044615 (GCS), AG057052 (GCS), HL96750 (GCS), and an Australian National Health & Medical Research Council CJ Martin Early Career Fellowship (MJF).

References

1. Liddell EGT, Sherrington CS. Recruitment and some other features of reflex inhibition. Proc R Soc Lond B. 1925;97:488–518.
2. Edgerton VR. Mammalian muscle fiber types and their adaptability. Am Zool. 1978;18:113–25.
3. Proctor DN, Sinning WE, Walro JM, Sieck GC, Lemon PWR. Oxidative capacity of human muscle fiber types: effects of age and training status. J Appl Physiol. 1995;78:2033–8.
4. Sieck GC, Roy RR, Edgerton VR, Harper RM, editors. Distribution of muscle fiber types in the diaphragm. In: Second Oxford meeting symposium: modelling and control of breathing. Lake Arrowhead, CA; 1982.
5. Sieck GC, Roy RR, Powell P, Blanco C, Edgerton VR, Harper RM. Muscle fiber type distribution and architecture of the cat diaphragm. J Appl Physiol. 1983;55(5):1386–92.
6. Sieck GC, Fournier M, Enad JG. Fiber type composition of muscle units in the cat diaphragm. Neurosci Lett. 1989;97(1-2):29–34.
7. Sieck GC, Zhan WZ, Prakash YS, Daood MJ, Watchko JF. SDH and actomyosin ATPase activities of different fiber types in rat diaphragm muscle. J Appl Physiol. 1995;79(5):1629–39.
8. Alvarez-Argote S, Gransee HM, Mora JC, Stowe JM, Jorgenson AJ, Sieck GC, et al. The impact of midcervical contusion injury on diaphragm muscle function. J Neurotrauma. 2016;33(5):500–9. https://doi.org/10.1089/neu.2015.4054.
9. Keswani NH, Hollinshead WH. The phrenic nucleus. III. Organization of the phrenic nucleus in the spinal cord of the cat and man. Proc Staff Meet Mayo Clin. 1955;30:566–77.
10. Mantilla CB, Zhan WZ, Sieck GC. Retrograde labeling of phrenic motoneurons by intrapleural injection. J Neurosci Methods. 2009;182:244–9. https://doi.org/10.1016/j.jneumeth.2009.06.016.
11. Prakash YS, Mantilla CB, Zhan WZ, Smithson KG, Sieck GC. Phrenic motoneuron morphology during rapid diaphragm muscle growth. J Appl Physiol. 2000;89(2):563–72.
12. Qiu K, Lane MA, Lee KZ, Reier PJ, Fuller DD. The phrenic motor nucleus in the adult mouse. Exp Neurol. 2010;226(1):254–8. https://doi.org/10.1016/j.expneurol.2010.08.026.
13. Rana S, Sieck GC, Mantilla CB. Diaphragm electromyographic activity following unilateral midcervical contusion injury in rats. J Neurophysiol. 2017;117(2):545–55. https://doi.org/10.1152/jn.00727.2016.
14. Song A, Ashwell KW, Tracey DJ. Development of the rat phrenic nucleus and its connections with brainstem respiratory nuclei. Anat Embryol (Berl). 2000;202(2):159–77.
15. Webber CL, Wurster RD, Chung JM. Cat phrenic nucleus architecture as revealed by horseradish peroxidase mapping. Exp Brain Res. 1979;35:395–406.
16. Prakash YS, Smithson KG, Sieck GC. Measurements of motoneuron somal volumes using laser confocal microscopy: comparisons with shape-based stereological estimations. NeuroImage. 1993;1(2):95–107.
17. Prakash YS, Smithson KG, Sieck GC. Application of the Cavalieri principle in volume estimation using laser confocal microscopy. NeuroImage. 1994;1(4):325–33.
18. Henneman E, Somjen G, Carpenter DO. Functional significance of cell size in spinal motoneurons. J Neurophysiol. 1965;28(3):560–80.
19. Sieck GC. Recruitment and frequency coding of diaphragm motor units during ventilatory and non-ventilatory behaviors. In: Swanson GD, Grodins FS, Hughson RL, editors. Respiratory control. New York: Plenum Press; 1989. p. 441–50.
20. Sieck GC. Conceptual model of ventilatory muscle recruitment and diaphragmatic fatigue. In: Khoo MCK, editor. Modeling and parameter estimation in respiratory control. New York: Plenum Press; 1990. p. 113–23.

21. Stuart DG, Enoka RM. Motoneurons, motor units, and the size principle. In: Rosenberg RN, editor. The clinical neurosciences. New York: Churchill Livingstone; 1983. p. 471–517.
22. Dick TE, Kong FJ, Berger AJ. Correlation of recruitment order with axonal conduction velocity for supraspinally driven diaphragmatic motor units. J Neurophysiol. 1987;57(1):245–59.
23. Jodkowski JS, Viana F, Dick TE, Berger AJ. Electrical properties of phrenic motoneurons in the cat: correlation with inspiratory drive. J Neurophysiol. 1987;58(1):105–24.
24. Mantilla CB, Seven YB, Zhan WZ, Sieck GC. Diaphragm motor unit recruitment in rats. Respir Physiol Neurobiol. 2010;173(1):101–6.
25. Seven YB, Mantilla CB, Sieck GC. Recruitment of rat diaphragm motor units across motor behaviors with different levels of diaphragm activation. J Appl Physiol. 2014;117(11):1308–16. https://doi.org/10.1152/japplphysiol.01395.2013.
26. Sieck GC, Fournier M. Diaphragm motor unit recruitment during ventilatory and nonventilatory behaviors. J Appl Physiol. 1989;66(6):2539–45.
27. Sieck GC. Organization and recruitment of diaphragm motor units. In: Roussos C, editor. The Thorax. 2nd ed. New York: Marcel Dekker; 1995. p. 783–820.
28. Sieck GC. Recruitment of diaphragm motor units during ventilatory and non-ventilatory behaviors. In: Stuart DG, Gantchev GN, Gurfinkel VS, Wiesendanger M, editors. Motor control VII. Proceedings of the VIIth international symposium on motor control, Borovets, Bulgaria. Tucson, AZ: Motor Control Press; 1996. p. 39–42.
29. Sieck GC, Prakash YS. The diaphragm muscle. In: Miller AD, Bianchi AL, Bishop BP, editors. Neural control of the respitatory muscles. Boca Raton, FL: CRC Press; 1997. p. 7–20.
30. Mantilla CB, Sieck GC. Phrenic motor unit recruitment during ventilatory and non-ventilatory behaviors. Respir Physiol Neurobiol. 2011;179(1):57–63. https://doi.org/10.1016/j.resp.2011.06.028.
31. Seven YB, Mantilla CB, Zhan WZ, Sieck GC. Motor unit recruitment order in diaphragm muscle following spinal cord injury. FASEB J. 2010;24(Meeting Abstract Supplement):1064.15.
32. Seven YB, Mantilla CB, Zhan WZ, Sieck GC. Non-stationarity and power spectral shifts in EMG activity reflect motor unit recruitment in rat diaphragm muscle. Respir Physiol Neurobiol. 2013;185(2):400–9. https://doi.org/10.1016/j.resp.2012.08.020.
33. Sieck GC. Neural control of the inspiratory pump. NIPS. 1991;6:260–4.
34. Kong FJ, Berger AJ. Firing properties and hypercapnic responses of single phrenic motor axons in the rat. J Appl Physiol. 1986;61(6):1999–2004.
35. Mantilla CB, Seven YB, Sieck GC. Convergence of pattern generator outputs on a common mechanism of diaphragm motor unit recruitment. Prog Brain Res. 2014;209:309–29. https://doi.org/10.1016/B978-0-444-63274-6.00016-3.
36. Elliott JE, Greising SM, Mantilla CB, Sieck GC. Functional impact of sarcopenia in respiratory muscles. Respir Physiol Neurobiol. 2016;226:137–46. https://doi.org/10.1016/j.resp.2015.10.001.
37. Sieck GC. Diaphragm muscle: structural and functional organization. Clin Chest Med. 1988;9(2):195–210.
38. Anderson CA, Dick TE, Orem J. Swallowing in sleep and wakefulness in adult cats. Sleep. 1995;18:325–9.
39. Umezaki T, Shiba K, Zheng Y, Miller AD. Upper airway motor outputs during vomiting versus swallowing in the decerebrate cat. Brain Res. 1998;781(1-2):25–36.
40. Zheng Y, Umezaki T, Nakazawa K, Miller AD. Role of pre-inspiratory neurons in vestibular and laryngeal reflexes and in swallowing and vomiting. Neurosci Lett. 1997;225(3):161–4.
41. Caccia MR, Harris JB, Johnson MA. Morphology and physiology of skeletal muscle in aging rodents. Muscle Nerve. 1979;2:202–12.
42. Hashizume K, Kanda K, Burke RE. Medial gastrocnemius motor nucleus in the rat: age-related changes in the number and size of motoneurons. J Comp Neurol. 1988;269(3):425–30.
43. Hashizume K, Kanda K. Differential effects of aging on motoneurons and peripheral nerves innervating the hindlimb and forelimb muscles of rats. Neurosci Res. 1995;22(2):189–96.

44. Ishihara A, Naitoh H, Katsuta S. Effects of ageing on the total number of muscle fibers and motoneurons of the tibialis anterior and soleus muscles in the rat. Brain Res. 1987;435(1-2):355–8.
45. Sieck GC, Roy RR, Powell P, Blanco C, Edgerton VR, Harper RM. Muscle fiber type distribution and architecture of the cat diaphragm. J Appl Physiol Respir Environ Exerc Physiol. 1983;55(5):1386–92.
46. Lance-Jones C. Motoneuron cell death in the developing lumbar spinal cord of the mouse. Dev Brain Res. 1982;4:473–9.
47. Allan DW, Greer JJ. Embryogenesis of the phrenic nerve and diaphragm in the fetal rat. J Comp Neurol. 1997;382(4):459–68.
48. Harris AJ, McCaig CD. Motoneuron death and motor unit size during embryonic development of the rat. J Neurosci. 1984;4(1):13–24.
49. Drey M, Krieger B, Sieber CC, Bauer JM, Hettwer S, Bertsch T, et al. Motoneuron loss is associated with sarcopenia. J Am Med Dir Assoc. 2014;15(6):435–9. https://doi.org/10.1016/j.jamda.2014.02.002.
50. Prakash YS, Sieck GC, editors. Morphometric analysis of phrenic motoneuron pools using confocal microscopy. Kemp station symposium on regulation of respiration; 1992.
51. Chakkalakal JV, Nishimune H, Ruas JL, Spiegelman BM, Sanes JR. Retrograde influence of muscle fibers on their innervation revealed by a novel marker for slow motoneurons. Development. 2010;137(20):3489–99. https://doi.org/10.1242/dev.053348.
52. Cameron WE, Brozanski BS, Guthrie RD. Postnatal development of phrenic motoneurons in the cat. Dev Brain Res. 1990;51:142–5.
53. Mantilla CB, Sieck GC. Key aspects of phrenic motoneuron and diaphragm muscle development during the perinatal period. J Appl Physiol. 2008;104(6):1818–27.
54. Dick TE, Oku Y, Romaniuk JR, Cherniack NS. Interaction between central pattern generators for breathing and swallowing in the cat. J Physiol. 1993;465:715–30.
55. Richter DW. Generation and maintenance of the respiratory rhythm. J Exp Biol. 1982;100:93–107.
56. Richter DW, Jordan D, Ballantyne D, Meesmann M, Spyer KM. Presynaptic depolarization in myelinated vagal afferent fibres terminating in the nucleus of the tractus solitarius in the cat. Pflugers Archiv Eur J Physiol. 1986;406(1):12–9.
57. Bellingham MC. Driving respiration: the respiratory central pattern generator. Clin Exp Pharmacol Physiol. 1998;25(10):847–56.
58. McKay LC, Janczewski WA, Feldman JL. Sleep-disordered breathing after targeted ablation of preBotzinger complex neurons. Nat Neurosci. 2005;8(9):1142–4. https://doi.org/10.1038/nn1517.
59. Smith JC, Ellenberger HH, Ballanyi K, Richter DW, Feldman JL. Pre-Botzinger complex: a brainstem region that may generate respiratory rhythm in mammals. Science. 1991;254(5032):726–9.
60. Koizumi H, Koshiya N, Chia JX, Cao F, Nugent J, Zhang R, et al. Structural-functional properties of identified excitatory and inhibitory interneurons within pre-Botzinger complex respiratory microcircuits. J Neurosci. 2013;33(7):2994–3009. https://doi.org/10.1523/JNEUROSCI.4427-12.2013.
61. Berger AJ. Phrenic motoneurons in the cat: subpopulations and nature of respiratory drive potentials. J Neurophysiol. 1979;42:76–90.
62. Gill PK, Kuno M. Excitatory and inhibitory actions on phrenic motoneurones. J Physiol. 1963;168:274–89.
63. Richter DW, Smith JC. Respiratory rhythm generation in vivo. Physiology (Bethesda). 2014;29(1):58–71. https://doi.org/10.1152/physiol.00035.2013.
64. Janczewski WA, Feldman JL. Distinct rhythm generators for inspiration and expiration in the juvenile rat. J Physiol. 2006;570(Pt 2):407–20. https://doi.org/10.1113/jphysiol.2005.098848.
65. Jiang C, Lipski J. Extensive monosynaptic inhibition of ventral respiratory group neurons by augmenting neurons in the Botzinger complex in the cat. Exp Brain Res. 1990;81(3):639–48.

66. Otake K, Sasaki H, Ezure K, Manabe M. Axonal projections from Botzinger expiratory neurons to contralateral ventral and dorsal respiratory groups in the cat. Exp Brain Res. 1988;72(1):167–77.
67. Dobbins EG, Feldman JL. Brainstem network controlling descending drive to phrenic motoneurons in rat. J Comp Neurol. 1994;347(1):64–86.
68. Ellenberger HH, Feldman JL. Monosynaptic transmission of respiratory drive to phrenic motoneurons from brainstem bulbospinal neurons in rats. J Comp Neurol. 1988;269:47–57.
69. Feldman JL, Loewy AD, Speck DF. Projections from the ventral respiratory group to phrenic and intercostal motoneurons in cat: an autoradiographic study. J Neurosci. 1985;5(8):1993–2000.
70. Lois JH, Rice CD, Yates BJ. Neural circuits controlling diaphragm function in the cat revealed by transneuronal tracing. J Appl Physiol. 2009;106(1):138–52.
71. Feldman JL, Cohen MI. Relation between expiratory duration and rostral medullary expiratory neuronal discharge. Brain Res. 1978;141:172–8.
72. Cohen MI, Piercey MF, Gootman PM, Wolotosky P. Synaptic connections between medullary inspiratory neurons and phrenic motoneurons as revealed by cross-correlation. Brain Res. 1974;81:319–24.
73. Davies JG, Kirkwood PA, Sears TA. The distribution of monosynaptic connexions from inspiratory bulbospinal neurones to inspiratory motoneurones in the cat. J Physiol. 1985;368:63–87.
74. Rybak IA, O'Connor R, Ross A, Shevtsova NA, Nuding SC, Segers LS, et al. Reconfiguration of the pontomedullary respiratory network: a computational modeling study with coordinated in vivo experiments. J Neurophysiol. 2008;100(4):1770–99. https://doi.org/10.1152/jn.90416.2008.
75. Hudson AL, Gandevia SC, Butler JE. Control of human inspiratory motoneurones during voluntary and involuntary contractions. Respir Physiol Neurobiol. 2011;179(1):23–33. https://doi.org/10.1016/j.resp.2011.06.010.
76. Ellenberger HH, Feldman JL. Brainstem connections of the rostral ventral respiratory group of the rat. Brain Res. 1990;513:35–42.
77. Lipski J, Zhang X, Kruszewska B, Kanjhan R. Morphological study of long axonal projections of ventral medullary inspiratory neurons in the rat. Brain Res. 1994;640(1-2):171–84.
78. Saji M, Miura M. Evidence that glutamate is the transmitter mediating respiratory drive from medullary premotor neurons to phrenic motoneurons: a double labeling study in the rat. Neurosci Lett. 1990;115(2-3):177–82.
79. Canning BJ, Chang AB, Bolser DC, Smith JA, Mazzone SB, McGarvey L, et al. Anatomy and neurophysiology of cough: CHEST guideline and expert panel report. Chest. 2014;146(6):1633–48. https://doi.org/10.1378/chest.14-1481.
80. Narula M, McGovern AE, Yang SK, Farrell MJ, Mazzone SB. Afferent neural pathways mediating cough in animals and humans. J Thorac Dis. 2014;6(Suppl 7):S712–9. https://doi.org/10.3978/j.issn.2072-1439.2014.03.15.
81. Berger AJ, Averill DB. Projection of single pulmonary stretch receptors to solitary tract region. J Neurophysiol. 1983;49(3):819–30.
82. Donoghue S, Garcia M, Jordan D, Spyer KM. The brain-stem projections of pulmonary stretch afferent neurones in cats and rabbits. J Physiol. 1982;322:353–63.
83. Sant'Ambrogio G, Tsubone H, Sant'Ambrogio FB. Sensory information from the upper airway: role in the control of breathing. Respir Physiol Neurobiol. 1995;102(1):1–16.
84. Aaron EA, Powell FL. Effect of chronic hypoxia on hypoxic ventilatory response in awake rats. J Appl Physiol (1985). 1993;74(4):1635–40.
85. Lahiri S, DeLaney RG. Relationship between carotid chemoreceptor activity and ventilation in the cat. Respir Physiol Neurobiol. 1975;24(3):267–86.
86. Lahiri S, DeLaney RG. Stimulus interaction in the responses of carotid body chemoreceptor single afferent fibers. Respir Physiol Neurobiol. 1975;24(3):249–66.
87. Vizek M, Pickett CK, Weil JV. Increased carotid body hypoxic sensitivity during acclimatization to hypobaric hypoxia. J Appl Physiol (1985). 1987;63(6):2403–10.

88. Zhang W, Carreno FR, Cunningham JT, Mifflin SW. Chronic sustained hypoxia enhances both evoked EPSCs and norepinephrine inhibition of glutamatergic afferent inputs in the nucleus of the solitary tract. J Neurosci. 2009;29(10):3093–102. https://doi.org/10.1523/JNEUROSCI.2648-08.2009.
89. Nattie E, Li A. Central chemoreception is a complex system function that involves multiple brain stem sites. J Appl Physiol (1985). 2009;106(4):1464–6. https://doi.org/10.1152/japplphysiol.00112.2008.
90. Pappenheimer JR, Fencl V, Heisey SR, Held D. Role of cerebral fluids in control of respiration as studied in unanesthetized goats. Am J Phys. 1965;208:436–50.
91. Haldane JS, Priestley JG. The regulation of the lung-ventilation. J Physiol. 1905;32(3-4):225–66.
92. Hilaire G, Voituron N, Menuet C, Ichiyama RM, Subramanian HH, Dutschmann M. The role of serotonin in respiratory function and dysfunction. Respir Physiol Neurobiol. 2010;174(1-2):76–88. https://doi.org/10.1016/j.resp.2010.08.017.
93. Lalley PM, Bischoff AM, Richter DW. 5-HT-1A receptor-mediated modulation of medullary expiratory neurones in the cat. J Physiol. 1994;476(1):117–30.
94. Lalley PM, Bischoff AM, Schwarzacher SW, Richter DW. 5-HT2 receptor-controlled modulation of medullary respiratory neurones in the cat. J Physiol. 1995;487(Pt 3):653–61.
95. Lindsay AD, Feldman JL. Modulation of respiratory activity of neonatal rat phrenic motoneurones by serotonin. J Physiol. 1993;461:213–33.
96. Morin D, Monteau R, Hilaire G. Compared effects of serotonin on cervical and hypoglossal inspiratory activities: an in vitro study in the newborn rat. J Physiol. 1992;451:605–29.
97. Hilaire G, Viemari JC, Coulon P, Simonneau M, Bevengut M. Modulation of the respiratory rhythm generator by the pontine noradrenergic A5 and A6 groups in rodents. Respir Physiol Neurobiol. 2004;143(2-3):187–97. https://doi.org/10.1016/j.resp.2004.04.016.
98. Tryba AK, Pena F, Lieske SP, Viemari JC, Thoby-Brisson M, Ramirez JM. Differential modulation of neural network and pacemaker activity underlying eupnea and sigh-breathing activities. J Neurophysiol. 2008;99(5):2114–25. https://doi.org/10.1152/jn.01192.2007.
99. Viemari JC, Hilaire G. Monoamine oxidase A-deficiency and noradrenergic respiratory regulations in neonatal mice. Neurosci Lett. 2003;340(3):221–4.
100. Viemari JC, Ramirez JM. Norepinephrine differentially modulates different types of respiratory pacemaker and nonpacemaker neurons. J Neurophysiol. 2006;95(4):2070–82. https://doi.org/10.1152/jn.01308.2005.
101. Proske U, Gandevia SC. The proprioceptive senses: their roles in signaling body shape, body position and movement, and muscle force. Physiol Rev. 2012;92(4):1651–97. https://doi.org/10.1152/physrev.00048.2011.
102. Duron B, Jung-Caillol MC, Marlot D. Myelinated nerve fiber supply and muscle spindles in the respiratory muscles of cat: quantitative study. Anat Embryol. 1978;152(2):171–92.
103. Corda M, von Euler C, Lennerstrand G. Proprioceptive innervation of the diaphragm. J Physiol. 1965;178:161–77.
104. Jammes Y, Arbogast S, De Troyer A. Response of the rabbit diaphragm to tendon vibration. Neurosci Lett. 2000;290(2):85–8.
105. Eldridge FL, Gill-Kumar P, Millhorn DE, Waldrop TG. Spinal inhibition of phrenic motoneurones by stimulation of afferents from peripheral muscles. J Physiol. 1981;311:67–79.
106. Remmers JE. Inhibition of inspiratory activity by intercostal muscle afferents. Respir Physiol Neurobiol. 1970;10(3):358–83.
107. Decima EE, von Euler C, Thoden U. Intercostal-to-phrenic reflexes in the spinal cat. Acta Physiol Scand. 1969;75(4):568–79.
108. Remmers JE. Extra-segmental reflexes derived from intercostal afferents: phrenic and laryngeal responses. J Physiol. 1973;233(1):45–62.
109. Bolser DC, Lindsey BG, Shannon R. Medullary inspiratory activity: influence of intercostal tendon organs and muscle spindle endings. J Appl Physiol (1985). 1987;62(3):1046–56.
110. Shannon R, Bolser DC, Lindsey BG. Medullary expiratory activity: influence of intercostal tendon organs and muscle spindle endings. J Appl Physiol (1985). 1987;62(3):1057–62.

111. Bellingham MC. Synaptic inhibition of cat phrenic motoneurons by internal intercostal nerve stimulation. J Neurophysiol. 1999;82(3):1224–32.
112. Bellingham MC, Lipski J. Respiratory interneurons in the C5 segment of the spinal cord of the cat. Brain Res. 1990;533(1):141–6.
113. Duffin J, Douse MA. Botzinger expiratory neurones inhibit propriobulbar decrementing inspiratory neurones. Neuroreport. 1993;4(11):1215–8.
114. Duffin J, Iscoe S. The possible role of C5 segment inspiratory interneurons investigated by cross-correlation with phrenic motoneurons in decerebrate cats. Exp Brain Res. 1996;112(1):35–40.
115. Lois JH, Rice CD, Yates BJ. Neural circuits controlling diaphragm function in the cat revealed by transneuronal tracing. J Appl Physiol (1985). 2009;106(1):138–52. https://doi.org/10.1152/japplphysiol.91125.2008.
116. Lane MA, Lee KZ, Fuller DD, Reier PJ. Spinal circuitry and respiratory recovery following spinal cord injury. Respir Physiol Neurobiol. 2009;169(2):123–32. https://doi.org/10.1016/j.resp.2009.08.007.
117. Zholudeva LV, Karliner JS, Dougherty KJ, Lane MA. Anatomical recruitment of spinal V2a interneurons into phrenic motor circuitry after high cervical spinal cord injury. J Neurotrauma. 2017;34(21):3058–65. https://doi.org/10.1089/neu.2017.5045.
118. Gandevia SC, Rothwell JC. Activation of the human diaphragm from the motor cortex. J Physiol. 1987;384:109–18.
119. Macefeild G, Gandevia SC. The cortical drive to human respiratory muscles in the awake state assessed by premotor cerebral potentials. J Physiol. 1991:1–14.
120. Shea SA. Behavioural and arousal-related influences on breathing in humans. Exp Physiol. 1996;81(1):1–26.
121. Fink BR. Influence of cerebral activity in wakefulness on regulation of breathing. J Appl Physiol. 1961;16:15–20.
122. Datta AK, Shea SA, Horner RL, Guz A. The influence of induced hypocapnia and sleep on the endogenous respiratory rhythm in humans. J Physiol. 1991;440:17–33.
123. Skatrud JB, Dempsey JA. Interaction of sleep state and chemical stimuli in sustaining rhythmic ventilation. J Appl Physiol Respir Environ Exerc Physiol. 1983;55(3):813–22.
124. Fournier M, Sieck GC. Mechanical properties of muscle units in the cat diaphragm. J Neurophysiol. 1988;59(3):1055–66.
125. Geiger PC, Cody MJ, Macken RL, Sieck GC. Maximum specific force depends on myosin heavy chain content in rat diaphragm muscle fibers. J Appl Physiol. 2000;89(2):695–703.
126. Geiger PC, Cody MJ, Sieck GC. Force-calcium relationship depends on myosin heavy chain and troponin isoforms in rat diaphragm muscle fibers. J Appl Physiol. 1999;87(5):1894–900.
127. Sieck GC, Ferreira LF, Reid MB, Mantilla CB. Mechanical properties of respiratory muscles. Compr Physiol. 2013;3(4):1553–67. https://doi.org/10.1002/cphy.c130003.
128. Sieck GC, Fournier M. Changes in diaphragm motor unit EMG during fatigue. J Appl Physiol. 1990;68(5):1917–26.
129. Sieck GC, Fournier M, Belman MJ. Physiological properties of motor units in the diaphragm. In: Bianchi AL, Denavit-Saubie M, editors. Neurogenesis of cntral respiratory rhythm. Hingham, MA: MTP; 1985. p. 227–9.
130. Sieck GC, Fournier M, Prakash YS, Blanco CE. Myosin phenotype and SDH enzyme variability among motor unit fibers. J Appl Physiol. 1996;80(6):2179–89.
131. Hamm TM, Nemeth PM, Solanki L, Gordon DA, Reinking RM, Stuart DG. Association between biochemical and physiological properties in single motor units. Muscle Nerve. 1988;11(3):245–54.
132. Nemeth PM, Hamm TM, Gordon DA, Reinking RM, Stuart DG. Application of cross-sectional single-fiber microchemistry to the study of motor-unit fatigability. In: Gantchev GN, Dimitrov B, Gatev P, editors. Motor Control. New York: Plenum; 1986.
133. Nemeth PM, Solanki L, Gordon DA, Hamm TM, Reinking RM, Stuart DG. Uniformity of metabolic enzymes within individual motor units. J Neurosci. 1986;6(3):892–8.

134. Enad JG, Fournier M, Sieck GC. Oxidative capacity and capillary density of diaphragm motor units. J Appl Physiol. 1989;67(2):620–7.
135. Johnson BD, Wilson LE, Zhan WZ, Watchko JF, Daood MJ, Sieck GC. Contractile properties of the developing diaphragm correlate with myosin heavy chain phenotype. J Appl Physiol. 1994;77:481–7.
136. Sieck GC, Lewis MI, Blanco CE. Effects of undernutrition on diaphragm fiber size, SDH activity, and fatigue resistance. J Appl Physiol. 1989;66:2196–205.
137. Lewis MI, Sieck GC. Effect of acute nutritional deprivation on diaphragm structure and function. J Appl Physiol. 1990;68:1938–44.
138. Miyata H, Zhan WZ, Prakash YS, Sieck GC. Myoneural interactions affect diaphragm muscle adaptations to inactivity. J Appl Physiol. 1995;79:1640–9.
139. Zhan WZ, Miyata H, Prakash YS, Sieck GC. Metabolic and phenotypic adaptations of diaphragm muscle fibers with inactivation. J Appl Physiol. 1997;82(4):1145–53.
140. Geiger PC, Cody MJ, Macken RL, Bayrd ME, Sieck GC. Mechanisms underlying increased force generation by rat diaphragm muscle fibers during development. J Appl Physiol. 2001;90:380–8.
141. Geiger PC, Cody MJ, Han YS, Hunter LW, Zhan WZ, Sieck GC. Effects of hypothyroidism on maximum specific force in rat diaphragm muscle fibers. J Appl Physiol. 2002;92(4):1506–14.
142. Sieck DC, Zhan WZ, Fang YH, Ermilov LG, Sieck GC, Mantilla CB. Structure-activity relationships in rodent diaphragm muscle fibers vs. neuromuscular junctions. Respir Physiol Neurobiol. 2012;180(1):88–96. https://doi.org/10.1016/j.resp.2011.10.015.
143. Greising SM, Mantilla CB, Gorman BA, Ermilov LG, Sieck GC. Diaphragm muscle sarcopenia in aging mice. Exp Gerontol. 2013; https://doi.org/10.1016/j.exger.2013.06.001.
144. Chamberlain S, Lewis DM. Contractile characteristics and innervation ratio of rat soleus motor units. J Physiol. 1989;412:1–21.
145. Kanda K, Hashizume K. Factors causing difference in force output among motor units in the rat medial gastrocnemius muscle. J Physiol (London). 1992;448:677–95.
146. Fournier M, Sieck GC. Topographical projections of phrenic motoneurons and motor unit territories in the cat diaphragm. In: Sieck GC, Gandevia SC, Cameron WE, editors. Respiratory muscles and their neuromotor control. New York: Alan R. Liss, Inc.; 1987. p. 215–26.
147. Sieck GC, Fournier M. Contractile and fatigue properties of diaphragm motor units. In: Sieck GC, Gandevia SC, Cameron WE, editors. Respiratory muscles and their neuromotor control. New York: Alan R. Liss, Inc.; 1987. p. 227–37.
148. Butler JE, McKenzie DK, Gandevia SC. Discharge properties and recruitment of human diaphragmatic motor units during voluntary inspiratory tasks. J Physiol. 1999;518(Pt 3):907–20.
149. Kernell D. The motoneurone and its muscle fibres. New York: Oxford University Press Inc.; 2006.
150. Gordon T, Thomas CK, Munson JB, Stein RB. The resilience of the size principle in the organization of motor unit properties in normal and reinnervated adult skeletal muscles. Can J Physiol Pharmacol. 2004;82(8-9):645–61.
151. Henneman E. Relation between size of neurons and their susceptibility to discharge. Science. 1957;126(3287):1345–7.
152. Henneman E, Olson CB. Relations between structure and function in the design of skeletal muscles. J Neurophysiol. 1965;28:581–98.
153. McPhedran AM, Wuerker RB, Henneman E. Properties of motor units in a homogeneous red muscle (soleus) of the cat. J Neurophysiol. 1965;28:71–84.
154. Gasser HS, Newcomer HS. Physiological action currents in the phrenic nerve. An application of the thermionic vacuum tube to nerve physiology. Am J Phys. 1921;57(1):1–26.
155. Gasser HS, Grundfest H. Axon diameters in relation to the spike dimensions and the conduction velocity in mammalian A fibers. Am J Phys. 1939;127:393–414.
156. Burke RE, Levine DN, Tsairis P, Zajac FE 3rd. Physiological types and histochemical profiles in motor units of the cat gastrocnemius. J Physiol. 1973;234(3):723–48.
157. Sypert GW, Munson JB. Basis of segmental motor control: motoneuron size or motor unit type? Neurosurg. 1981;8(5):608–21.

158. Mendell LM. The size principle: a rule describing the recruitment of motoneurons. J Neurophysiol. 2005;93(6):3024–6. https://doi.org/10.1152/classicessays.00025.2005.
159. Zajac FE, Faden JS. Relationship among recruitment order, axonal conduction velocity, and muscle-unit properties of type-identified motor units in cat plantaris muscle. J Neurophysiol. 1985;53(5):1303–22.
160. Sieck GC. Diaphragm motor units and their response to altered use. Sem Respir Med. 1991;12:258–69.
161. Gill LC, Mantilla CB, Sieck GC. Impact of unilateral denervation on transdiaphragmatic pressure. Respir Physiol Neurobiol. 2015;210:14–21. https://doi.org/10.1016/j.resp.2015.01.013.
162. Greising SM, Sieck DC, Sieck GC, Mantilla CB. Novel method for transdiaphragmatic pressure measurements in mice. Respir Physiol Neurobiol. 2013;188(1):56–9. https://doi.org/10.1016/j.resp.2013.04.018.
163. Greising SM, Mantilla CB, Medina-Martinez JS, Stowe JM, Sieck GC. Functional impact of diaphragm muscle sarcopenia in both male and female mice. Am J Physiol Lung Cell Mol Physiol. 2015;309(1):L46–52. https://doi.org/10.1152/ajplung.00064.2015.
164. Khurram OU, Sieck GC, Mantilla CB. Compensatory effects following unilateral diaphragm paralysis. Respir Physiol Neurobiol. 2017;246:39–46. https://doi.org/10.1016/j.resp.2017.07.007.
165. Sieck GC. Physiological effects of diaphragm muscle denervation and disuse. Clin Chest Med. 1994;15(4):641–59.
166. Sieck GC, editor. Recruitment and frequency coding of diaphragm motor units during ventilatory and non-ventilatory behaviors. Oxford Meeting: Respiratory Control Conference; 1988.
167. Sieck GC, Prakash YS. The diaphragm muscle. In: Miller AD, Bianchi AL, Bishop BP, editors. Neural control of the respiratory muscles. Boca Raton: CRC Press; 1996. p. 7–20.
168. Sieck GC (1997) Diaphragm muscle neuromotor control: adaptations to disuse. Anesthesiology and Intensive Care (Kazakhstan). 1–11
169. Sieck GC, Mantilla CB. Role of neurotrophins in recovery of phrenic motor function following spinal cord injury. Respir Physiol Neurobiol. 2009;169(2):218–25.
170. Steier J, Kaul S, Seymour J, Jolley C, Rafferty G, Man W, et al. The value of multiple tests of respiratory muscle strength. Thorax. 2007;62(11):975–80. https://doi.org/10.1136/thx.2006.072884.
171. Sieck GC, Mantilla CB. Effect of mechanical ventilation on the diaphragm. N Engl J Med. 2008;358(13):1392–4.
172. Buller AJ, Eccles JC, Eccles RM. Interactions between motoneurones and muscles in respect of the characteristic speeds of responses. J Physiol. 1960;150:417–39.
173. Dubowitz V. Cross-innervated mammalian skeletal muscle: histochemical, physiological, and biochemical observations. J Physiol (London). 1967;193:481–96.
174. Guth L, Watson PK, Brown WC. Effects of cross-reinnervation on some chemical properties of red and white muscles of rat and cat. Exp Neurol. 1968;20(1):52–69.
175. Karpati G, Engel WK. Transformation of the histochemical profile of skeletal muscle by "foreign" innervation. Nature. 1967;215(109):1509–10.
176. Prewitt MA, Salafsky B. Effect of cross innervation on biochemical characteristics of skeletal muscles. Am J Phys. 1967;213(1):295–300.
177. Aravamudan B, Mantilla CB, Zhan WZ, Sieck GC. Denervation effects on myonuclear domain size of rat diaphragm fibers. J Appl Physiol. 2006;100(5):1617–22.
178. Argadine HM, Hellyer NJ, Mantilla CB, Zhan WZ, Sieck GC. The effect of denervation on protein synthesis and degradation in adult rat diaphragm muscle. J Appl Physiol. 2009;107(2):438–44.
179. Geiger PC, Cody MJ, Macken RL, Bayrd ME, Sieck GC. Effect of unilateral denervation on maximum specific force in rat diaphragm muscle fibers. J Appl Physiol. 2001;90(4):1196–204.
180. Geiger PC, Bailey JP, Zhan WZ, Mantilla CB, Sieck GC. Denervation-induced changes in myosin heavy chain expression in the rat diaphragm muscle. J Appl Physiol. 2003;95(2):611–9.
181. Gosselin LE, Prakash YS, Masters DB, Sieck GC. Effect of aging on diaphragm neuromuscular junction morphology. Neurosci Abstr (Abstract). 1995;21:1664.

182. Mantilla CB, Rowley KL, Zhan WZ, Fahim MA, Sieck GC. Synaptic vesicle pools at diaphragm neuromuscular junctions vary with motoneuron soma, not axon terminal, inactivity. Neuroscience. 2007;146(1):178–89.
183. Prakash YS, Zhan WZ, Miyata H, Sieck GC. Adaptations of diaphragm neuromuscular junction following inactivity. Acta Anat. 1995;154(2):147–61.
184. Prakash YS, Miyata H, Zhan WZ, Sieck GC. Inactivity-induced remodeling of neuromuscular junctions in rat diaphragmatic muscle. Muscle Nerve. 1999;22(3):307–19.
185. Sieck GC, Zhan WZ. Denervation alters myosin heavy chain expression and contractility of developing rat diaphragm muscle. J Appl Physiol. 2000;89(3):1106–13.
186. Sieck GC, Zhan WZ, Han YS, Prakash YS. Effect of denervation on ATP consumption rate of diaphragm muscle fibers. J Appl Physiol. 2007;103(3):858–66.
187. Zhan WZ, Prakash YS, Miyata H, Sieck GC. Morphological adaptations of diaphragm neuromuscular junction to prolonged inactivity. Neurosci Abstr (Abstract). 1995;21:1663.
188. Prakash YS, Miyata H, Zhan WZ, Sieck GC. Inactivity alters structural and functional properties of the neuromuscular junction. In: Steinacker JM, Ward SA, editors. The physiology and pathophysiology of exercise tolerance. New York: Plenum Press; 1996. p. 59–66.
189. Blanco CE, Zhan WZ, Fang YH, Sieck GC. Exogenous testosterone treatment decreases diaphragm neuromuscular transmission failure in male rats. J Appl Physiol. 2001;90(3):850–6.
190. Elliott JE, Omar TS, Mantilla CB, Sieck GC. Diaphragm muscle sarcopenia in Fischer 344 and Brown Norway rats. Exp Physiol. 2016;101(7):883–94. https://doi.org/10.1113/EP085703.
191. Farkas GA, Gosselin LE, Zhan WZ, Schlenker EH, Sieck GC. Histochemical and mechanical properties of diaphragm muscle in morbidly obese Zucker rats. J Appl Physiol. 1994;77(5):2250–9.
192. Fournier M, Alula M, Sieck GC. Neuromuscular transmission failure during postnatal development. Neurosci Lett. 1991;125(1):34–6.
193. Geiger PC, Bailey JP, Mantilla CB, Zhan WZ, Sieck GC. Mechanisms underlying myosin heavy chain expression during development of the rat diaphragm muscle. J Appl Physiol. 2006;101(6):1546–55.
194. Gosselin LE, Johnson BD, Sieck GC. Age-related changes in diaphragm muscle contractile properties and myosin heavy chain isoforms. Am J Respir Crit Care Med. 1994;150:174–8.
195. Greising SM, Gransee HM, Mantilla CB, Sieck GC. Systems biology of skeletal muscle: fiber type as an organizing principle. Wiley Interdiscip Rev Syst Biol Med. 2012;4(5):457–73.
196. Greising SM, Medina-Martínez JS, Vasdev AK, Sieck GC, Mantilla CB. Analysis of muscle fiber clustering in the diaphragm muscle of sarcopenic mice. Muscle Nerve. 2015;52(1):76–82.
197. Howell S, Maarek JM, Fournier M, Sullivan K, Zhan WZ, Sieck GC. Congestive heart failure: differential adaptation of the diaphragm and latissimus dorsi. J Appl Physiol. 1995;79(2):389–97.
198. Howell S, Zhan WZ, Sieck GC. Diaphragm disuse reduces Ca2+ uptake capacity of sarcoplasmic reticulum. J Appl Physiol. 1997;82(1):164–71.
199. Lewis MI, LoRusso TJ, Zhan W-Z, Sieck GC. Interactive effects of denervation and malnutrition on diaphragm structure and function. J Appl Physiol. 1996;81:2165–72.
200. Lewis MI, Monn SA, Sieck GC. Effect of corticosteroids on diaphragm fatigue, SDH activity, and muscle fiber size. J Appl Physiol. 1992;72(1):293–301.
201. Lewis MI, Sieck GC, Fournier M, Belman MJ. Effect of nutritional deprivation on diaphragm contractility and muscle fiber size. J Appl Physiol. 1986;60:596–603.
202. Lewis MI, Zhan WZ, Sieck GC. Adaptations of the diaphragm in emphysema. J Appl Physiol. 1992;72(3):934–43.
203. Mantilla CB, Greising SM, Zhan WZ, Seven YB, Sieck GC. Prolonged C2 spinal hemisection-induced inactivity reduces diaphragm muscle specific force with modest, selective atrophy of type IIx and/or IIb fibers. J Appl Physiol. 2013;114(3):380–6. https://doi.org/10.1152/japplphysiol.01122.2012.
204. Mantilla CB, Sieck GC. Neuromotor control in chronic obstructive pulmonary disease. J Appl Physiol. 2013;114:1246–52. https://doi.org/10.1152/japplphysiol.01212.2012.

205. Ottenheijm CA, Heunks LM, Sieck GC, Zhan WZ, Jansen SM, Degens H, et al. Diaphragm dysfunction in chronic obstructive pulmonary disease. Am J Respir Crit Care Med. 2005;172(2):200–5. https://doi.org/10.1164/rccm.200502-262OC.
206. Prakash YS, Fournier M, Sieck GC. Effects of prenatal undernutrition on developing rat diaphragm. J Appl Physiol. 1993;75:1044–52.
207. Prakash YS, Gosselin LE, Zhan WZ, Sieck GC. Alterations of diaphragm neuromuscular junctions with hypothyroidism. J Appl Physiol. 1996;81:1240–8.
208. Rowley KL, Mantilla CB, Sieck GC. Respiratory muscle plasticity. Respir Physiol Neurobiol. 2005;147(2-3):235–51.
209. Watchko JF, Sieck GC. Respiratory muscle fatigue resistance relates to myosin phenotype and SDH activity during development. J Appl Physiol. 1993;75:1341–7.
210. Mantilla CB, Sieck GC. Impact of diaphragm muscle fiber atrophy on neuromotor control. Respir Physiol Neurobiol. 2013;189(2):411–8. https://doi.org/10.1016/j.resp.2013.06.025.
211. Mantilla CB, Stowe JM, Sieck DC, Ermilov LG, Greising SM, Zhang C, et al. TrkB kinase activity maintains synaptic function and structural integrity at adult neuromuscular junctions. J Appl Physiol. 2014;117(8):910–20. https://doi.org/10.1152/japplphysiol.01386.2013.
212. Sieck GC, Gransee HM. Respiratory muscles: structure, function & regulation, Colloquium series on integrated systems physiology: from molecule to function to disease, vol. 34. Morgan & Claypool Life Sciences; 2012.
213. Cruz-Jentoft AJ, Baeyens JP, Bauer JM, Boirie Y, Cederholm T, Landi F, et al. Sarcopenia: European consensus on definition and diagnosis: report of the European working group on Sarcopenia in older people. Age Ageing. 2010;39(4):412–23. https://doi.org/10.1093/ageing/afq034.
214. Doherty TJ. Invited review: aging and sarcopenia. J Appl Physiol. 2003;95(4):1717–27. https://doi.org/10.1152/japplphysiol.00347.2003.
215. Greising SM, Ermilov LG, Sieck GC, Mantilla CB. Ageing and neurotrophic signalling effects on diaphragm neuromuscular function. J Physiol. 2015;593(2):431–40. https://doi.org/10.1113/jphysiol.2014.282244.
216. Enright PL, Kronmal RA, Manolio TA, Schenker MB, Hyatt RE. Respiratory muscle strength in the elderly. Correlates and reference values. Cardiovascular Health Study Research Group. Am J Respir Crit Care Med. 1994;149(2 Pt 1):430–8.
217. Polkey MI, Harris ML, Hughes PD, Hamnegard CH, Lyons D, Green M, et al. The contractile properties of the elderly human diaphragm. Am J Respir Crit Care Med. 1997;155(5):1560–4.
218. Tolep K, Higgins N, Muza S, Criner G, Kelsen SG. Comparison of diaphragm strength between healthy adult elderly and young men. Am J Respir Crit Care Med. 1995;152(2):677–82.
219. Gawel M, Kostera-Pruszczyk A. Effect of age and gender on the number of motor units in healthy subjects estimated by the multipoint incremental MUNE method. J Clin Neurophysiol. 2014;31(3):272–8. https://doi.org/10.1097/WNP.0000000000000066.
220. Greising SM, Stowe JM, Sieck GC, Mantilla CB. Role of TrkB kinase activity in aging diaphragm neuromuscular junctions. Exp Gerontol. 2015;72:184–91. https://doi.org/10.1016/j.exger.2015.10.013.
221. Greising SM, Vasdev AK, Zhan WZ, Sieck GC, Mantilla CB. Chronic TrkB agonist treatment in old age does not mitigate diaphragm neuromuscular dysfunction. Physiol Rep. 2017;5(1) https://doi.org/10.14814/phy2.13103.
222. Kadhiresan VA, Hassett CA, Faulkner JA. Properties of single motor units in medial gastrocnemius muscles of adult and old rats. J Physiol. 1996;493(Pt 2):543–52.
223. Kanda K. Effects of food restriction on motoneuronal loss with advancing age in the rat. Microsc Res Tech. 2002;59(4):301–5. https://doi.org/10.1002/jemt.10208.
224. Lexell J, Taylor CC, Sjostrom M. What is the cause of the ageing atrophy? Total number, size and proportion of different fiber types studied in whole vastus lateralis muscle from 15- to 83-year-old men. J Neurol Sci. 1988;84(2-3):275–94.
225. McNeil CJ, Doherty TJ, Stashuk DW, Rice CL. Motor unit number estimates in the tibialis anterior muscle of young, old, and very old men. Muscle Nerve. 2005;31(4):461–7. https://doi.org/10.1002/mus.20276.

226. Pettigrew FP, Gardiner PF. Changes in rat plantaris motor unit profiles with advanced age. Mech Ageing Dev. 1987;40(3):243–59.
227. Piasecki M, Ireland A, Coulson J, Stashuk DW, Hamilton-Wright A, Swiecicka A, et al. Motor unit number estimates and neuromuscular transmission in the tibialis anterior of master athletes: evidence that athletic older people are not spared from age-related motor unit remodeling. Physiol Rep. 2016;4(19) https://doi.org/10.14814/phy2.12987.
228. Piasecki M, Ireland A, Jones DA, McPhee JS. Age-dependent motor unit remodelling in human limb muscles. Biogerontology. 2016;17(3):485–96. https://doi.org/10.1007/s10522-015-9627-3.
229. Piasecki M, Ireland A, Stashuk D, Hamilton-Wright A, Jones DA, McPhee JS. Age-related neuromuscular changes affecting human vastus lateralis. J Physiol. 2016;594(16):4525–36. https://doi.org/10.1113/JP271087.
230. Power GA, Dalton BH, Behm DG, Doherty TJ, Vandervoort AA, Rice CL. Motor unit survival in lifelong runners is muscle dependent. Med Sci Sports Exerc. 2012;44(7):1235–42. https://doi.org/10.1249/MSS.0b013e318249953c.
231. Prakash YS, Sieck GC. Age-related remodeling of neuromuscular junctions on type-identified diaphragm fibers. Muscle Nerve. 1998;21(7):887–95.
232. Sugiura M, Kanda K. Progress of age-related changes in properties of motor units in the gastrocnemius muscle of rats. J Neurophysiol. 2004;92(3):1357–65. https://doi.org/10.1152/jn.00947.2003.
233. Larsson L, Sjodin B, Karlsson J. Histochemical and biochemical changes in human skeletal muscle with age in sedentary males, age 22–65 years. Acta Physiol Scand. 1978;103(1):31–9. https://doi.org/10.1111/j.1748-1716.1978.tb06187.x.
234. Kawamura N, Gotoda Y, Yoshikura H. The rise in medical care expenditures in Japan, trends in disease patterns: 1977-81. Am J Public Health. 1985;75(12):1442–4.
235. Tomlinson BE, Irving D. The numbers of limb motor neurons in the human lumbosacral cord throughout life. J Neurol Sci. 1977;34(2):213–9.
236. Hashizume K, Kanda K. Neuronal dropout is greater in hindlimb motor nuclei than in forelimb motor nuclei in aged rats. Neurosci Lett. 1990;113(3):267–9.
237. Jacob JM. Lumbar motor neuron size and number is affected by age in male F344 rats. Mech Ageing Dev. 1998;106(1-2):205–16.
238. Zhang C, Goto N, Suzuki M, Ke M. Age-related reductions in number and size of anterior horn cells at C6 level of the human spinal cord. Okajimas Folia Anat Jpn. 1996;73(4):171–7.
239. Balice-Gordon RJ. Age-related changes in neuromuscular innervation. Muscle Nerve Suppl. 1997;5:S83–7.
240. Courtney J, Steinbach JH. Age changes in neuromucular junction morphology and acetylcholine receptor distribution on rat skeletal muscle fibres. J Physiol. 1981;320:435–47.
241. Fahim MA, Holley JA, Robbins N. Scanning and light microscopic study of age changes at a neuromuscular junction in the mouse. J Neurocytol. 1983;12:13–25.
242. Kelly SS, Robbins N. Statistics of neuromuscular transmitter release in young and old mouse muscle. J Physiol. 1987;385:507–16.
243. Robbins N. Compensatory plasticity of aging at the neuromuscular junction. Exp Gerontol. 1992;27:75–81.
244. Rosenheimer JL, Smith DO. Differential changes in the endplate architecture of functionally diverse muscles during aging. J Neurophysiol. 1985;53:1567–81.
245. Ruff RL. Sodium channel slow inactivation and the distribution of sodium channels on skeletal muscle fibres enable the performance properties of different skeletal muscle fibre types. Acta Physiol Scand. 1996;156(3):159–68.
246. Smith DO. Muscle-specific decrease in presynaptic calcium dependence and clearance during neuromuscular transmission in aged rats. J Neurophysiol. 1988;59(4):1069–82.
247. Wokke JH, Jennekens FG, van den Oord CJ, Veldman H, Smit LM, Leppink GJ. Morphological changes in the human end plate with age. J Neurol Sci. 1990;95(3):291–310.

Imaging of the Spinal Cord

3

Owen D. M. Stechishin, Manraj K. S. Heran,
Jason R. Shewchuk, A. Talia Vertinsky, and Cornelia Laule

Contents

Anatomical Imaging Techniques

Radiography

Due to the poor soft tissue contrast inherent to radiography, spinal radiographs cannot directly evaluate the spinal cord. The primary utility of radiography in cases of myelopathy is to evaluate potential anatomic abnormalities of the spinal column that may contribute to the underlying pathology. In cases of myelopathy in the post-operative spine, radiographs are the preferred initial modality to assess spinal hardware integrity, and to evaluate for signs of instability, including changes in osseous

O. D. M. Stechishin · M. K. S. Heran · J. R. Shewchuk · A. T. Vertinsky
Department of Radiology, The University of British Columbia, Vancouver, BC, Canada

C. Laule (✉)
Department of Radiology, The University of British Columbia, Vancouver, BC, Canada

Department of Pathology & Laboratory Medicine, Department of Physics & Astronomy, International Collaboration on Repair Discoveries (ICORD), The University of British Columbia, Vancouver, BC, Canada
e-mail: claule@physics.ubc.ca

B. Greenberg (ed.), *Myelopathy*, https://doi.org/10.1007/978-3-030-99906-3_3

alignment between upright and supine views, or subluxation on flexion and extension views (Fig. 3.1).

Computed Tomography

Computed tomography (CT) also has relatively limited capacity to directly assess the spinal cord as it provides suboptimal soft tissue contrast between the spinal cord, cerebrospinal fluid (CSF) within the thecal sac, and the epidural space. Administration of intravenous iodinated contrast can opacify the epidural venous plexus, and may be helpful to distinguish the epidural and intradural spaces, particularly in the cervical spine where there is little epidural fat. However, intravenous contrast does not significantly improve visualization of the spinal cord itself (Fig. 3.2).

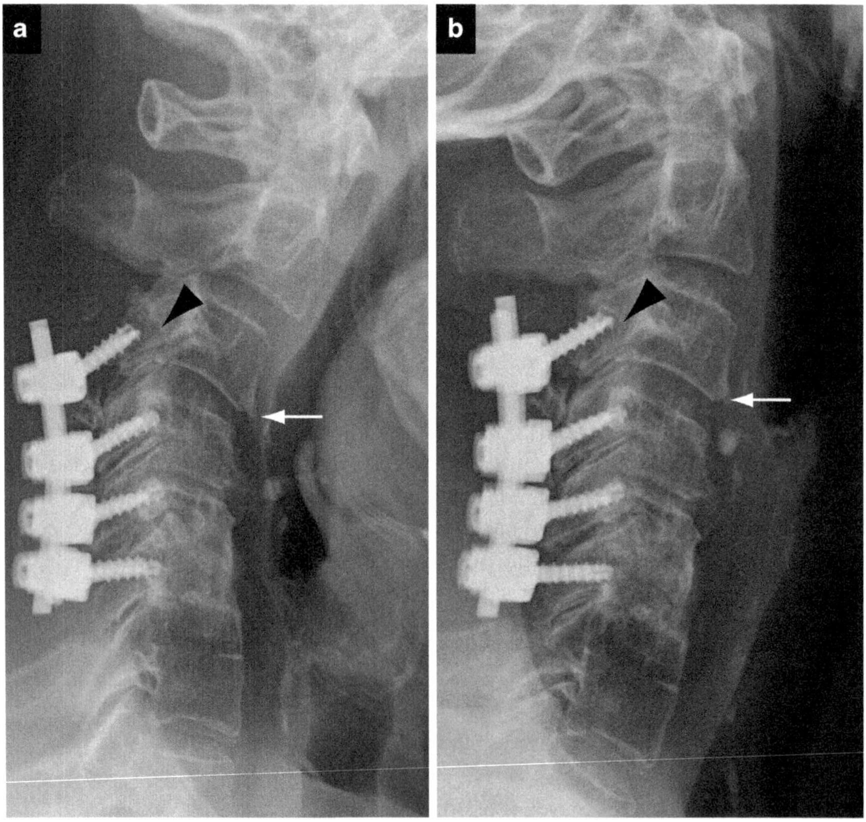

Fig. 3.1 Radiographic evaluation of spinal instability in a patient with prior C3–6 laminectomy and posterior fusion. On the radiograph obtained with the neck in flexion (**a**), there is 4 mm of anterolisthesis of C3 on C4 (white arrow), which completely reduces on the radiograph with the neck in extension (**b**). Lucency around the C3 pedicle screws (black arrowhead), which partially pull out of the pedicles on the flexion view, is indicative of screw loosening

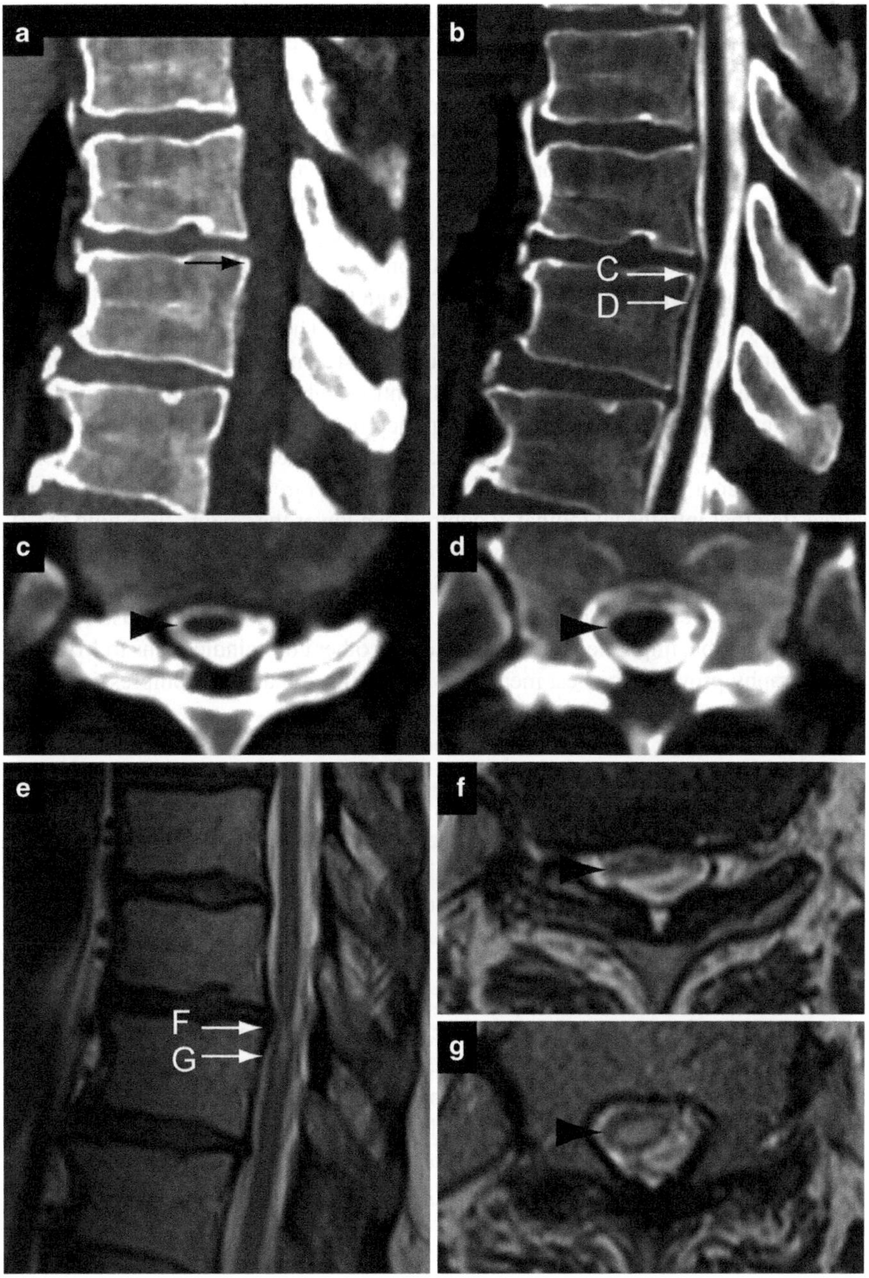

Fig. 3.2 Multimodality imaging of a patient with intrathecal adhesions deforming the spinal cord. (**a**) Intravenous contrast enhanced CT is unable to discern the spinal cord from the CSF in the thecal sac and does not demonstrate an apparent abnormality at the level of T10–11 disc space (arrow). (**b–d**) CT myelogram demonstrates focal anterior displacement and deformity of the spinal cord outlined by high attenuation intrathecal contrast. Axial images confirm focal deformity of the spinal cord (black arrowhead) in the anterior-posterior direction (**c**) compared to a more normal appearing level more caudally (**d**). (**e–g**) T2W MR images demonstrate increased T2 signal in the spinal cord at the level of the T10–11 disc space (**f**) that extends inferiorly for a short distance (**g**)

Nonetheless, CT can play an important role in the evaluation of compressive myelopathy. Due to the speed and relatively widespread availability of CT, it is particularly useful in the acute setting if MRI is not immediately available. CT is also often complementary to MRI as osseous structures are much better assessed by CT than MRI. In spinal trauma, CT is superior to MRI in characterizing bony abnormalities, especially when considering surgical management. In compressive myelopathy due to disc disease, CT can better distinguish disc osteophyte complexes from disc protrusions. Similarly, ossification of the posterior longitudinal ligament (OPLL) is much easier to identify on CT than MRI (Fig. 3.3).

In order to better resolve the spinal cord from the surrounding CSF in the thecal sac, CT myelography can be performed (Fig. 3.2). The main disadvantage of CT myelography is the need for dural puncture (most commonly done in the lumbar region) to administer intrathecal iodinated contrast, which may limit the availability of this examination. Moreover, any dural puncture has inherent small risks of iatrogenic spinal infection, hemorrhage and post-procedure headache or CSF leak. There have also been a few case reports in the literature of rare post-myelogram seizures suggesting that intrathecal iodinated contrast can lower the seizure threshold [1, 2].

In CT myelography, iodinated contrast opacifies the CSF space within the thecal sac, therefore providing indirect visualization of the spinal cord. However, in patients who cannot undergo MRI because of severe claustrophobia, MR-incompatible implanted medical devices or other contraindications to MRI, CT myelography provides the best means for evaluating spinal cord compression.

Magnetic Resonance Imaging

MRI is the workhorse for imaging in myelopathy as it is the only modality able to achieve sufficient soft tissue contrast to directly evaluate the spinal cord. A combination of sequences with varying degrees of T1 and T2 weighting are performed for in vivo tissue characterization. In order to adequately visualize the anatomy of the spinal cord, in-plane spatial resolution of 1 mm × 1 mm and thin slices (1–2 mm) are usually used.

T2 weighted (T2W) sequences are the most important sequences for evaluation of the spinal cord due to inherent high sensitivity for water, and hence can detect spinal cord edema associated with myelopathy (Fig. 3.2e–g). However, it should be noted that not all increased T2 signal within the spinal cord necessarily represents potentially reversible edema, as irreversible gliosis will also result in increased T2 signal in the spinal cord. T2W sequences also allow for visualization of the CSF in the thecal sac surrounding the spinal cord and nerve roots. High resolution three dimensional T2W sequences such as 3D Constructive Interference in Steady State (CISS), 3D True Fast Imaging with Steady-state free Precession (True-FISP) and Fast Imaging Employing STeady-state Acquisition (FIESTA) permit reconstruction of images with high spatial resolution in multiple planes. These techniques can be particularly useful for visualizing the inner structure of cysts or cystic tumors, the walls of arachnoid cysts or arachnoid webs, spinal cord herniations,

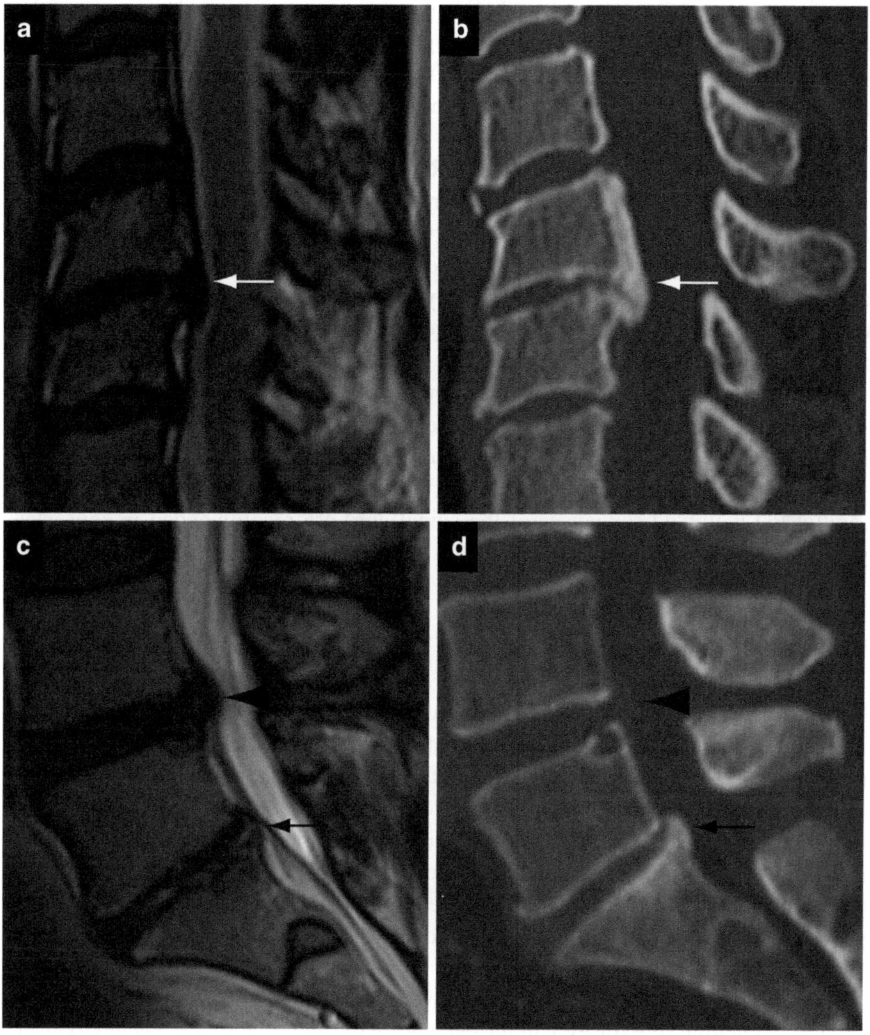

Fig. 3.3 CT can be complementary to MRI in evaluation of compressive myelopathy due to degenerative disc disease or other pathologies. On T2W MRI (**a**), low T2 signal is seen indenting the thecal sac posterior to the C4–5 disc space (white arrow), which can be confidently diagnosed as focal ossification of the posterior longitudinal ligament (OPLL) on CT (**b**). Similarly, low T2 signal is seen posterior to the L4–5 (black arrowhead) and L5-S1 (black arrow) disc spaces indenting the thecal sac (**c**). Integrating the appearances on MRI (**c**) and CT (**d**), a disc extrusion at L4–5 and a disc-osteophyte complex at L5-S1 with a large osteophyte arising off the superior endplate of S1 can be confidently diagnosed

pseudomeningoceles, dural leaks in intracranial hypotension, and the abnormal vessels in spinal cord vascular malformations [3–8].

T1 weighted (T1W) sequences allow for detection of substances with inherent high T1 signal such as methemoglobin in subacute hemorrhage or melanin in melanoma metastases. However, T1W sequences are particularly important for detecting enhancement with intravenous gadolinium, indicating disruption of the blood-spinal cord barrier commonly seen in aggressive inflammatory and neoplastic processes. Chemical fat suppression techniques are often used to increase the conspicuity of subtle enhancement.

Short Tau-Inversion Recovery (STIR) sequences provide a mix of T1 and T2 weighting with suppression of the signal from fat, allowing for superior detection of abnormal fluid within the spinal cord, vertebral bodies and paraspinal soft tissues. STIR sequences are particularly useful in cases of traumatic myelopathy to confirm and evaluate the extent of traumatic injury as they provide superior sensitivity for edema in the bone marrow and soft tissues associated with acute spinal fractures and ligamentous disruption.

Proton density (PD) weighted sequences reflect the density of water and are mainly used to non-specifically evaluate areas of damage. In multiple sclerosis (MS), PD weighted sequences have been reported to be superior to fast spin-echo T2W sequences for detecting lesions in the cervical spinal cord [9]. As such, axial and sagittal PD weighted sequences of the spinal cord are recommended in consensus guidelines for MS imaging [10].

Nuclear Medicine

Nuclear medicine imaging techniques have a limited role in spinal cord imaging and are usually restricted to excluding spinal infection or metastasis as a cause for myelopathy. With PET and SPECT cameras having a spatial resolution on the order of several millimeters, they can only provide limited detail in the spinal cord. A few reports characterizing ^{18}Fluoro-deoxyglucose metabolism in the human spinal cord in normal and pathological states have been published. Several studies have suggested that the ^{18}Fluoro-deoxyglucose metabolic pattern of the cervical cord may predict a patient's clinical outcome after decompressive surgery for cervical spine stenosis, but evaluation of the spinal cord by PET is not routine in clinical practice [11–14]. However, with the increasing availability of fusion imaging with PET/MRI, the potential role for PET in the evaluation of myelopathy is expected to grow.

Vascular Imaging Techniques

CT Angiography

CT angiography (CTA) allows for assessment of the larger vascular structures supplying the spine. Its main advantages are its rapid acquisition time and widespread availability. It should be noted though that CT does impart a significant dose of ionizing radiation to the patient. A single phase CT covering the thoracic and lumbar spine has an average dose of 15.6 mSv, which is the equivalent of 5 years of background radiation [15]. Another disadvantage of CTA is that it lacks the spatial resolution to reliably assess small caliber vessels, including the anterior and posterior spinal arteries, or even the radicular arteries in many cases. Sensitivity of CTA for detecting and characterizing spinal vascular abnormalities is generally considered inferior to MRI. However, CTA has been reported to identify up to three quarters of spinal arteriovenous dural fistulas [16, 17]. In patients who cannot undergo MR angiography, and in situations of known vascular abnormalities limited to a confined area of the spine, CTA is particularly useful for initial evaluation of the spinal vasculature in a non-invasive manner as a means to limit the extent of subsequent catheter angiography (Fig. 3.4).

MR Angiography

There are several MRI techniques that allow for non-invasive vascular imaging without the need for iodinated contrast or ionizing radiation. **Flow voids within vessels on T2W sequences** are the simplest method for assessing the vasculature on MRI as nearly all acquisitions will have at least one T2W sequence. Low signal within vessels on T2W images results from out-of-plane flow signal loss and provides a means to confirm patency in fast flowing, large caliber vascular structures. This technique relies on the direction of flow being perpendicular to the plane of the MRI slice and cannot assess in-plane vascular flow. The spatial resolution achieved on typical acquisitions also usually limits assessment to medium size vessels such as the vertebral arteries, and precludes assessment of the anterior or posterior spinal arteries.

Time of flight (TOF) angiography is a second MRI method to assess vascular flow without the need for intravenous contrast administration. In contrast to T2W flow voids, this technique uses flow-related "enhancement", with unsaturated protons in blood flowing into a slice resulting in high signal. TOF angiography can be acquired as a series of parallel slices (2D TOF) or as a 3D volume (3D TOF), which has the advantage of isotropic voxels allowing for multiplanar reconstructions. Decreased signal is seen in vessels with slow, turbulent, in-plane, or retrograde flow. The disadvantages of this technique are the relatively long acquisition times and inability to dynamically image blood flow [18].

Contrast enhanced MR angiography (MRA) techniques provide both anatomical and temporal information about the spinal vasculature. The simplest technique for performing contrast enhanced MRA is multiphase imaging of the area of interest, typically with arterial, venous and delayed phases. However, the temporal resolution achieved with this method is usually on the order of 1 min. Newer time-resolved sequences such as Time Resolved Imaging of Contrast KineticS (TRICKS) or Time-resolved angiography With Interleaved Stochastic Trajectories (TWIST) allow for contrast bolus tracking and can achieve temporal resolution on the order of 1 s [19].

In general, MRA lacks the spatial and temporal resolution to reliably assess small caliber vessels, and catheter angiography is still considered the gold standard for vascular imaging in the spine. As such, MRA has been traditionally used for

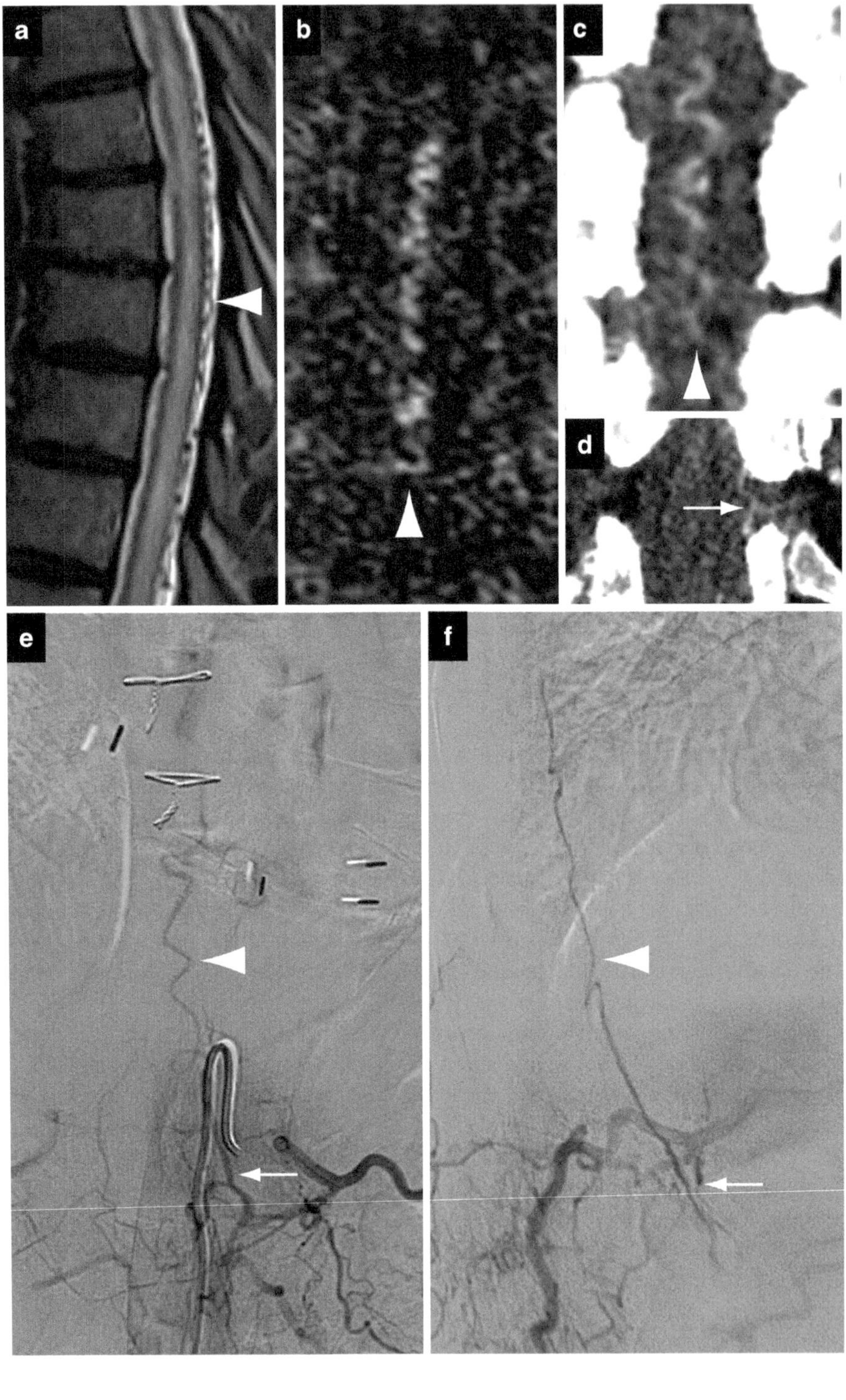
a
b
c
d
e
f

initial evaluation, to decrease the extent of catheter angiography required when assessing a spinal dural AV fistula or AVM (Fig. 3.4). However, several recent reports indicate improved performance of contrast enhanced MRA at 3 T field strength capable of accurately identifying and characterizing the vascular anatomy of spinal dural arteriovenous fistulas in many cases [17, 20].

Catheter Angiography

Digital subtraction catheter angiography remains the gold standard for spinal vascular imaging due to the superior spatial and temporal resolution compared to CTA and MRA. Vessel-specific selective angiography with microcatheters provides the best characterization of complex vascular anatomy (Fig. 3.4). Catheter angiography can also allow for endovascular treatment in those situations where it is deemed technically feasible and appropriate. The issues associated with it are quite small, but include potential access site-related complications, such as infection, local hematoma and pseudoaneurysm formation, as well as those associated with ionizing radiation exposure during fluoroscopy. There is also an extremely small risk of iatrogenic stroke or spinal cord infarct.

Pitfalls

Spinal Hardware Artifacts

Metallic spinal hardware is a source of significant artifact on both CT and MRI. Beam hardening artifact in CT is related to atomic number, with tantalum resulting in more artifact than stainless steel, and titanium resulting in the least artifact. Beam hardening artifact can be reduced by increasing the kilovolt peak and tube charge, although this results in an increased radiation dose to the patient. Iterative reconstruction techniques and dual energy acquisition with post-processing of virtual monoenergetic images allow for greater metallic artifact reduction with less of an increase in the radiation dose to the patient (Fig. 3.5) [21].

Fig. 3.4 Multimodality characterization of a spinal dural arteriovenous fistula (dAVF). (**a**) T2W MRI demonstrates extensive serpentine low T2 signal flow voids (arrowhead) posterior to the thoracic spinal cord consistent with a spinal dAVF. A long segment of high T2 signal is seen within the thoracic spinal cord. (**b–d**) Coronal images from a time resolved MR angiogram (**b**) and CT angiogram (**c**) demonstrate a serpentine vessel (arrowhead) posteriorly in the spinal canal representing the pathologically enlarged dorsal draining vein of the affected spinal cord. On the CT angiogram, a feeding artery (arrow) is seen arising from the left T11 radicular artery (**d**). Digital subtraction catheter angiography in anterior-posterior (**e**) and lateral (**f**) projections from a selective left T11 radicular artery injection confirm the arterial supply arising from the left T11 radicular artery (arrow) to the dAVF (arrowhead)

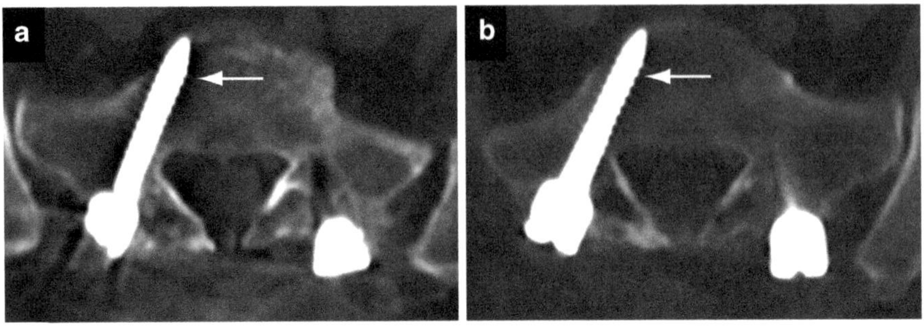

Fig. 3.5 Spinal hardware metal artifact reduction on dual energy CT. Beam hardening artifact results in apparent lucency (arrow) around the right S1 pedicle screw (**a**) on a polyenergetic image at 120 kVp, but is demonstrated to be artifact on a virtual monoenergetic image at 135 kVp (**b**). Streak artifact around the pedicle screws is also significantly reduced in the virtual monoenergetic image allowing for better evaluation of osseous and soft tissue detail

With respect to MRI, metallic hardware disrupts the homogeneity of the local magnetic field, thereby accelerating spin dephasing, leading to decreased signal and spatial distortion in the resulting image (Fig. 3.6). Metallic artifact is worst with alloys that contain ferromagnetic elements, such as stainless steel. The severity of the artifact also depends on the type of sequence. Gradient echo and echo planar sequences have significantly more artifact than spin-echo sequences due to the lack of a 180° refocusing pulse. Similarly, chemical fat suppression can fail due to the metal hardware perturbing the local magnetic environment and altering the Larmor frequency of protons in fat (Fig. 3.6). Fat saturation by inversion recovery techniques is much less affected by metallic elements, and STIR sequences are recommended over chemical fat saturation in patients with spinal hardware.

Gibbs Artifact

Gibbs artifact refers to a series of parallel lines adjacent to an abrupt change in signal intensity [22]. This artifact is usually most apparent clinically on sagittal images of the spine where Gibbs artifact due to the abrupt transition between the CSF and the spinal cord can create the appearance of a syrinx. The absence of a syrinx in images of the corresponding region acquired in the transverse plane confirms this finding as artifact (Fig. 3.7). As such, in spinal imaging studies, at least one sequence not acquired in the sagittal plane should be obtained. Gibbs artifact can occur in both the phase and frequency encoding directions, although it is usually most apparent in the phase encoding direction as the number of phase encoding steps is minimized to decrease acquisition time. Gibbs artifact can be reduced by increasing the image matrix size, although any increase in the phase encoding direction will directly increase image acquisition time.

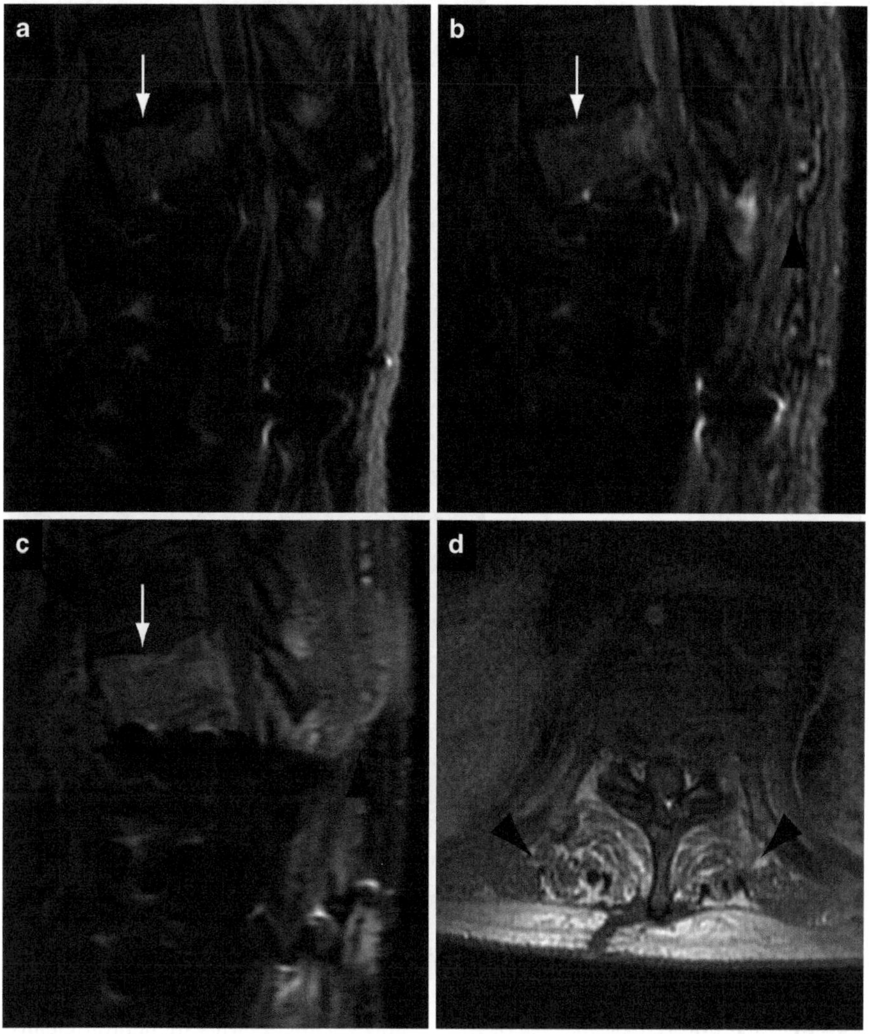

Fig. 3.6 Spinal hardware metal artifact on MRI. Extensive susceptibility artifact from bilateral posterior rods and pedicle screws results in signal drop out on T2W (**a**), STIR (**b**) and T1W fat saturated post-gadolinium (**c**) images. Increased STIR signal and enhancement is seen in the T11 vertebral body with anterior paraspinal inflammation (arrow) consistent with vertebral osteomyelitis. Increased signal within the posterior paraspinal soft tissues extending to the skin surface seen in the T1W post-gadolinium image but not the STIR image (arrowheads), is artifact due to failure of chemical fat saturation from the adjacent metallic hardware. Heterogeneous fat suppression (arrowheads) is confirmed in a corresponding location of an axial T1W fat saturated pre-gadolinium image (**d**)

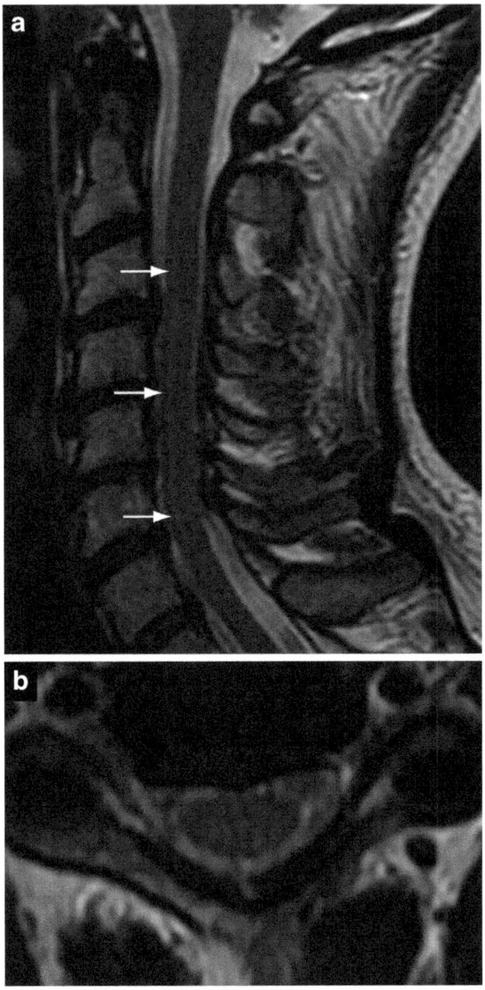

Fig. 3.7 Gibbs artifact manifests as thinlinear high T2 signal projected over the spinal cord from C3–6 on sagittal T2W images (arrows in **a**), which is not reproduced on axial T2W images (**b**)

CSF Flow Artifact

The flow of CSF can result in foci of decreased signal on T2W images, which can mimic an intradural mass or abnormal dilated blood vessel. This usually is seen in the posterior aspect of the thecal sac, but can occur lateral to the spinal cord as well. This artifact results from CSF flowing out of the slice plane prior to the 180° refocusing pulse resulting in decreased signal. If there is turbulent flow of CSF within the thecal sac, this can also contribute to CSF signal loss due to spin dephasing. This finding can be confirmed as artifact on a gradient echo sequence as the shorter time to echo minimizes flow related phenomena (Fig. 3.8). Additionally, most vendors include flow compensation techniques in their software packages that employ a gradient pulse to suppress CSF flow artifacts on T2W sequences [8].

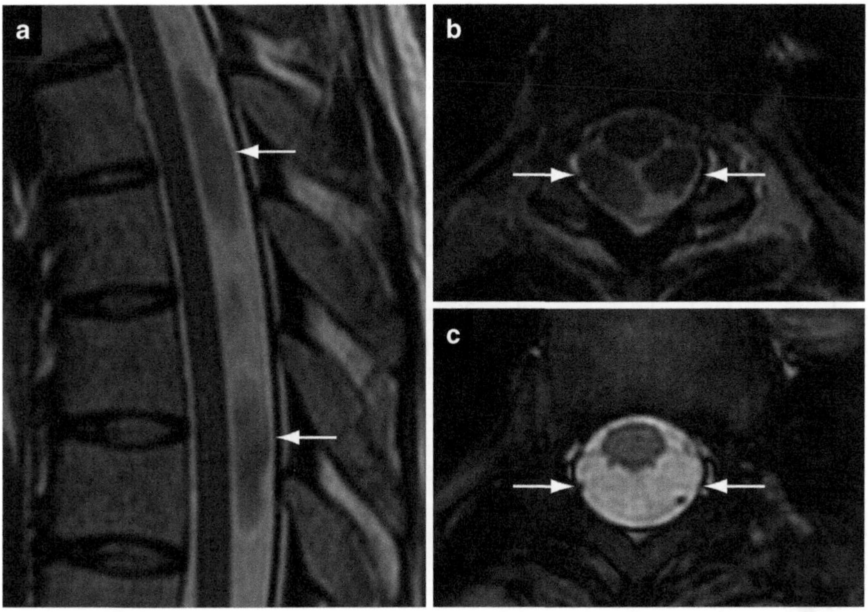

Fig. 3.8 CSF flow artifact manifests as low T2 signal (arrows) within the thecal sac dorsal to the spinal cord on T2W fast spin echo images in the sagittal (**a**) and axial planes (**b**), which is not reproduced on a gradient recalled echo image (**c**)

Motion Artifact

Artifacts created by motion are most apparent in the phase encoding direction and can project over the spinal canal if the image acquisition parameters are not carefully selected. Suppression pulses can be applied to the viscera anterior to the spine to decrease motion artifacts related to the pharynx, lungs and heart. The phase and frequency encoding directions can also be flipped to remove motion artifact projecting over the spine.

Advanced Imaging Techniques

There are several advanced MRI techniques that have been routinely used for research applications and have become relatively common in clinical imaging of the brain. Many of these techniques are also starting to be employed in clinical imaging of the spinal cord, and likely will play an increasing role in the future. However, while most advanced imaging techniques can achieve adequate image quality in the brain at 1.5 T field strength, the results in the spinal cord at 1.5 T are often suboptimal and ideally a 3 T system should be used in the spinal cord.

CSF Flow Imaging

CSF flow can be measured using a phase contrast technique [23, 24]. Two phase encoding pulses are sequentially applied in opposite directions. In protons that are stationary, these two pulses cancel each other out and result in no signal. Conversely protons that move between the two pulses will experience different gradients and emit signal. The velocity encoding gradient determines the greatest velocity that can be measured without aliasing artifacts occurring. A velocity encoding gradient of at least 10 cm/s is suggested based on measurement of CSF flow in healthy volunteers and may need to be set at greater than 20 cm/s if there is significant acceleration due to CSF flowing through a narrow channel [25].

Imaging of CSF flow can be helpful in differentiating spinal cord herniation from an arachnoid cyst (Fig. 3.9) [8, 26]. In both cases, the cord will be deviated anteriorly with an apparent enlarged dorsal CSF space. In cases of a dorsal arachnoid cyst, CSF flow should not be present within the cyst as it is not in direct communication with the thecal sac. Conversely, in spinal herniation, flow of CSF can be demonstrated in the dorsal CSF space as it is simply CSF filling the empty space in the dorsal portion of the thecal sac.

Diffusion Weighted Imaging and Diffusion Tensor Imaging

Diffusion weighted imaging (DWI) measures the relative differences in diffusion of water between tissues. DWI sequences begin with an initial T2* weighted image (B = 0 image) followed by a strong gradient applied symmetrically on either side of a 180° pulse, which alters the phase of the water molecules. In water molecules that are stationary, the gradients before and after the 180° pulse counteract each other, maintaining T2*signal. Conversely, in water molecules that have moved between the application of the first and second gradients, the gradients do not completely counteract each other, resulting in loss of signal. Tissues with restricted diffusion will therefore have high signal on the high B value images relative to normal tissue [27].

There are two important pitfalls with DWI. Firstly, diffusion cannot be assessed in tissues that are inherently T2 dark as they have very low signal on the B = 0 image. Secondly, T2 shine-through is a potential false positive on DWI sequences. True restricted diffusion will be low signal on the apparent diffusion coefficient (ADC) map, whereas T2 shine-through will have high signal.

Diffusion tensor imaging (DTI) (i.e. white matter "tractography") allows for the in vivo visualization of axonal tracts (Fig. 3.10). In the spine, water molecules primarily diffuse in the cranio-caudal direction because the majority of the axonal tracts in the spinal cord run in this orientation and therefore limit lateral diffusion of water molecules. By using the data from multidimensional vector algorithms with six or more gradient directions, the axonal connectivity of the spinal cord can be modeled [27].

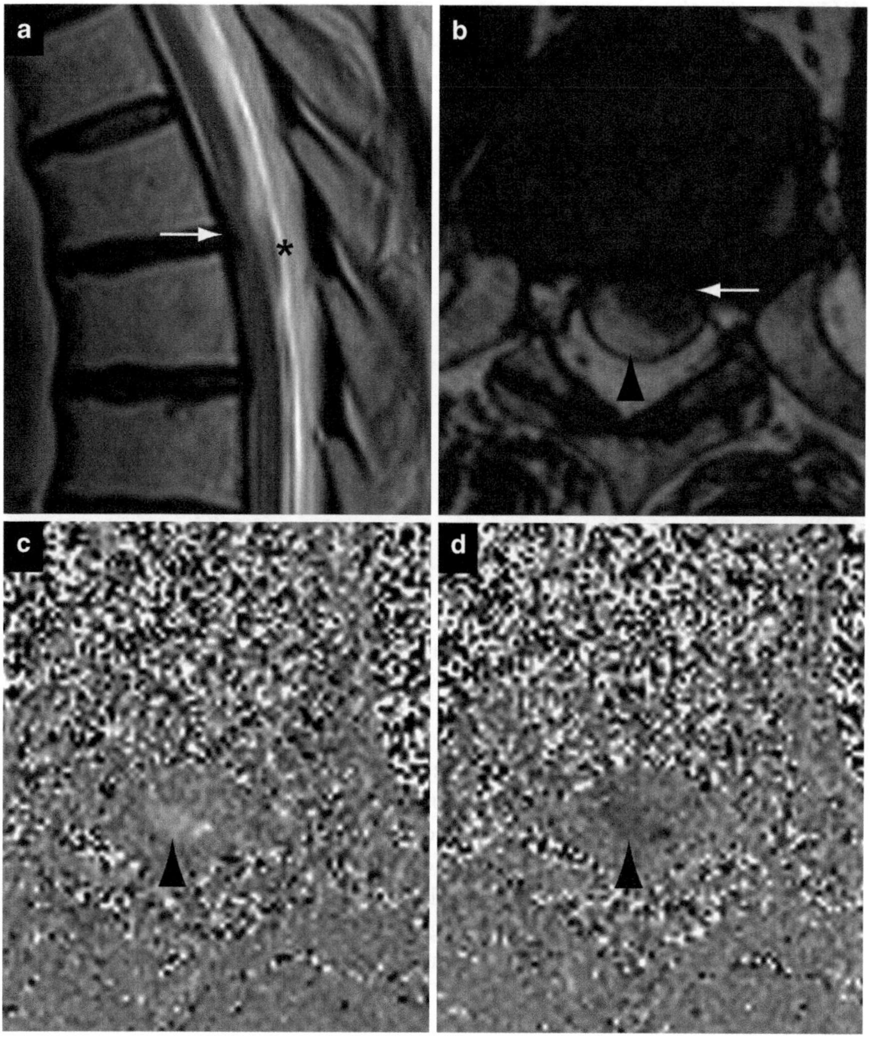

Fig. 3.9 Evaluation of idiopathic spinal cord herniation with CSF flow imaging. (**a**, **b**) Sagittal T2W image (**a**) and axial high resolution 3D CISS image (**b**) demonstrate focal anterior displacement of the spinal cord at the level of the T6–7 disc space, with no CSF seen anterior to the spinal cord (white arrow). A low T2 signal flow void (asterisk in **a**) indicates flow of CSF within the expanded dorsal CSF space. (**c**, **d**) Phase contrast axial images at the same level demonstrate periodically alternating high and low signal within the expanded dorsal CSF space (black arrowhead) indicating biphasic CSF flow, which confirms an anterior spinal cord herniation and excludes a dorsal arachnoid cyst

DWI and DTI are echo planar sequences that have the advantage of rapid acquisition as all of k space can be filled in one or a small number of echo trains. However, the disadvantage of such long echo trains is significant spatial distortion that can result from motion or susceptibility differences between adjacent tissues. This is

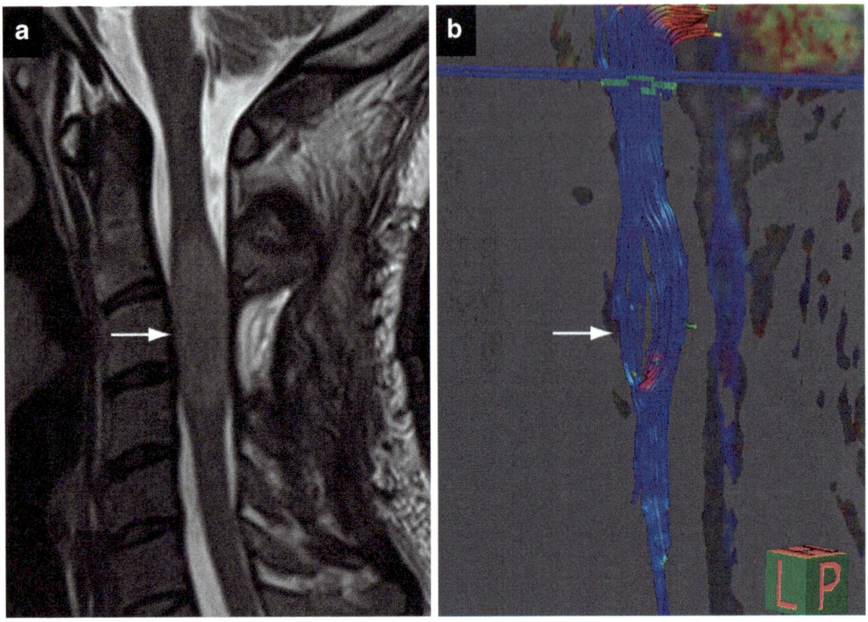

Fig. 3.10 DTI tractography in the spinal cord. (**a**) T2W MRI demonstrates an expansile mildly T2 high signal astrocytoma in the cervical cord at the level of C3. (**b**) DTI tractography demonstrates lateral displacement of the white matter tracts around the tumor

particularly problematic in the spine compared to the brain given the small size of the spinal cord, susceptibility artifact from the bone-soft tissue interface, and respiratory and cardiac motion. Spatial distortion can be decreased by reducing the readout bandwidth, although this results in decreased signal. Imaging in the transverse, rather than the sagittal, plane can also reduce distortion, although this significantly increases image acquisition time if a large cranio-caudal extent of the spinal cord needs to be imaged [28]. Advanced DWI techniques such as Readout Segmentation Of Long Variable Echo trains (RESOLVE) and Periodically Rotated overlapping ParallEL Lines with Enhanced Reconstruction (PROPELLER) have less susceptibility artifact and distortion compared to single shot echo planar DWI [29, 30].

MR Perfusion

MR perfusion allows for interrogation of blood flow through the microvasculature of a particular tissue. There are several MRI perfusion techniques that are used in the brain and other organs, which are starting to also be applied in the spine. However, poor spatial resolution within the spinal cord and significant image distortion due to susceptibility artifacts from the adjacent spinal column remain substantial limitations to MR perfusion imaging in the spinal cord.

In **dynamic susceptibility contrast (DSC)** MR perfusion, local magnetic field susceptibility due to the presence of gadolinium is used to measure tissue perfusion.

An echo planar sequence is used to rapidly image the first pass of the gadolinium bolus into the tissue of interest, with the amount of T2* signal loss proportional to the amount of gadolinium in the microvasculature. The inherent susceptibility artifacts due to the adjacent bone in the vertebral column and aerated lung make DSC much more difficult to perform in the spinal cord versus in the brain. Nonetheless, there are a few reports of successful use of DSC to assess perfusion in cervical spine tumors [31, 32].

In **dynamic contrast-enhanced (DCE)** MR perfusion, the increased T1 signal due to T1 shortening caused by gadolinium is used to calculate perfusion parameters by computational modeling [33, 34]. A 3D T1 spoiled gradient recalled echo sequence is used as it provides sufficient temporal resolution of 2–15 s over at least 5 min required for dynamically imaging contrast enhancement and washout. DCE MR perfusion has been used in the spine to characterize the vascularity of extradural spinal metastases as a means to help select patients amenable to endovascular therapy [35]. Preclinical studies have also looked at DCE MR perfusion for assessment of spinal cord injury [36, 37].

In **arterial spin labelling (ASL)** MR perfusion, water protons in arterial blood are magnetically labeled with a radiofrequency pulse. A control image is obtained prior to labeling and subtracted from the labeled image, with the remaining signal proportional to blood flow. Unlike DSC and DCE MR perfusion, ASL perfusion does not require intravenous gadolinium, and must be performed prior to any gadolinium administration as gadolinium will reduce the signal obtained. Echo planar sequences are usually used for ASL perfusion, which are challenging in the spinal cord due to the inherent susceptibility artifacts from the bone in the vertebral column and aerated lung. ASL perfusion has been used in the mouse spinal cord, but there is little published on its use in the human spinal cord [38].

Susceptibility Weighted Imaging

Susceptibility weighted imaging (SWI) detects subtle inhomogeneities in the local magnetic field. A gradient recalled echo T2* weighted sequence is used as the lack of a 180° refocusing pulse makes it highly sensitive to the accelerated dephasing of transverse magnetization induced by magnetic field inhomogeneity. This technique is routinely used in the brain to detect microhemorrhage and hemosiderin deposition, as well as foci of mineralization. SWI is not routinely used in clinical practice in the spinal cord as it is difficult to identify pathological susceptibility artifacts amongst the significant inherent susceptibility artifacts resulting from the bone-soft tissue interface as well as respiratory and cardiac motion artifact.

Spectroscopy

Spectroscopy allows for the identification and relative quantification of normal and abnormal metabolites in vivo. Spectroscopy is much more technically challenging in the spinal cord than in the brain due to the small physical dimensions of the spinal cord, CSF flow artifact, respiratory and cardiac motion artifacts, and local magnetic field inhomogeneity due to bone-soft tissue interfaces. Careful shimming of B0 is necessary to minimize magnetic field inhomogeneity. Saturation bands and pulse triggering are used to reduce CSF flow artifacts.

There are a few reports in the literature of the use of spectroscopy to differentiate spinal cord tumors from inflammatory lesions, as well as to evaluate amyotrophic lateral sclerosis [39, 40]. Spectroscopy has also been reported as a means to predict outcome in cervical spondylotic myelopathy after surgery [41].

Functional Imaging

Functional imaging (fMRI) allows for in vivo real time interrogation of neuronal function by measuring regional changes in blood flow and blood oxygen content. The small size of the spinal cord makes fMRI more challenging to perform than in the brain. Currently, fMRI is only used in the spine for research applications. Potentially, fMRI could be used to evaluate residual motor function in spinal cord injury patients, monitor changes in function in multiple sclerosis and amyotrophic lateral sclerosis and plan treatment for tumors near key neuronal tracts in the spinal cord [42].

Magnetization Transfer

Magnetization transfer (MT) methods detect the exchange of magnetization between non-aqueous tissue and water [43] following off resonance excitations. The premise of the MT approach is that (1) compared to hydrogens attached to water, hydrogens attached to non-aqueous molecules (i.e. all lipids and proteins in myelin and glial cells) have a much broader range of MR frequencies and that (2) hydrogens within myelin preferentially exchange magnetization with water molecules [44, 45]. Thus, following off-resonance excitations, decreases in the MR signal indirectly probe the non-aqueous component of the tissue.

Although not yet used in day-to-day clinical settings, there is an extensive research literature on the use of MT to characterize various types of spinal cord myelopathy [46], and quantitative MR methods including MT show high sensitivity to detect myelopathy progression [47]. An exciting new approach to MT is the inhomogeneous MT (ihMT) technique [48, 49], where the contrast is proposed to be generated by long-lived dipolar couplings between protons in lipid molecules. Initial work on this technique suggests that it is preferentially sensitive to the signal from hydrogens in lipids in CNS tissue. Given that 70–80% of myelin is lipid, ihMT may prove to be a marker for myelin, and more research is warranted on this variant of MT.

Myelin Water Imaging

Myelin water imaging (MWI) measures water trapped within the myelin bilayers, based on the property that myelin water has a faster relaxation time than water in other physical spaces. A number of approaches exist, including gradient echo decay curve T2* [50–53], T1 methods [54], and multi-component driven equilibrium single pulse observation of T1 and T2 (mcDESPOT) [55]. However, the most common approach is the Carr-Purcell-Meiboom-Gill (CPMG) or spin echo method [56–62], which has been validated in human brain [63, 64] and spinal cord [65] as specific to myelin. While not yet used clinically, myelin water imaging can successfully be implemented in the spinal cord in vivo to measure myelin-loss pathology in MS and cervical spondylotic myelopathy, as well as to monitor changes over time [57, 66–70]. An in-depth review of myelin water in the cord can be found elsewhere [71].

Conclusion

Imaging is a crucial component in the clinical evaluation and management of spinal cord myelopathy. While radiography, CT and nuclear medicine each have a role, MRI is the main modality used for spinal cord imaging. Imaging the cord is challenging for a number of reasons including its small size, physical location adjacent to bony structures and CSF, as well as close proximity to moving anatomy of the lungs, heart and neck. A number of strategies can be employed to minimize these challenges and other pitfalls commonly encountered in spinal cord imaging. Emerging techniques like DWI, DTI tractography, MR perfusion, and advanced quantitative MR techniques are expected to play an increasing role in the clinical evaluation of myelopathy in the future.

References

1. Fedutes BA, Ansani NT. Seizure potential of concomitant medications and radiographic contrast media agents. Ann Pharmacother. 2003;37:1506–10.
2. Singh S, Rajpal C, Nannapeneni S, Venkatesh S. Iopamidol myelography-induced seizures. Med Gen Med. 2005;7:11.
3. Ferré JC, Carsin-Nicol B, Hamlat A, Carsin M, Morandi X. MR imaging features of idiopathic thoracic spinal cord herniations using combined 3D-fiesta and 2D-PC cine techniques. J Neuroradiol. 2005;32:125–30.
4. Morris JM, Kaufmann TJ, Campeau NG, Cloft HJ, Lanzino G. Volumetric myelographic magnetic resonance imaging to localize difficult-to-find spinal dural arteriovenous fistulas. J Neurosurg Spine. 2011;14:398–404. https://doi.org/10.3171/2010.11.SPINE10328.
5. Nakagawa A, Kusaka Y, Jokura H, Shirane R, Tominaga T. Usefulness of constructive interference in steady state (CISS) imaging for the diagnosis and treatment of a large extradural spinal arachnoid cyst. Minim Invasive Neurosurg. 2004;47:369–72.
6. Roser F, Ebner FH, Danz S, Riether F, Ritz R, Dietz K, et al. Three-dimensional constructive interference in steady-state magnetic resonance imaging in syringomyelia: advantages

over conventional imaging. J Neurosurg Spine. 2008;8:429–35. https://doi.org/10.3171/SPI/2008/8/5/429.
7. Sakoda A, Yamashita KI, Hayashida M, Iwamoto Y, Yamasaki R, Kira JI. A case of superficial siderosis ameliorated after closure of dural deficit detected by MRI-CISS (constructive interference in steady state) imaging. Rinsho Shinkeigaku. 2017;57:180–3. https://doi.org/10.5692/clinicalneurol.cn-000960.
8. Honey CM, Martin KW, Heran MKS. Syringomyelia fluid dynamics and cord motion revealed by serendipitous null point artifacts during cine MRI. AJNR Am J Neuroradiol. 2017;38:1845–7. https://doi.org/10.3174/ajnr.A5328.
9. Chong AL, Chandra RV, Chuah KC, El R, Stuckey SL. Proton density MRI increases detection of cervical spinal cord multiple sclerosis lesions compared with T2-weighted fast spin-echo. AJNR Am J Neuroradiol. 2016;37:180–4. https://doi.org/10.3174/ajnr.A4476.
10. Simon JH, Li D, Traboulsee A, Coyle PK, Arnold DL, Barkhof F, et al. Standardized MR imaging protocol for multiple sclerosis: consortium of MS centers consensus guidelines. AJNR Am J Neuroradiol. 2006;27:455–61.
11. Do BH, Mari C, Tseng JR, Quon A, Rosenberg J, Biswal S. Pattern of 18F-FDG uptake in the spinal cord in patients with non-central nervous system malignancy. Spine (Phila Pa 1976). 2011;36:E1395–401. https://doi.org/10.1097/BRS.0b013e31820a7df8.
12. Taralli S, Leccisotti L, Mattoli MV, Castaldi P, de Waure C, Mancuso A, et al. Physiological activity of spinal cord in children: an 18F-FDG PET-CT study. Spine (Phila Pa 1976). 2015;40:E647–52. https://doi.org/10.1097/BRS.0000000000000895.
13. Patel NJ, Gupta V, Vibhute PG, Jain MK, Accurso JM. A large cohort study of 18F fluorodeoxy-glucose uptake in normal spinal cord: quantitative assessment of the contamination from adjacent vertebral marrow uptake and validity of normalizing the cord uptake against the lumbar thecal sac. J Comput Assist Tomogr. 2017;41:125–30. https://doi.org/10.1097/RCT.0000000000000479.
14. Eicker SO, Langen KJ, Galldiks N, Stoffels G, Herdmann J, Steiger HJ, et al. Clinical value of 2-deoxy-[18F]fluoro-D-glucose positron emission tomography in patients with cervical spondylotic myelopathy. Neurosurg Focus. 2013;35:E2. https://doi.org/10.3171/2013.3.FOCUS1379.
15. Richards PJ, George J, Metelko M, Brown M. Spine computed tomography doses and cancer induction. Spine (Phila Pa 1976). 2010;35:430–3. https://doi.org/10.1097/BRS.0b013e3181cdde47.
16. Morris JM. Imaging of dural arteriovenous fistula. RadiolClin North Am. 2012;50:823–39. https://doi.org/10.1016/j.rcl.2012.04.011.
17. Oda S, Utsunomiya D, Hirai T, Kai Y, Ohmori Y, Shigematsu Y, et al. Comparison of dynamic contrast-enhanced 3T MR and 64-row multidetector CT angiography for the localization of spinal dural arteriovenous fistulas. AJNR Am J Neuroradiol. 2014;35:407–12. https://doi.org/10.3174/ajnr.A3660.
18. Wheaton AJ, Miyazaki M. Non-contrast enhanced MR angiography: physical principles. J Magn Reson Imaging. 2012;36:286–304. https://doi.org/10.1002/jmri.23641.
19. Hadizadeh DR, Marx C, Gieseke J, Schild HH, Willinek WA. High temporal and high spatial resolution MR angiography (4D-MRA). Rofo. 2014;186:847–59. https://doi.org/10.1055/s-0034-1366661.
20. Zhou G, Li MH, Lu C, Yin YL, Zhu YQ, Wei XE, et al. Dynamic contrast-enhanced magnetic resonance angiography for the localization of spinal dural arteriovenous fistulas at 3T. J Neuroradiol. 2017;44:17–23. https://doi.org/10.1016/j.neurad.2016.10.002.
21. Katsura M, Sato J, Akahane M, Kunimatsu A, Abe O. Current and novel techniques for metal artifact reduction at CT: practical guide for radiologists. Radiographics. 2018;38:450–61. https://doi.org/10.1148/rg.2018170102.
22. Levy LM, Di Chiro G, Brooks RA, Dwyer AJ, Wener L, Frank J. Spinal cord artifacts from truncation errors during MR imaging. Radiology. 1988;166:479–83.
23. Levy LM. MR imaging of cerebrospinal fluid flow and spinal cord motion in neurologic disorders of the spine. Magn Reson Imaging Clin N Am. 1999;7:573–87.

24. Bae YJ, Lee JW, Lee E, Yeom JS, Kim KJ, Kang HS. Cervical compressive myelopathy: flow analysis of cerebrospinal fluid using phase-contrast magnetic resonance imaging. Eur Spine J. 2017;26:40–8. https://doi.org/10.1007/s00586-016-4874-9.
25. Bunck AC, Kroger JR, Juttner A, Brentrup A, Fiedler B, Schaarschmidt F, et al. Magnetic resonance 4D flow characteristics of cerebrospinal fluid at the craniocervicaljunction and the cervical spinal canal. EurRadiol. 2011;21:1788–96. https://doi.org/10.1007/s00330-011-2105-7.
26. Haber MD, Nguyen DD, Li S. Differentiation of idiopathic spinal cord herniation from CSF-isointense intraspinal extramedullary lesions displacing the cord. Radiographics. 2014;34:313–29. https://doi.org/10.1148/rg.342125136.
27. Tanenbaum LN. Clinical applications of diffusion imaging in the spine. Magn Reson Imaging Clin N Am. 2013;21:299–320. https://doi.org/10.1016/j.mric.2012.12.002.
28. Vargas MI, Delattre BMA, Boto J, Gariani J, Dhouib A, Fitsori A, et al. Advanced magnetic resonance imaging (MRI) techniques of the spine and spinal cord in children and adults. Insights Imaging. 2018; https://doi.org/10.1007/s13244-018-0626-1.
29. Hayes LL, Jones RA, Palasis S, Aguilera D, Porter DA. Drop metastases to the pediatric spine revealed with diffusion-weighted MR imaging. Pediatr Radiol. 2012;42:1009–13. https://doi.org/10.1007/s00247-011-2295-9.
30. Andre JB, Bammer R. Advanced diffusion-weighted magnetic resonance imaging techniques of the human spinal cord. Top Magn Reson Imaging. 2010;21:367–78. https://doi.org/10.1097/RMR.0b013e31823e65a1.
31. Liu X, Germin BI, Ekholm S. A case of cervical spinal cord glioblastoma diagnosed with MR diffusion tensor and perfusion imaging. J Neuroimaging. 2011;21:292–6. https://doi.org/10.1111/j.1552-6569.2009.00459.x.
32. Liu X, Kolar B, Tian W, Germin BI, Huang Y, Hu R, et al. MR perfusion-weighted imaging may help in differentiating between nonenhancing gliomas and nonneoplastic lesions in the cervicomedullary junction. J Magn Reson Imaging. 2011;34:196–202. https://doi.org/10.1002/jmri.22594.
33. Sourbron SP, Buckley DL. Classic models for dynamic contrast-enhanced MRI. NMR Biomed. 2013;26:1004–27. https://doi.org/10.1002/nbm.2940.
34. Leach MO, Morgan B, Tofts PS, Buckley DL, Huang W, Horsfield MA, et al. Imaging vascular function for early stage clinical trials using dynamic contrast enhanced magnetic resonance imaging. Eur Radiol. 2012;22:1451–64. https://doi.org/10.1007/s00330-012-2446-x.
35. Mazura JC, Karimi S, Pauliah M, Banihashemi MA, Gobin YP, Bilsky MH, et al. Dynamic contrast enhanced magnetic resonance perfusion compared with digital subtraction angiography for the evaluation of extradural spinal metastases: a pilot study. Spine (Phila Pa 1976). 2014;39:E950–4. https://doi.org/10.1097/BRS.0000000000000409.
36. Bilgen M, Narayana PA. A pharmacokinetic model for quantitative evaluation of spinal cord injury with dynamic contrast enhanced magnetic resonance imaging. Magn Reson Med. 2001;46:1099–106.
37. Tatar I, Chou PC, Desouki MM, El Sayed H, Bilgen M. Evaluating regional blood spinal cord barrier dysfunction following spinal cord injury using longitudinal dynamic contrast-enhanced MRI. BMC Med Imaging. 2009;9:10. https://doi.org/10.1186/1471-2342-9-10.
38. Duhamel G, Callot V, Decherchi P, Le Fur Y, Margueste T, Cozzone PJ, et al. Mouse lumbar and cervical spinal cord blood flow measurements by arterial spin labeling: sensitivity optimization and first application. Magn Reson Med. 2009;62:430–9. https://doi.org/10.1002/mrm.22015.
39. Hock A, Henning A, Boesiger P, Kollias SS. (1)H-MR spectroscopy in the human spinal cord. AJNR Am J Neuroradiol. 2013;34:1682–9. https://doi.org/10.3174/ajnr.A3342.
40. Carew JD, Nair G, Pineda-Alonso N, Usher S, Hu X, Benatar M. Magnetic resonance spectroscopy of the cervical cord in amyotrophic lateral sclerosis. Amyotroph Lateral Scler. 2011;12:185–91. https://doi.org/10.3109/17482968.2010.515223.
41. Holly LT, Ellingson BM, Salamon N. Metabolic imaging using proton magnetic spectroscopy as a predictor of outcome following surgery for cervical spondylotic myelopathy. Clin Spine Surg. 2017;30:E615–9. https://doi.org/10.1097/BSD.0000000000000248.

42. Leitch JK, Figley CR, Stroman PW. Applying functional MRI to the spinal cord and brainstem. Magn Reson Imaging. 2010;28:1225–33. https://doi.org/10.1016/j.mri.2010.03.032.
43. Wolff SD, Balaban RS. Magnetization transfer contrast (MTC) and tissue water proton relaxation in vivo. Magn Reson Med. 1989;10:135–44.
44. Henkelman RM, Stanisz GJ, Graham SJ. Magnetization transfer in MRI: a review. NMR Biomed. 2001;14:57–64.
45. Stanisz GJ, Kecojevic A, Bronskill MJ, Henkelman RM. Characterizing white matter with magnetization transfer and T(2). Magn Reson Med. 1999;42:1128–36.
46. Smith SA, Pekar JJ, van Zijl PC. Advanced MRI strategies for assessing spinal cord injury. Handb Clin Neurol. 2012;109:85–101.
47. Martin AR, De Leener B, Cohen-Adad J, Kalsi-Ryan S, Cadotte DW, Wilson JR, et al. Monitoring for myelopathic progression with multiparametric quantitative MRI. PLoS One. 2018;13:e0195733.
48. Varma G, Girard OM, Prevost VH, Grant AK, Duhamel G, Alsop DC. Interpretation of magnetization transfer from inhomogeneously broadened lines (ihMT) in tissues as a dipolar order effect within motion restricted molecules. J Magn Reson. 2015;260:67–76.
49. Varma G, Duhamel G, de Bazelaire C, Alsop DC. Magnetization transfer from inhomogeneously broadened lines: a potential marker for myelin. Magn Reson Med. 2015;73:614–22.
50. Du YP, Chu R, Hwang D, Brown MS, Kleinschmidt-DeMasters BK, Singel D, et al. Fast multislice mapping of the myelin water fraction using multicompartment analysis of T2* decay at 3T: a preliminary postmortem study. Magn Reson Med. 2007;58:865–70.
51. Sati P, van Gelderen P, Silva AC, Reich DS, Merkle H, de Zwart JA, et al. Micro-compartment specific T2* relaxation in the brain. NeuroImage. 2013;77:268–78.
52. Nam Y, Lee J, Hwang D, Kim DH. Improved estimation of myelin water fraction using complex model fitting. NeuroImage. 2015;116:214–21.
53. Lenz C, Klarhofer M, Scheffler K. Feasibility of in vivo myelin water imaging using 3D multigradient-echo pulse sequences. Magn Reson Med. 2012;68:523–8. https://doi.org/10.1002/mrm.23241.
54. Labadie C, Lee JH, Rooney WD, Jarchow S, Aubert-Frecon M, Springer CS Jr, et al. Myelin water mapping by spatially regularized longitudinal relaxographic imaging at high magnetic fields. Magn Reson Med. 2014;71:375–87.
55. Deoni SC, Rutt BK, Arun T, Pierpaoli C, Jones DK. Gleaning multicomponent T1 and T2 information from steady-state imaging data. Magn Reson Med. 2008;60:1372–87.
56. MacKay A, Whittall K, Adler J, Li D, Paty D, Graeb D. In vivo visualization of myelin water in brain by magnetic resonance. Magn Reson Med. 1994;31:673–7.
57. Wu Y, Alexander AL, Fleming JO, Duncan ID, Field AS. Myelin water fraction in human cervical spinal cord in vivo. J Comput Assist Tomogr. 2006;30:304–6.
58. Prasloski T, Rauscher A, MacKay AL, Hodgson M, Vavasour IM, Laule C, et al. Rapid whole cerebrum myelin water imaging using a 3D GRASE sequence. NeuroImage. 2012;63:533–9.
59. Oh J, Han ET, Lee MC, Nelson SJ, Pelletier D. Multislice brain myelin water fractions at 3T in multiple sclerosis. J Neuroimag. 2007;17:156–63.
60. Oh J, Han ET, Pelletier D, Nelson SJ. Measurement of in vivo multi-component T2 relaxation times for brain tissue using multi-slice T2 prep at 1.5 and 3 T. Magn Reson Imaging. 2006;24:33–43.
61. Nguyen TD, Wisnieff C, Cooper MA, Kumar D, Raj A, Spincemaille P, et al. T(2) prep three-dimensional spiral imaging with efficient whole brain coverage for myelin water quantification at 1.5 tesla. Magn Reson Med. 2012;67:614–21.
62. Nguyen TD, Deh K, Monohan E, Pandya S, Spincemaille P, Raj A, et al. Feasibility and reproducibility of whole brain myelin water mapping in 4 minutes using fast acquisition with spiral trajectory and adiabatic T2prep (FAST-T2) at 3T. Magn Reson Med. 2016;76:456–65. https://doi.org/10.1002/mrm.25877.
63. Laule C, Leung E, Lis DK, Traboulsee AL, Paty DW, MacKay AL, et al. Myelin water imaging in multiple sclerosis: quantitative correlations with histopathology. Mult Scler. 2006;12:747–53.

64. Laule C, Kozlowski P, Leung E, Li DK, Mackay AL, Moore GR. Myelin water imaging of multiple sclerosis at 7 T: correlations with histopathology. NeuroImage. 2008;40:1575–80.
65. Laule C, Yung A, Pavolva V, Bohnet B, Kozlowski P, Hashimoto SA, et al. High-resolution myelin water imaging in post-mortem multiple sclerosis spinal cord: a case report. Mult Scler. 2016;22:1485–9.
66. Minty EP, Bjarnason TA, Laule C, Mackay AL. Myelin water measurement in the spinal cord. Magn Reson Med. 2009;61:883–92.
67. Laule C, Vavasour IM, Zhao Y, Traboulsee AL, Oger J, Vavasour JD, et al. Two-year study of cervical cord volume and myelin water in primary progressive multiple sclerosis. Mult Scler. 2010;16:670–7.
68. MacMillan EL, Madler B, Fichtner N, Dvorak MF, Li DK, Curt A, et al. Myelin water and T(2) relaxation measurements in the healthy cervical spinal cord at 3.0T: repeatability and changes with age. NeuroImage. 2011;54:1083–90.
69. Kolind SH, Deoni SC. Rapid three-dimensional multicomponent relaxation imaging of the cervical spinal cord. Magn Reson Med. 2011;65:551–6.
70. Liu H, MacMillian EL, Jutzeler CR, Ljungberg E, MacKay AL, Kolind SH, et al. Assessing structure and function of myelin in cervical spondylotic myelopathy: evidence of demyelination. Neurology. 2017;89:602–10.
71. Laule C, MacKay AL. T2 relaxation. In: Cohen-Adad J, Wheeler-Kingshott CA, editors. Quantitative MRI of the spinal cord. Elsevier; 2014. p. 179–204.

Traumatic Disorders: Surgical Treatment of Myelopathy Secondary to Trauma

4

Zach Pennington, A. Karim Ahmed, Camilo Molina, C. Rory Goodwin, and Daniel M. Sciubba

Contents

Z. Pennington
Department of Neurosurgery, The Johns Hopkins Hospital, Baltimore, MD, USA

Department of Neurosurgery, Mayo Clinic, Rochester, MN, USA
e-mail: pennington.zachary@mayo.edu

A. K. Ahmed
Department of Neurosurgery, The Johns Hopkins Hospital, Baltimore, MD, USA
e-mail: aahmed33@jhmi.edu

C. Molina
Department of Neurosurgery, Washington University in St Louis, St Louis, MO, USA
e-mail: cmolina@wustl.edu

C. R. Goodwin
Department of Neurosurgery, Duke University Medical Center, Durham, NC, USA
e-mail: rory.goodwin@duke.edu

D. M. Sciubba (✉)
Department of Neurosurgery, The Johns Hopkins Hospital, Baltimore, MD, USA

Department of Neurosurgery, Northwell Health/Donald and Barbara Zucker School of Medicine, Manhasset, NY, USA
e-mail: dsciubba1@northwell.edu

B. Greenberg (ed.), *Myelopathy*, https://doi.org/10.1007/978-3-030-99906-3_4

Introduction

Each year more than 2.1 million Americans are involved in some form of accident, including falls, motor vehicle collisions, assaults, and ballistic trauma, accounting for nearly 21% of all years of potential life lost (Table 4.1). Of these, nearly 10% of patients will die, most commonly secondary to motor vehicle accidents, falls, and assault. Many others will be left with permanent injury, including spinal cord injury, which affects 11,000–15,000 Americans annually [1–5] and 10.4–83 per million population worldwide. The rate of spinal cord injury has steadily increased since the 1960s [5], perhaps due to the increased ownership of personal vehicles. It disproportionately affects males 16–24 and males >65, with a rate of 87–144 per million and 84–131 per million population, respectively, most commonly occurring secondary to motor vehicle accident (31–43%), fall (18.5–40.4%), sports injury (7.3–11.3%), and firearm injury or other violence (5.4–18.5%) [6–8]. It is also more common among those sustaining cervical spine injuries (55% of the SCI population) than among thoracic (15%), thoracolumbar (15%), and lumbosacral (15%) injuries [5, 9].

Of those with SCI, 30% of patients die before reaching the hospital and another 4.4–16.7% die within the hospital [5]. The rate of death prior to arrival is highest for those with violence as the primary mechanism of injury (OR = 1.53), those with C-spine injuries (OR = 2.3), those who are ventilator-dependent (OR = 39.5) and those with more severe neurological injuries (OR: Frankel A = 6.46, B = 4.5, C = 3.22) [5, 7, 10]. Frankel score, which has since been superseded by the American Spinal Injury Association (ASIA) Impairment Scale, defines the severity of spinal cord based upon motor and sensory function. Frankel E is defined as normal function (with possible reflex abnormalities), Frankel D denotes patients with useful motor function below the level of injury, and Frankel C denotes patients with residual motor function, but which is so too severe to allow practical application. Frankel B denotes patients with only sensory preservation below the level of injury and Frankel A denotes patients with no neurological function below the level of injury. The most common reason for death in those with complete spinal cord injury, which

Table 4.1 Most common causes of unintentional injury in the United States, 2001–2015

	Non-fatal		Fatal	
Mechanism	(per 100,000/year)	%	(per 100,000)	%
Fall	186.1	28	8.13	13.4
Struck By/Against Object	97.4	15	0.34	0.6
Overexertion	73.1	11	0.00	0.0
MVC (car or motorcycle)	65.4	10	13.35	22.1
Cut/Puncture Wound	47.5	7	0.88	1.5
Assault	36.5	5	5.75	9.5
Bite/String	31.3	5	n.g.	n.g.
Poisoning	17.8	3	13.03	21.6
Unknown	15.9	2	2.80	4.6
Total	665.8	100.0	60.35	100.0

Source: https://www.cdc.gov/injury/index.html
Key: *n.g.* not given

comprises 45% of the SCI patient population [5], are respiratory complications (28%), cardiac complications (23%), and pulmonary embolism (9.7%) [7]. Even when patients are successfully discharged from the hospital, they are burdened by the sequelae of their injury, and the costs of caring for it, which is estimated to be between $9.7 and $12.6 billion dollars annually in the US [4, 6].

Mechanisms of Injury

The Pathophysiology of Cord Injury

Spinal cord injury can be divided into primary and secondary phases [4, 5]. Primary injury is the mechanical damage done at the time of traumatic injury, including initial cord damage (e.g. transection) and persistent compression [5]. Secondary injury, by contrast, shows delayed onset and is caused by cord ischemia, excitotoxic neuronal death, immunological injury, hemorrhage, or neurogenic shock [4]. Those with pre-existing central stenosis are thought to be at higher risk for both the primary and secondary injury, as increased central stenosis secondary to injury is more poorly tolerated.

The exact mechanism of secondary injury is still unknown; though multiple etiologies have been proposed. These include changes in cord perfusion, ionic derangements (including Ca^{2+} influx), neurotransmitter accumulation (especially glutamate), arachidonic acid release and free radical production, edema, apoptosis, loss of ATP-dependent processes, and inflammation [5, 11]. Of note, recent studies have shown that the acute inflammatory response following traumatic injury is greater in the spinal cord, compared to the cerebral cortex [12, 13] Current evidence suggests that many, if not all, of these mechanisms may be involved in generating secondary spinal cord injury, however no consensus exists among the literature regarding which is the key mediator of damage.

The first pathological agents proposed were free radicals, which were thought to cause damage through peroxidation of membrane lipids, leading to ion gradient disruption and membrane lysis [5]. This was supported by *in vivo* experiments on mice and rats, where high-dose methylprednisolone limited the extent of spinal cord injury following cord impaction by inhibiting the prostaglandin-dependent production of hydroxyl free radicals [14, 15]. The authors concluded that these agents abrogated the injury by improving blood flow and inhibiting lipid peroxidation. However, clinical trials in humans, notably the NASCIS II and NASCIS III trials showed minimal benefit to the use of methylprednisolone, outweighed by negative side effects in a medically ill trauma patient population, suggesting that perhaps free radical damage is not the sole contributing cause of secondary cord injury in humans [16].

Other mechanisms proposed included reactive vasospasm, hemorrhage, decreased sympathetic tone, and Wallerian degeneration, which occurs as a result of the shearing of axons during primary trauma. The proposal that changes in cord perfusion contribute to secondary injury has becoming increasingly popular since the early 2000s. Early studies showed that cord injury was commonly characterized by hemorrhagic necrosis and central myelomalacia at the site of injury. This was accompanied by disruption of the capillaries and smaller arteries that perfuse the cord – the microcirculation. Later studies have shown that this microcirculation hypoperfusion is compounded by decreased sympathetic flow and pericyte activation, which causes capillary constriction [17]. This hypoperfusion in turn has been shown to cause degeneration of spinal cord axons [18], which results in the clinical symptoms of myelopathy, including numbness, paresthesia, balance disturbance and gait ataxia, and UMN signs including hyperreflexia and spasticity.

Classifying the Injury

Systems of Classification

Multiple classification systems have been developed to classify traumatic spine injuries, including the Allen system [19], Harris system [20] and Subaxial Cervical Injury Classification System (SLIC) [21, 22] for cervical spine injuries, and the Thoracolumbar Injury Classification and Severity Score (TLICS) for thoracolumbar injuries [23]. These classifications use a combination of neurological injury and radiographic description of the vertebral column damage to categorize the injury. The Allen and Harris scales rely more heavily on radiological findings and attempt to describe the mechanism of injury in cervical spine trauma, whereas the SLIC and TLICS place stronger evidence on the neurological status of the patient and are intended to guide the management of spine injury. Though the 2013 AANS/CNS guidelines for management of cervical spine injury have advised the use of SLIC system for the classification of C spine injuries [24], no consensus exists among providers. In fact, a recent survey of members of the Spine Trauma Study Group demonstrated that the TLICS and Allen systems are the most popular classification systems [25].

SCI Syndromes

In addition to classifying the radiographic appearance of the injury, SCI can also be categorized as syndromic or non-syndromic depending upon whether the confluence of symptoms and radiographic findings has previously been named. Named SCI syndromes include syringomyelia, spinal shock, anterior cord syndrome, central cord syndrome, Brown-Séquard Syndrome, conus medullaris syndrome, cauda equina syndrome, and subacute post-traumatic ascending myelopathy (SPAM). Some of these syndromes, including central cord syndrome and cauda equina syndrome, are far more common than other (e.g. SPAM), but overall the minority of patients (21%) have syndromic SCI [1]. The results of select large case series are reported in Table 4.2.

Syringomyelia

Syringomyelia is characterized by the accumulation of CSF within the spinal canal and post-traumatic syringomyelia is thought to occur secondary to disruption in CSF flow [26, 27]. Syrinxes most commonly extend cephalad in cases of trauma, as the cervical cord expands more easily than does the thoracic cord [26, 28, 29]. Syringomyelia, also known as progressive posttraumatic cystic myelopathy[29], is documented in 0.5–7.3% of SCI cases [29–34], though some radiologic and autopsy

Table 4.2 Select series describing syndromic SCI patients

Series	Patients	Findings and conclusions
Ahn et al. (2000) [54]	Meta-analysis of 322 patients with cauda equina syndrome (all causes) treated w/ surgical decompression	62% of cauda equina cases secondary to trauma
	Sex: 58% ♂; Age: 42.3	Surgical decompression provide improvement in pain (83%), motor function (75%), urinary continence (73%), sexual function (67%), rectal function (64%), and sensation (56%)
Aito et al. (2007) [61]	82 patients w/ traumatic CCS	58% of patients had no evidence of bony injury
	Sex: 88% ♂; Age: 52	Cervical injuries are more common
	ASIA: 2.4% A, 14.6% B, 45.1% C, 37.8% D	Functional outcomes of surgery are worst for those > 65y.o.
Chen et al. (2009) [66]	49 patients w/traumatic CCS following C spine injury	Timing of surgery has no effect on neurological improvement
	Sex: 81.6% ♂; Age: 55.9	Younger patients (< 65y.o.) more likely to improve motor function and ambulation w/ surgery
Daniels et al. (2007) [255]	24,098 patients from Nationwide Inpatient Sample w/ thoracolumbar fractures	Only 8.3% of patients had neurological injury
		Patients more likely to be treated surgically if they have neurological injury, are treated at high-volume center or treated at academic center
Dvorak et al. (2005) [63]	70 patients with traumatic CCS secondary to C spine injury	Patients have better motor function (ASIA motor scale) post-intervention if they are younger and have higher AMS at presentation
	Sex: 81% ♂; Age: 51	
Falci et al. (1999) [256]	70 patients w/ traumatic syringomyelia	Surgery produces functional improvement in 64% of patients; pain improvement in 56%
	Sex: 83.1% ♂; Age: 26	96% of patients satisfied w/ outcomes of surgery
	Level: C1-6 (41%); C6-T1 (34%); T (22%), conus (3%)	Motor and sensory loss are most common presenting symptoms
	ASIA: A (90%), B (2%), C (5%), D (3%)	
Guest et al. (2002) [257]	50 patients w/ traumatic CCS Age: 45 54% of patients w/ associated TBI	Patients surgically decompressed in less than 24 h have shorter ICU and hospital stay
Klekamp et al. (1997) [258]	52 patients w/ traumatic syringomyelia	Recurrence in 92–100% of patients; stabilization of neurological status in 83% of surgical group
	Sex: 73.6% ♂; Age: 46 Complete SCI in 28.8%; incomplete in 44.2%	Decompression is preferable treatment v. shunting

(continued)

Table 4.2 (continued)

Series	Patients	Findings and conclusions
Klekamp et al. (2012) [26]	137 patients w/ traumatic syringomyelia Age 47; 22.6% C; 65.7% T; 11.7% conus 40.1% w/ incomplete SCI; 32.8% w/ complete SCI Surgery in 44.5%	51% of patients report symptom improvement Recurrence in 18% of surgical patients Surgical decompression recommended as treatment; cordectomy highly effective
Krebs et al. (2016) [259]	138 patients w/ traumatic syringomyelia Sex: 79.7% ♂; Age: 42 Level: 13.8% C; 42% C/T; 36.2% T; 3.6% conus ASIA: 78.3% A, 8.7% B, 2.2% C, 2.9% D	Syringomyelia is more common in patients with complete CI Symptomatic syringomyelia may develop decades after trauma (median 15 year in this series) Younger patients have shorter prodrome
McKinley et al. (2007) [1]	175 patient w/ syndromic SCI of cohort of 839 SCI patients; 29.4% ASIA A-C Syndrome: CCS = 44.0%; CES = 25.1%; BSS = 17.1%; CMS = 8%; ACS = 5%; PCS = 1% Sex: 77.1% ♂; Race: 57.1% black, 34.9% white, 7.4% other Level: C4-8 (59.6%); T1-10 (4.7%); T11-L1 (10.9%); L2-S2 (25.8%)	Patients with CCS, CES, and ACS were generally oldest; BSS patients were generally youngest MOI varies by syndrome: MVC most common MOI for BSS and CCS; Fall most common for CCS and CMS CCS and BSS most common in C spine; CES is most common syndrome in T12-S2. Functional improvement worst for patients with PCS and CES; rehab stay longest for ACS
Peacock et al. (1977) [40]	450 patients w/ stab wound to spine Sex: 84% ♂; Age: < 30y.o. Level: 29.6% C; 63.8% T; 6.7% L BSS in 69.5% of incomplete SCI	BSS occurs in majority of cases w/ spinal cord stabwound Patients w/ BSS have good recovery – 65.6% recover ambulation
Rahimi-Movaghar et al. (2006) [260]	Cohort of 24 patients w/ traumatic conus medullaris syndrome treated w/ decompression Sex: 87% ♂; Age: 27 Severity: 67% w/ complete deficit pre-op	41.6% of patients have improvement of cord function, 63.6% had improvement in bladder function, and 83.3% had improvement in root function Time to decompression not related to degree of neurological improvement
Roth et al. (1991) [42]	38 patients w/ BSS or BSS plus syndrome Sex: 79% ♂; Age: 21.1; Level: 76% C; 74% T; 4% L;4% S Frankel: 97.4% D	All patients w/ incomplete SCI causing BSS improved Patients w/ BSS plus have greater recovery Predominate UE v. LE weakness is positive predictor of recovery of unassisted ambulation

Table 4.2 (continued)

Series	Patients	Findings and conclusions
Sgouros and Williams (1996) [261]	57 patients w/ syringomyelia	Syringomyelia may take years to present (mean 10.4 year in this study)
	Sex: 84% ♂; Age: 23.6; Frankel: 72% A Level: 22.8% C; 43.9% upper T; 22.8% lower T; 10.5% L	Arachnoid reconstruction more likely to produce improvement than shunting/drain placement
Stevens et al. (2010) [3]	126 patients w/ traumatic CCS	Surgically treated patients had better neurological outcome, but intervention timing did not matter
	Sex: 80.2% ♂; Age: 52.6 67 treated surgically	LOS shorter for those operated <24 h post-injury
Vannemreddy et al. (2002) [34]	58 patients w/ traumatic syringomyelia	Complete SCI more common in syringomyelia than general SCI population
	Sex: 79.3% male; Age: 42.2 Level: 48.3% C; 51.7% T or L Complete SCI in 69%	Prodrome is shorter for C and T spine injuries

Key: *ACS* anterior cord syndrome, *Age* mean age of cohort, *BSS* Brown-Séquard Syndrome, *CCS* central cord syndrome, *CES* cauda equina syndrome, *CMS* conus medullaris syndrome, *GSW* gunshot wound, *MOI* mechanism of injury, *MVC* motor vehicle crash, *PCS* posterior cord syndrome

studies have suggested that it may occur in more than 25% of cases [30, 33, 35, 36]. Multiple series have suggested that post-traumatic syringomyelia is more common in those with complete versus incomplete SCI [26, 30] and may be preventable with early post-traumatic decompression of the spinal canal [37]. Patients most commonly present with sensory disturbances, pain, and motor weakness [28, 30]. The diagnosis is made radiographically through demonstration of an intraparenchymal T2-hyperintense mass consistent with fluid accumulation [29] and cord displacement consistent with arachnopathy [26]. Cine MRI may be useful in demonstrating the level of CSF flow obstruction, especially in previously operated patients, who are likely to have already had arachnoid scarring prior to trauma [26]. Patients often show a delayed symptom onset, with a series of 20 patients reported by Hayashi and colleagues showing an average latency of 126 months [31]. Various treatments have been tried, including shunting of CSF across the defect, spinal cordectomy, and surgical decompression, with a recent systematic review by Bonfield and colleagues giving a weak recommendation of cord untethering and expansile duraplasty without addressing the cyst [30]. They found insufficient evidence to suggest treatment of asymptomatic syrinxes and recommended that these be treated with observation.

Brown-Séquard Syndrome

Classically occurring secondary to spinal cord stab injuries, Brown-Séquard Syndrome (BSS) is characterized by unilateral lesioning of the dorsal columns or complete cord hemisection. Due to the fact that it generally occurs secondary to penetrating trauma, BSS most commonly occurs following thoracic spine trauma (64–74%), though it may also occur with cervical (30–32%) and lumbar cord injury (4–7%) [38–40]. Patients with classical BSS present with ipsilateral loss of large fiber inputs below the level of the lesion (vibration sense and proprioception) and contralateral loss of small fiber inputs below the level of the lesion (temperature, itch, nociception). More modern examinations of BSS have begun to examine Brown-Séquard Plus Syndrome, which presents with ipsilateral hemiparesis or hemiparalysis below the level of the lesion, in addition to the symptoms of classical BSS [41].

In some cases reported in the literature, BSS has been associated with a post-traumatic Horner's syndrome, generally ipsilateral to the side of large fiber findings [43–49]. This phenomenon can occur from either compressive [43, 45, 48, 50–52] or penetrating injuries [44, 46, 47]. In the case of the former, unilateral compression of the cord produces a dorsal column palsy, leading to the BSS finding as well as a palsy of the ciliospinal tract, producing the ipsilateral Horner's. Alternatively, as can occur in a large penetrating wound, the damage may occur to the post-spinal portion of the second order neurons as they ascend in the sympathetic chain [51, 52]. Both injuries appear to have the potential for improvement with conservative management alone [50–53], but the number of reported post-traumatic cases is too sparse to reach definitive conclusions.

Cauda Equina Syndrome and Conus Medullaris Syndrome

Cauda equina syndrome is one of the most well-documented syndromic sequelae of traumatic spine injury, occurring exclusively secondary to lumbar spine trauma, most commonly between L3 and S1 [54]. Cauda equina syndrome is an acute radiculopathy treated with emergent surgical decompression, like other post-traumatic compressive myelopathies. Patients most commonly present with bilateral lower extremity weakness or radicular pain, saddle anesthesia, and urinary and/or fecal incontinence [54]. The largest study to date studying this syndrome was presented by Ahn and colleagues in 2000. They found that patients had significantly better recovery of motor function, fecal continence, urinary continence, and perineal sensation if treated within the first 48 h following injury [54]. Other studies have had similar results, leading to current guidelines suggesting emergent decompression in these patients [55–58].

Conus medullaris syndrome (CMS) presents similarly to cauda equina syndrome, but results from compression of the conus medullaris, as opposed to the cauda equina, which makes it a true myelopathy. Patients initially present with absent lower-limb deep tendon reflexes, saddle anesthesia, urinary retention, and variable lower extremity weakness—eventually patients demonstrate hyperreflexia from upper motor tract deficits. Due to the smaller craniocaudal extension of the conus, conus medullaris syndrome is a rarer entity than cauda equina syndrome [1], with only one moderately-sized series reported to date specifically examining post-traumatic CMS. This study, reported by Rahimi-Movaghar and colleagues, examined 24 patients with CMS who were treated with surgical decompression. Seventy-five percent of patients experienced neurological improvement (Frankel scale) and 64% experienced improvement in bladder function, leading the authors to conclude that CMS patients should be treated with surgical decompression. The study size was too small to examine the effect of the timing of surgical decompression on neurological recovery, but consensus among the field is that there is benefit to emergent decompression.

Central Cord Syndrome

Central cord syndrome (CCS) is the most common post-traumatic myelopathy, accounting for 44% of all patients in the series by McKinley and colleagues [1]. Early studies suggested that the key driver of neurological deficits was extensive gray matter damage at the level of injury. Concomitant, lesser injury to the surrounding white matter tracts was thought to result in other associated features, including urinary retention, variable sensory loss below the level of the lesion, and motor weakness in the lower extremities. However, as the principal injury was to the cervical spinal cord gray matter, deficits were more extensive in the distal upper extremities versus the lower extremities. Though this theory appears consistent with imaging that shows T2 hyperintensity within the cord parenchyma [59], histological studies have suggested that the key pathological feature is destruction of the corticospinal tract bilaterally [60], with central gray destruction being secondary. These studies also demonstrate variable axon damage in the ventral and dorsal columns, which helps to explain the variable sensory deficits observed clinically [60].

Functional recovery is often good in patients with CCS, though the degree of recovery is thought to be poorer in older adults [1], who show lower rates of ambulation and independent bladder function [61]. Treatment for central cord syndrome has historically been nonoperative [62], but more recent studies have indicated that patients treated with surgery may have superior outcomes [63]. Nonoperative management consists of immobilizing the cervical spine and maintaining the mean arterial pressure (MAP from 85–90 mmHg to prevent cord hypoperfusion [59, 64]. Surgery is indicated in cases where the patient is deteriorating neurologically or there is impending instability [59, 64]. Anterior approaches are often preferred for lesions involving only one or two levels and posterior approaches are preferred for lesions that are more extensive. Posterior approaches are also indicated in cases of ossified PLL due to the increased risk of CSF leak seen in cases treated with an anterior approach [59]. For those cases that can feasibly be treated with either approach, the surgeon must decide based upon the patient's risk profile, as anterior approaches are more commonly associated with dysphagia and hoarseness, whereas posterior approaches are more commonly associated with wound dehiscence and surgical site pain. There is no consensus regarding the timing of surgery, as some studies have suggested that decompression within 24 h provides better neurological recovery [3, 65], whereas others have found no association between neurological recovery and the timing of surgery [66].

Spinal Shock

Spinal shock describes the confluence of severe hypotension and bradycardia that often occur secondary to loss of sympathetic output [4, 67]. It most commonly occurs secondary to cervical spine injury (19% of all cervical spine injuries present with neurogenic shock) [68], and patients present with flaccid paralysis and areflexia below the level of injury [69, 70]. Patients are treated with sympathomimetics and antidiuretics to maintain perfusion pressure and prevent further spinal cord damage [4]. Patients are also monitored for signs of infection or thromboembolism, as pneumonia and venous thromboembolism are two of the most common complications in this patient population [67].

Subacute Post-traumatic Ascending Myelopathy

Subacute post-traumatic ascending myelopathy is a rare neurological deterioration occurring days to weeks following SCI [71, 72]. It is defined as progressive neurological deterioration at least 4 levels above index lesion [73–75]. Some groups suggest that SPAM may result from alterations in CSF dynamics [72], but to date, the exact cause and pathophysiology of this condition are unknown at present [76]. As a result, the condition is defined clinically as a progressive neurological deterioration that cannot be explained by mechanical instability or syringomyelia [75].

The overall number of cases reported in the literature is quite small. Two large series of patients with traumatic spinal cord injury [77, 78] documented SPAM in 5–6% of all patients with SCI. These patients showed T2-hyperintensity and cord edema in areas superior to cord lesion, peaking an average of 18 days post-injury [79]. Most patients experience moderate neurological recovery, but almost all patients have residual neurological deficit following resolution of the cord edema.

Imaging

Though specific imaging recommendations for each type of spine trauma are specified later in this chapter, it is important to outline the objectives of imaging in the setting of spine trauma. The two main goals are: (1) to assess the osseoligamentous damage to the vertebral column, and (2) to assess the damage to the neurological elements comprising the cord and associated roots. As reported in numerous places throughout the literature, the osseous injury is best assessed with CT, as this can show both impending structural instability, as well as bone quality in cases where operative management is being considered [80–82]. By contrast, MRI provides the best assessment of both the ligamentous and neurological injuries [83]. Though assessment of the ligamentous injury is important for trauma at every level, it is perhaps most important in patients suffering trauma to the craniocervical junction, the intricate structure of which relies heavily on ligamentous attachments. Injury to these elements is often accompanied by intra-ligamentous edema that is readily detected using STIR sequencing [83]

Assessment of the neurological injury must account for the size, severity, and evolution of the injury [83]. MR imaging is the single best way of making these assessments [84], as regions of cord damage are edematous, T1-isointense, T2 hyperintense lesions on MR [36], but are undetectable on other imaging modalities. These myelomalacia changes on MR represent edematous changes in the cord parenchyma, which become more common with increasing time post-injury [85]. In the acute injury state, these edematous changes are occasionally obfuscated by intraparenchymal hemorrhage, which is seen in 18.5% of patients. It is a particularly worrisome finding, as previous studies have identified intraparenchymal hemorrhage as a negative predictor of neurological recovery [86].

The extent of the lesion can easily be delineated by making measurements of the T2 hyperintensity in the sagittal and axial planes [85]. Determination of the chronicity of the cord injury is slightly more difficult, though one common method of doing so involves assessing cord atrophy [36, 84, 87]. Normally the spinal cord has an anteroposterior dimension greater than 7 mm in the cervical region and 6 mm in the thoracic region [36, 84]. However, in instances of chronic post-traumatic myelopathy – those cases with histories longer than 2 years – the cord experiences axon dropout, resulting in a decrease in cord size [84]. The importance of these findings is that patients with acute cord injuries have a much higher probability of recovering function than do those with chronic injuries. Lastly, MR imaging allows the cord to be evaluated for post-traumatic cyst and syrinx formation. Both types of fluid-filled masses can compress the cord and exacerbate the symptomatology of the post-traumatic myelopathy.

The T2 signal changes seen in cases of post-traumatic myelopathy are not unique to this pathology. Also, in the differential are degenerative spondylosis resulting in SCC and inflammatory pathologies of the spinal cord, including idiopathic transverse myelitis and multiple sclerosis. Distinguishing between these pathologies relies heavily upon the patient's history, but there are some radiographic differences between these etiologies. Key among these differences is the enhancement seen with use of a gadolinium contrast agent. The lesion seen in post-traumatic myelopathy will show enhancement only within the region of maximal compression, whereas the idiopathic transverse myelitis lesion will often show diffuse enhancement throughout the lesion, and the lesions of multiple sclerosis will often show either no enhancement, if chronic, or peripheral enhancement, if acute [88]. Ultimately, if suspicion for an inflammatory myelitis exists, a neurological consult should be sought to avoid providing surgical management to an inflammatory pathophysiology.

Management of Spinal Trauma

Treatment of traumatic myelopathy constitutes just one part of the management of traumatic spine injuries. When designing treatment for this, the surgeon must consider several things, including damage to the bony elements, discoligamentous injury, the extent of neurological damage, the type of neurological damage (compressive, penetrating, or ischemic), and the potential for neurological recovery.

Cervical Spine Trauma

In 2013, the AANS and CNS published an updated set of guidelines describing recommendations for the treatment of patients with traumatic cervical spine injuries [16, 24, 64, 68, 82, 89–103]. Though these guidelines are by no means a definitive guide for the treatment of cervical spine trauma, owing to the low quality of evidence supporting many of the recommendations, they form a useful decision which may improve patient outcomes.

Pre-hospital Care

Immediately following the occurrence of cervical spine trauma, patients should be triaged at the scene by trained EMS personnel, as previous studies have suggested that this may reduce the proportion of patients who present with complete neurological compromise [104, 105]. Per the Fresno/Kings/Madera EMS protocol, shown to be 99% sensitive for the detection of cervical spine injury [106], cervical spine immobilization is recommended for all patients suffering cervical spine injury or spinal cord injury, or sustaining trauma capable of causing cervical spine injury. Immobilization should be performed with a rigid cervical collar in the adult population or a Kendrick extraction device in pediatric cases, and the patient should be transferred to a rigid backboard using either a high arm spine method or fireman lift method; the log-roll technique should not be used [90]. The combination of immobilization with a rigid collar and fixation on a backboard limit motion of the injured segments and thus reduce the risk of further injury. Patients who are neurologically intact, awake, alert, sober, without neck pain or tenderness, and without a painful distracting injury that might interfere with evaluation need not be immobilized [107, 108].

Once securely immobilized on the backboard, patients should be expediently and carefully transported to the nearest facility capable of providing definitive care, with preference for SCI specialty centers where possible [90]. Treatment at such facilities has previously been associated with better neurological outcomes and shorter hospitalizations [109]. An emphasis should be placed on the urgency of transportation, as previous studies by groups in Switzerland have shown that the best neurological outcomes are achieved in patients who reach a definitive care center within 12 h of injury [110, 111]. The means of transportation does not affect overall outcome, as a previous study by Burney and colleagues comparing patients transferred by ground and those transferred by air had statistically indiscernible outcomes so long as patients received treatment within the first 24 h following injury [112].

In-hospital Care

Once in hospital, patients with suspected cervical spine trauma should be assessed clinically and radiographically. Patients that have sustained traumatic injury should first undergo primary and secondary trauma surveys to identify impending life-threatening injuries. Current recommendations are that patients be clinically evaluated using the ASIA impairment and motor scales for neurological assessment, Spinal Cord Independence Measure III (SCIM III) for functional assessment, and the International Spinal Cord Injury Basic Pain Data Set for the assessment of pain, physical functioning, and emotional functioning [91]. Some reports suggest that the ASIA motor scale, which uses separate 50 point scales for the upper and lower extremities, has low sensitivity in paraplegic and quadriplegic studies, but several large studies have suggested that is the best standardized neurological examination that is currently available [113, 114].

In the acute setting, the American Spinal Injury Association (ASIA) scale can be utilized to assess function. Long-term assessment may involve the SCIM III, which contains three domains describing patient function – room and toilet, indoors mobility, and outdoors mobility [115, 116]. Because of its assessment of patients across multiple domains, some groups describe it as the best assessment of global disability in those with SCI [117]. It has also been shown by several groups to have a high degree of inter-rater reliability and to be superior to the competing Functional Independent Measure (FIM).

Multiple previous guidelines have been established regarding appropriateness of radiographic evaluation in trauma patients, including the NEXUS and Canadian C-Spine rules. Like these guidelines, those put forth by the CNS/AANS group rely heavily upon the patient's level of function at initial assessment when evaluating the need for radiographic assessment [82]. In awake, sober, asymptomatic patients without distracting injuries and who have a full functional range of motion in the neck, radiographic assessment is not required and the patient may be discharged from cervical spine immobilization. In patients who are awake, yet symptomatic, patients should be imaged with a high-quality CT of the cervical spine. CT has been shown to be superior to 3-view radiograph for the evaluation of C-spine trauma, with a sensitivity of 99–100% compared to 36-64% for conventional 3-view cervical spine radiographs. However, in instances were CT is not available, 3-view cervical spine radiographs should be obtained. MRI is likely to add little to the assessment of osseous injury in this population [118] and patients should remain immobilized until asymptomatic. In patients who obtunded and have suspected cervical spine injury, a high-quality CT of the neck should be ordered, as it has a high sensitivity (97.4–98.1%) and positive predictive value (100%) for the detection of cervical spine injury. All obtunded patients should remain immobilized until they become asymptomatic or a normal MRI is obtained, which should be ordered within 48 h of injury to assess spinal cord compression and ligamentous injury [119].

Following radiographic evaluation of the injury, a decision must then be made as to whether the injury should be treated operatively or nonoperatively. Current guidelines from the CNS are based upon level III evidence, but recommend that patients should initially be treated non-operatively using closed reduction with Gardner-Wells tongs [92]. This method is effective at reducing the injury in up to 80% of cases, with the associated risk of neurological deterioration being quite low – only 2–4% of patients. Additionally, most of the neurological deterioration seen in patients treated with nonoperative management are transient, with only 15% of patients having permanent neurological deficits because of closed reduction, most commonly secondary to epidural hematoma, overdistraction, disk herniation, or an unrecognized lesion rostral to the reduced level.

Though the CNS/AANS joint group recommended preliminary closed reduction for the treatment of minimally displaced odontoid fractures, C1/2 rotatory subluxations, facet dislocations, hangman fractures, and subaxial fractures with malalignment, they acknowledge that many patients may benefit from operative treatment of their injury [92]. The recommendations made by the group were made based upon the type of osseoligamentous injury, though in most cases, conservative management with external immobilization is recommended as first line therapy, with operative management being indicated only in cases of severe trauma, instability, or a previous failure of conservative management.

Occipital Condyle Fractures

Occipital condyle fractures are an uncommon sequela of trauma, occurring in 1.7 per 1000 trauma patients per year [120]. They are most commonly associated with atlas and axis fractures and are readily detected using CT [93]. Nearly 40% of patients with OC fractures have neurological deficits, but an additional 30% are neurologically intact. The CNS/AANS group recommends that all OC fractures be treated nonoperatively with external C spine immobilization, however the quality of evidence is low. As a result, the decision of whether or not to treat these injuries operatively is largely based upon the perceived stability of the injury. Type I fractures - comminuted fractures of the condyle – and type II fractures – extended linear basilar skull fractures – are both treated conservatively in most cases [120, 121]. Type III injuries by contrast – avulsion fractures with alar ligament attachment – are potentially unstable and patients may benefit from open reduction of the injury [122] Operative management may reasonably be achieved through a posterior occipitocervical fusion. The patient is first radiographed to verify the sagittal alignment and determine any correction in cervical lordosis that needs to be achieved. Additionally, it allows for assessment of injuries at other of the cervical spine. The patient is then placed prone with the head positioned in natural alignment, correcting any kyphosis present in the cervical spine. A posterior midline incision is made and subperiosteal dissection is performed over the occiput and cervical vertebrae, extending wide to also expose the lateral masses. Care must be taken during this dissection to avoid injury to the vertebral artery above the C1 arch and the C2 nerve roots between the C1 and C2 posterior elements. C1 lateral mass screws are placed, followed by placement of C2 pedicle screws. Alternatively, translaminar screws may be placed if there is concern for vertebral artery injury, which is more common in pedicle screw instrumentation. However, this technique cannot be employed when decompression is to be performed at this level. Additional levels may be instrumented with lateral mass screws depending upon the patient's bone quality, the number of injured levels, and the degree of sagittal correction that is necessary. If the injury has compressed the cord, laminectomies may be performed at the involved levels to reduce pressure on the cord. After placement of the cervical instrumentation, an occipital plate is placed. Rods are contoured to the correction desired and fixed to the plate and cervical screws.

Atlanto-Occipital Dislocation Injuries

The majority of patients with atlanto-occipital dislocation are symptomatic, with 48% of patients having a cranial nerve deficit, 42% being paretic, and nearly 30% being hemiplegic or quadriplegic [123]. Additionally, this injury has a high associated mortality, with 15–38% of patients dying within 90 days of injury, and so proper assessment and treatment of this injury are of paramount importance in patients with cervical spine injury [123–125]. Persons with suspected atlanto-occipital dislocation injuries should be imaged with CT where possible and lateral C spine radiographs when CT is unavailable. A number of methods have been developed to assess atlanto-occipital dislocation on these radiographic studies, including the basion-dens interval [126], basion-atlas interval [127, 128], Powers ratio [129], and Sun ratio [130]. However, the most sensitive and user-friendly measure for assessing craniocervical instability is the condyle-C_1 interval introduced by Pang et al. which should be under 4 mm under normal conditions. Unilateral or bilateral increase in this measurement above 4 mm is indicative of craniocervical instability, which requires immediate management.

Internal fixation is recommended in all patients with atlanto-occipital dislocation injuries, and conservative treatment with traction is contraindicated due to the approximately 10% risk of neurological deterioration with this intervention [123]. Either anterior or posterior approaches may be utilized for surgical intervention, however posterior approaches are preferred, as they allow for superior reduction of the dislocation and better stabilization of the craniocervical junction [131]. Posterior fixation has historically been achieved with C1-2 cable wiring and occipital bone wiring. But current practice is to utilize occipitocervical fusion with screw and occipital plate fixation [131]. If traumatic changes to the spine are confined to the craniocervical junction, patients may reasonably be treated with O-C1 or O-C2 fusions. Patients presenting with subaxial injuries in addition to occipitocervical junction pathology should be treated with longer constructs. These constructs require pre-operative assessment of sagittal alignment – C2 to C7 lordosis – in order to ensure that surgery does not fuse the patient into a non-physiologic alignment.

Isolated Atlas Fractures

The treatment of isolated atlas fractures is determined by the type of fracture and the integrity of the transverse atlantal ligament [94]. Any fracture with extension to the lateral mass, containing the vertebral artery foramen, should be followed with vascular imaging to rule out injury. Fractures without associated ligamentous rupture should be treated with cervical immobilization, whereas those with ligamentous rupture should be treated with open fracture reduction and fixation. Type I (simple anterior or posterior arch fractures) and type II fractures (burst fractures of anterior or posterior arch) are usually not associated with transverse ligament injury and so can be treated with closed reduction. Case reports have suggested that such treatment is a highly effective means of treating the injury [132–134]. Type III fractures however – those with lateral mass fracture – are often associated with transverse ligament injury and are considered unstable. They are unlikely to heal with traction or closed reduction alone (less than 70% of cases heal this way). As a result, it is recommended that they be treated with C1-2 stabilization and fusion. Diagnosis of ligamentous rupture can be made using an odontoid view cervical radiograph, as atlas fractures with ligamentous rupture are associated with lateral displacement of C1 on C2 that exceeds 7 mm – the so called "Rule of Spence"[135]. However, the most sensitive means of assessing ligamentous injury is MRI [136].

Isolated Axis Fractures

Axis fractures can be coarsely divided into odontoid and vertebral body fractures and fractures of the posterior elements. Vertebral body and odontoid fractures constitute the majority of these lesions, with a recent series by Robinson and colleagues examining 233 patients with axis fractures revealed that 78.5% of axial fractures involve the odontoid, compared with only 11.2% being hangman's fractures – fractures through the bilateral pars interarticularis [137]. Each of these groups can be further classified radiographically using CT or cervical radiographs.

Posterior element fractures are divided into hangman fractures and atypical axial fractures, such as those of the lamina. The former uncommonly cause neurological injury (6.5% in the series of Fielding) and are classified using either the Francis or Effendi/Levine grading scales, which use cervical radiographs to assess instability and the C2/3 angulation. The Francis scale divides lesions into five grades. Grade I-III lesions are considered to show mild-to-moderate C2/3 angulation and should be treated preliminarily with external immobilization, as up to 95% of conservatively managed patients are successfully treated in this fashion [24, 138, 139]. They should only be treated operatively in cases of progressive instability or failure of conservative management. By contrast, grade IV lesions – those with C2/3 angulation >11° and vertebral body displacement between 3.5 mm and half of C3 vertebral width – and grade V lesion – those with complete C2/3 disk disruption – should be treated operatively in all cases [24, 95]. The Effendi/Levine scale makes similar divisions, with type 1, 2 and 2A lesions demonstrating mild-to-moderate angulation, and type 3 lesions showing severe angulation and bilateral C2/3 facet dislocation. And similar recommendations apply to this grading system, with type 3 lesions being immediately surgical and the other types being indicated for preliminary conservative management.

Most anterior element fractures occur through the odontoid and can be classified as type I (fracture through upper dens), II (fracture at base/neck of dens), or III (fracture through dens and body of axis) [140]. Type II fracture comprise 58–65% of all odontoid fractures [141, 142] and can be further subdivided into type IIA, IIB, and IIC based upon the angle of the fracture plane and displacement of fracture [140]. Current CNS/AANS guidelines recommend external immobilization as first line therapy for all odontoid fracture subtypes, unless there is suggestion of severe ligamentous injury or craniocervical instability [95]. However nonunion occurs in 28–35% of cases treated with halo immobilization and 57% of cases treated with traction [142]. These rates may be even higher for older patients, those with greater fracture displacement, and those with greater delays in treatment [143, 144]. In cases where operative management is indicated, patients can be treated with either an anterior odontoid screw, or posterior fixation. Anterior odontoid screw is an excellent option for type IIC fractures due to the fracture angulation, but the technique is technically demanding. As a result, posterior instrumentation may be preferable, especially for those with a disrupted transverse ligament. Case series examining the technique have demonstrated good results, achieving fusion in 87–100% of cases [142].

Combined Atlas-Axis Fractures

Combined atlantoaxial fractures are seen in 5–53% of cases with fracture of either the atlas or axis [96], but comprise only 4–26.7% of all cervical spine injuries [145, 146]. Halo-vest immobilization is considered first line therapy in most cases, with the chief exception being combined C1-type II odontoid fractures with an atlanto-dens interval exceeding 5 mm and combined C1-hangman fractures with C2/3 angulation exceeding 11°. These injuries should be treated operatively, preferable with posterior fusion, which achieves successful fusion in 90% or more of cases.

Atlanto-Axial Dislocation

Though not explicitly covered by the CNS/AANS guidelines, another important set of pathologies of the craniovertebral junction are atlantoaxial dislocations. Like atlanto-occipital dislocations, instability at the atlantoaxial joint has a high associated morbidity, and can cause myelopathy or even death in some cases [147]. Evaluation of the injury is made radiographically through a combination of dynamic films and high quality CT. Using these studies along with applied traction, the clinician can categorize the injury based upon the nature of the dislocation – rotatory, vertical, or horizontal – and the reducibility of the deformity. Multiple metrics exist for the diagnosis of atlantoaxial subluxation, including the anterior atlanto-dens interval (ADI) and posterior atlas-dens interval for the assessment of horizontal subluxation, and the dens-atlas interval (DAI) and Ranawat value for vertical subluxation [148, 149]. The DAI is defined as the vertical distance between the tip of the dens and the transverse line connecting the inferior edges of the anterior and posterior atlantal arches. The Ranawat value is defined as the length of the line from the midpoint of the base of the axis inferior endplate to the transverse axis of the atlas (the transversely-orienting line connecting the midpoints of the anterior and posterior atlantal arches in the mid-sagittal plane). Normal values for these metrics are: ADI <3 mm in adults or <5 mm in children [150], a posterior atlanto-dens interval <19 mm [151], a Ranawat value ≥13 mm, and a DAI <13 mm [148]. Rotatory subluxation is also assessed radiographically, and can be classified using the Fielding classification system, which characterizes the subluxation based upon the relative displacement of the atlantal and axial lateral masses [152]. Type I subluxations show rotatory fixation without horizontal translation, type II injuries show rotatory fixation with anterior atlantal displacement between 3 and 5 mm and unilateral facet disarticulation, type III injuries show the same displacement with bilateral facet joint disarticulation, and type IV injuries show rotatory fixation with posterior displacement. Unlike purely translation dislocations, which can be effectively assayed using plain cervical radiographs, rotatory atlantoaxial subluxations are most effectively assayed using CT imaging.

Most atlantoaxial subluxations must be treated surgically. Many authors recommend the use of pre-operative traction to reduce the deformity. The deformity is then completely reduced through open fixation, which can be accomplished via anterior-only, posterior-only, or combined approaches Several instrumentation options are available, including C1 lateral mass-C2 pedicle screw fixation, C1/2 transarticular screw fixation, and C1 lateral mass-C2 translaminar screw instrumentation [147, 153]. The latter has become the most popular technique due to the significant overlap with techniques used to instrument the subaxial spine. That being said, all three instrumentation methods show good fixation strength [154, 155] and no high-quality biomechanical evidence exists to support one instrumentation method relative one another, though C2 pedicle and C1/2 transarticular screws appear superior to C2 laminar screws with respect to lateral bending [156–158]. There is also no high-quality evidence to support the superiority of an anterior versus a posterior-only approach for decompression and reduction of the deformity, and so the approach chosen should be selected based upon the location of associated pathologies, the need to instrument the occiput or subaxial levels, and surgeon preference. In cases with associated odontoid injury or persistent cord compression despite reduction of the subluxation, an anterior stage may be required to decompress the cord, while in cases were subaxial instrumentation will be required, a posterior approach is often preferable [150].

Subaxial Cervical Spine Injuries

Subaxial cervical spine injuries comprise over two-thirds of cervical spine trauma and may produce tetraplegia in up to 87% of cases with jumped facets [159, 160]. Patients should be treated preliminarily with closed reduction and bed rest in order to reduce cord compression [92, 98]. Risk factors for failing conservative management are vertebral height loss greater than 40%, kyphosis greater than 15%, and vertebral subluxation greater than 20%. Patients who fail conservative management should be treated with open reduction of the fracture, which can be accomplished with either anterior or posterior approaches. The advantages of an anterior approach are that positioning is straightforward, dissection occurs along defined tissue planes, fusion is achieved in 90–100% of cases and complications are less frequent. Additionally, the anterior approach may allow for better clearance of bony fragments in comminuted fractures, which improves neurological recovery. Anterior approaches offer poorer stabilization and correction of kyphosis however, and are associated with an increased risk for transient dysphasia. Posterior approaches by contrast allow for effective reduction of subluxation, better correction of kyphosis, and lower rates of hardware failure [161], though they are associated with more significant muscle disruption and perioperative complications in up to 37% of patients. Both groups provide similar improvement of neurological function, with a series by Lambiris and colleagues reporting an average improvement of 1 ASIA grade for each approach.

Spinal Cord Injury Without Radiographic Abnormality (SCIWORA)

Though most patients suffering spine trauma will have radiographic evidence of spinal column injury, upward of 35% of patients will have no such radiographic findings [162]. These patients are clinically myelopathic and have non-focal CT and radiographs, a condition known as SCIWORA or spinal cord concussion. Though multiple injuries and age groups can be implicated in this phenomenon, patients are most commonly children with incomplete SCI secondary to motor vehicle collision or sports injury [162–164]. Because SCIWORA is, by definition, without radiographic findings, the joint CNS/AANS guidelines recommend that patients with SCIWORA have a total spine MRI and flexion-extension radiographs in the acute setting to investigate for both neurologic damage and the ligamentous injury [100], though these findings may still be negative in up to 78% of patients [163]. Patients should be initially treated with external immobilization, unless there is evidence of gross instability. In this small subset of cases (6–13%), operative management may be considered [163]. In cases where conservative management is used, the patient may be immobilized for up to 12 weeks, with discontinuation of the collar when patients become asymptomatic or have clean flexion-extension films [100]. After being cleared, patients should continue to avoid high-risk activities such as contact sports for 6 months, as they are at increased risk of injury [100]. Recovery from SCIWORA is generally quite good, with up to 94% of children making a complete recovery [163]. Recurrence of symptoms has been documented in both pediatric and adult populations, but is far more common in the pediatric population, where it may occur in 11% of cases [165]. Negative predictors of neurological recovery include hematomyelia, cord transection, and ASIA A status at presentation [162, 165, 166]

Steroid Use

Current recommendations regarding the use of methylprednisolone in patients with post-traumatic spinal cord injury are controversial. The guidelines published by the CNS/AANS joint group found class 1 evidence recommending against the use of methylprednisolone, but standard of care at many centers is to provide steroids in order to reduce cord swelling and promote neurological recovery [16].

The strongest level evidence for the use of methylprednisolone usage in acute spinal cord injury comes from the National Acute Spinal Cord Injury series of studies (NASCIS I-III). The first of these studies was conducted in the 1980s and compared two ten day regimens of methylprednisolone, with a high dose group receiving a 1000 mg loading dose and a low dose group receiving a 100 mg loading dose; both groups received a 100 mg q6h maintenance dose for the remainder of the period [167] The investigators observed no difference in neurological recovery, but did note higher rates of wound infection and death in the high dose group. A follow-up study was then conducted comparing a 24-h methylprednisolone regimen (30 mg/kg loading dose followed by 5.4 mg/kg/hr maintenance dose for 23 hours) to a naloxone placebo and found that patients started on the methylprednisolone dose within 8 h of injury had slightly greater motor function improvement at discharge [168]. Interestingly, patients receiving the steroid dose more than 8 h post-injury showed worse neurological improvement than the naloxone group, suggesting that the timing of the steroid administration may significantly impact the results. As with the prior study though, the methylprednisolone group had a higher complication rate, with a 2 times higher risk of wound infection and three times higher risk of pulmonary embolism [16, 168]. The final phase of the NASCIS series compared methylprednisolone use to a "super steroid" – tirilazad mesylate – and found no significant difference in neurological improvement [169–171]. However, it was observed that a 48-h course of methylprednisolone produced superior motor recovery to a 24-h could if started within 8 h of injury, again suggesting that the benefits of steroids may be tied to the timing of administration.

The AANS/CNS group interpreted these results, along with other class II and class III evidence to indicate that methylprednisolone increases the complication profile of patients with spinal cord injury, without providing significant benefit in terms of neurological improvement. Given that only the NASCIS II trial compared methylprednisolone to placebo, it may be reasonable to make conclusions based upon this study, which did observe a small benefit to steroid administration, if treatment begins within 8 h of injury. However, the risk profile of this treatment is significant and so the decision to use IV steroids in patients with post-traumatic spinal cord injury should be made at the institutional level.

Thoracolumbar Spine Trauma

Unlike cervical spine trauma, no guidelines had been issued by either the AANS or CNS for the treatment of thoracic spine trauma at the time of the writing of this chapter [172]. However, many of the principles for the treatment of patients with cervical spine trauma causing neurological dysfunction also hold for symptomatic thoracolumbar trauma. Stable, asymptomatic lesions are first referred for conservative management and highly unstable injuries and injuries causing neurological deterioration are treated operatively [173].

As with cervical trauma, multiple systems have been proposed for classifying thoracolumbar trauma, though no classification system has been universally accepted. The AOSpine Thoracolumbar Spine Injury Classification System, published by the Spine Trauma Study Group in 2005 and updated in 2013, is the most recent classification system and comes from the same cohort that produced the SLIC system recommended by the AANS/CNS group for the classification of cervical injury. It classifies injuries based upon the morphology of the injury (indicating immediate mechanical stability), integrity of the posterior ligamentous complex (indicating long-term stability), and neurological status of the patient. Furthermore, it seeks to predict the neurological outcome of patient and so guide the treatment of patients sustaining thoracolumbar trauma. The initial rendition of the scale assigned patients an overall score and based the decision to pursue operative management based upon that score [23]. However, the most recent revision classifies injuries based upon the different levels for each of the three factors and bases the decision to pursue operative management on the patient's individual pathology [174]. Additionally, they recommend that surgical candidates should be treated with an anterior approach when neurological injury is present, a posterior approach when the posterior ligamentous complex has been compromised, and a combined anterior-posterior approach where both issues are present. The simplicity of use of the TLICS system and moderate-to-excellent interobserver reliability have led to become the most commonly used system for the classification of thoracolumbar trauma [25, 175, 176].

Recently, the American Association for the Surgery of Trauma TL-Spine Multicenter Study Group published the results of prospective study of more than 3000 patients treated at 14 US trauma centers. All patients were evaluated with diagnostic imaging of the thoracolumbar spine and clinical examination, which revealed TL-spine injury in 16.3% of patients and clinically significant TL-spine injury in 8.6% of patients. Based upon the radiographic and clinical findings in these patients, they developed a clinical rule for the thoracolumbar spine evaluation in trauma patients. The authors argued that imaging is indicated for all patients who are alert and evaluable and who have pain, tenderness to palpation, deformity, or neurological deficit, or who were subjected to a high-risk injury mechanism (MVA, crush injury, or fall) and were older than 60 years of age. In patients who are indicated for radiographic evaluation, CT is considered the modality of choice and is recommended by the Eastern Association for the Surgery of Trauma [173, 177].

Currently, no high-quality evidence exists to describe the surgical indications for surgery in thoracolumbar spine trauma [178], though the goals of surgery are anatomical reconstruction, functional improvement, and neurological improvement. Several level III studies have been published comparing the benefits of operative and conservative management of thoracolumbar trauma. In patients with thoracolumbar spine trauma without neurological deficit or overt instability, multiple studies, including several randomized trials have shown no long-term benefit to operative management with regards to pain, disability, or overall health [179, 180], Similarly, no benefit has been shown to the use of clinical orthosis in patients suffering thoracolumbar burst fractures without associated neurological deficit with regards to long-term improvement of pain or function [181]. However, in patients with neurological dysfunction secondary to traumatic thoracolumbar spinal fractures, there may be a benefit to operative management. A recent retrospective cohort study with blinded inclusion was published by Stadhourder and colleagues comparing neurologic recovery, disability improvement, pain improvement, and overall health improvement in patients treated operatively versus nonoperatively for traumatic thoracic or lumbar fractures. Patients treated operatively were more likely to have a neurological deficit pre-operatively (ASIA D or worse), but were also more likely to experience neurological recovery by 1-year post-operatively and by last follow-up. These differences only approached significance though due to the small size of the cohort with pre-operative neurological deficit. Because of this, the group reached no conclusions regarding the indications for operative management.

Though less common than burst fractures, chance fractures – axial fractures through the vertebral body and posterior elements secondary to extreme flexion-distraction forces – also deserve mention [182]. These injuries are thought to be most common in the thoracolumbar spines (T10-L2) of adults involved in motor vehicle accidents, leading them to also be known as seat belt fracture [183]. In such cases, the lap belt portion of the restraint serves as a fixed fulcrum over which the spine is forced to flex, distracting and dividing the posterior tension band. This plane then propagates forward to involve the vertebral body, creating the axial chance fracture [182, 183]. Though most common in adults, case reports of children sustaining chance fractures also exist [184–186], as do reports of chance fractures secondary to other mechanisms of injury, including falls from height and extreme sports injuries [182, 187, 188]. Diagnosis of these injuries can be made with good AP and lateral radiographs, and treatment usually involves closed reduction and immobilization of the fracture with a TLSO brace or hyperextension cast. Recovery is generally quite good following treatment, but in untreated patients the injury will frequently progress to a focal kyphotic deformity causing significant back pain and requiring operative management [183]. Surgery with instrumented fusion may also be required in cases where displacement is too great to be achieved with closed reduction alone [189] and cases where the posterior ligamentous complex is compromised, as such an injury will not heal [182].

Both anterior and posterior approaches can be successfully used to treat thoracolumbar trauma[173]. A recent meta-analysis of the available literature by Xu and colleagues examined the outcomes of anterior versus posterior approaches for thoracolumbar burst fractures [178]. The authors observed no differences between the groups with regards to return to work, complications, or degree of corrections. However, patients treated with an anterior approach were slightly more likely to experience neurological improvement (46.7% v. 29.9%, $p < 0.06$), albeit at the expense of greater intraoperative blood loss, higher cost, and longer operative times. Because of the higher intraoperative morbidity and nonsignificant difference in outcomes, the authors recommend the use of a posterior approach for the treatment of thoracolumbar trauma. Additionally, given the advancements in expandable interbody devices, corpectomy and anterior column reconstruction can be accomplished via a single stage posterior transpedicular or extreme-lateral, transpsoas approach [173, 190, 191]. In fact, many groups have begun to treat thoracolumbar trauma with minimally invasive techniques, using percutaneous kyphoplasty [192, 193] or corpectomy through an expandable retractor, and percutaneous short segment instrumentation to help stabilize the affected level and prevent progressive kyphosis at this level [193–197]. Corpectomy of the involved level provides more effective decompression of the spinal canal and may provide superior anterior column reconstruction. However, it is associated with higher morbidity and may not be indicated in all patients [192]. Studies comparing the minimally invasive approaches have noted no difference in long-term patient reported outcomes, but patients treated by minimally invasive techniques have significantly lower intraoperative blood loss and so may have faster recoveries post-operatively [198].

Risk Factors for Post-traumatic Myelopathy

As previously touched upon in this chapter, not every trauma patient will experience post-traumatic myelopathy. In fact, the majority of trauma patients will show no signs of myelopathy. Multiple studies have been done in order to determine the risk factors for the development of post-traumatic myelopathy. These findings can be broadly grouped into two categories – those associated with pre-traumatic stenosis [37], and those associated with pre-traumatic spinal column instability. In the case of the former, which is defined as a canal diameter of less than 10 mm, it is thought that the pre-existing stenosis decreases the CSF cushion around the cord and so may allow for more direct transfer of energy to the cord [199]. This results in the cavitation – seen in post-traumatic syringomyelia – and direct contusion of the cord, which is detectable as T2-hyperintensity on post-traumatic MRI [200]. Reasons for pre-existing stenosis include yellow ligament hypertrophy, age-related spondylosis, ossification of the posterior longitudinal ligament [199–203], disc protrusions and herniations [200], diffuse idiopathic skeletal hyperostosis (DISH)[200], and congenitally short pedicles, like those seen in achondroplasia [204]. Diagnosis of those patients who are at increased risk for SCI secondary to canal stenosis can be made using the absolute anteroposterior diameter of the canal, the Torg-Pavlov ratio, or the spinal cord occupation ratio. Previous papers have identified patients with canal diameters less than 10–13 mm, Torg-Pavlov ratios less than 0.80–0.82 [205], and spinal canal occupation ratios greater than 70–80% are indicative of an increased risk of SCI secondary to trauma [206]. Each of these metrics has its own relative benefits, with the sagittal AP canal diameter being the easiest to measure and the spinal cord occupation ratio being the only one to account for cord diameter. Additionally, each metric has been shown to have high sensitivity, but low specificity in the diagnosis of myelopathy secondary to canal stenosis [207]. As a result, the metric employed should be based upon the familiarity of the consulting clinician with each of these values.

The second set of risk factors – those creating pre-traumatic vertebral column instability – are in large part made up of connective tissue disorders, such as Morquio syndrome [208–214] Hurler Syndrome, Hunter Syndrome, Sly Syndrome [214], os odontoideum [215–217], osteogenesis imperfecta [210, 218–220], rheumatoid arthritis [221–224], Marfan syndrome [225], and Ehlers-Danlos syndrome, though Down Syndrome [226, 227] has also been associated with cranial settling. The decreased stability seen in these conditions means that the vertebral column is less able to tolerate the significant forces exerted upon it during trauma. As a result, the column is more susceptible to flexion-distraction injuries, rotatory subluxations, and vertebral subluxations, which stretch the axons of the spinal cord, producing axonal damage and subsequent myelopathy [228]. Similarly, increased rigidity of the vertebral column, as is seen in ankylosing spondylitis and autofusion, is also associated with an increased risk for post-traumatic myelopathy. Fractures through the fused anterior and middle columns creates a single fulcrum in the bony spine, over which the cord is stretched, producing axonal injury and subsequent post-traumatic edema, which produce an acute-onset myelopathy.

In general, it is not suggested that patients with any of the above conditions undergo prophylactic decompression or stabilization, except in cases of craniocervical instability, cord signal changes or gross instability. In this small subset of cases, internal fixation should be applied due to the high mortality associated with such conditions [200, 204, 217, 229]. Rather, patients with the above risk factors should be closely monitored and should be advised to avoid scenarios in which they might be exposed to significant traumatic forces, owing to their increased risk profile.

Surgical Techniques

Though the vast majority of spinal trauma patients are treated nonoperatively, a significant number of patients have surgical indications and are best treated through operative management. The techniques employed to address cervical trauma vary by level and can accordingly be divided into cervical, thoracic, and lumbar approaches.

Cervical Spine

Cervical approaches include the traditional posterior midline approach, which is most effective for occipitocervical fusions, the anterior, Smith-Robinson approach, which is familiar to most surgeons, and the direct lateral approach, which has been used by some groups to address trauma of the craniocervical junction. Other approaches include endonasal and transoral approaches, but these may involve the use of an access surgeon and are seldom, if ever, employed for traumatic etiologies.

Posterior approaches generally provide superior correction for cervical fractures, especially when the fracture is accompanied by dislocation. They have higher associated complication rates though, with post-op wound infections and wound dehiscence being of greatest concern. Anterior cervical approaches reduce the risk of wound dehiscence and may improve spinal canal decompression in cases of comminuted fracture. However, they are associated with poorer post-operative correction of deformity and are more commonly associated with swallowing difficulty post-operatively, though this deficit is usually transient. Both approaches offer similar neurological recovery though and so the approach chosen should be made on a case-by-case basis depending upon surgeon preference and the relative importance of deformity reduction.

Anterior Odontoid Screw Placement

Anterior odontoid screw placement is one effective means of addressing type II odontoid fractures. It serves as an alternative to both the Gallie and Brooks-type fusions involving sublaminar wiring, as well as the posterior Harms-type C1-2 fusion and C1-2 transarticular screw fixation. The procedure has been previously described by multiple groups and is best used in patients with type IIB odontoid fractures – those with posteroinferior fracture planes [140]. The procedure begins by placing the patient supine and securing their head in a table-mounted Mayfield clamp. A rolled towel is placed underneath the patient's shoulders to introduce cervical lordosis and facilitate placement of the screw. The patient's head is also flexed at the atlanto-occipital junction to reduce the displaced odontoid fragment. At this point, intraoperative imaging is used to localize the pathological level, with some groups now reporting the use of an O-Arm (Medtronic) in order to provide imaging for intraoperative navigation. The patient's neck is incised at the level of C5-6, just superior to the thyroid cartilage and the platysma is divided in the sagittal plane. The platysma is then retracted and dissection continues along the medial aspect of the sternocleidomastoid until the carotid artery is palpable. A retractor is then introduced to laterally retract the carotid sheath and contents, while another is used to medially retract the trachea and esophagus. The longus colli muscles are then mobilized from the anterior vertebral faces and a spinal needle is used to localize the C2/3 disc space. In cases where intra-operative CT-guided navigation is being used, the O-arm is again introduced to obtain a new set of images for alignment. The trajectory of the odontoid screw is then plotted with a probe and verifying with imaging. A pneumatic drill is used to bore through the superior aspect of C3 and inferior aspect of C2, targeting the displaced tip of the odontoid. During this process, it is recommended that fluoroscopy be used to verify drill positioning. After drilling the C2 and C3 bodies, a lag screw is introduced – it should be long enough to traverse the C3 and C2 vertebral bodies and involve the odontoid fragment, but should not be so long as to overhang the surface of the vertebral body. Once the screw is inserted, the fracture is reduced, and the positioning is verified radiographically, the wound is closed.

The chief advantage of this type of instrumentation relative to posterior atlanto-axial fusion is that it preserves motion at the craniocervical junction, which is responsible for more than half of the mobility in the cervical spine. Additionally, it is non-load bearing and so is less affected by poor bone quality than is posterior fusion. On the downside, this technique requires significant intraoperative radiation and ha a steep learning curve. Additionally, it cannot be used in patients with more extensive cervical spine trauma, which is observed in a nontrivial number of patients.

Anterior Cervical Corpectomy and Fusion

The anterior cervical corpectomy is an effective means of addressing subaxial cervical trauma, especially in patients with highly comminuted fractures of the vertebral body [230, 231]. In addition to effectively addressing anterior column damage, this approach makes use of the same Smith-Robinson approach that is utilized in the omnipresent anterior cervical discectomy and fusion, may provide superior functional outcomes in patients being treated for compressive myelopathy, and has a lower incidence of post-operative C5 palsy compared to posterior approaches [232, 233]. As discussed above in the anterior odontoid instrumentation, this procedure has the downside of increased risk of esophageal dysmotility postoperatively. It also offers poorer correction of deformity in patients with focal kyphosis and has an increased risk of requiring reoperation [232].

Briefly, the patient is placed prone with their head fixed in a table-mounted Mayfield clamp. Care should be taken to ensure that the proper amount of cervical lordosis is induced, though in patients with comminuted fractures, it may be beneficial to simultaneously monitor EMGs or SSEPs to ensure that the induction of lordosis does not exacerbate cord compression. The lesion level is then localized, the patient is draped, and a Smith-Robinson approach is employed to expose the involved levels. Caspar pins are placed above and below the lesion level to maintain distraction, and a high-speed drill is used to corpectomize the damaged level, leaving the posterior margin in place [234]. The posterior margin is then removed with Kerrison rongeurs to complete the corpectomy. Osseous fragments within the canal are removed and the neural foramina are decompressed if they are implicated in the vertebral damage. The drill is then used to prepare the superior and inferior endplates and an autograft titanium mesh cage is placed. PEEK cages and fibular allograft have also been used effectively [234–236]. Caspar distraction is released and cage positioning is confirmed on radiograph. A titanium retaining plate is then placed and the wound is closed in the usual fashion.

Posterior Cervical Fusion

Posterior midline approaches to address cervical trauma are extremely popular for cervical spine trauma as they provide high overall rates of fusion [142, 237] and when combined with laminectomy, they can provide both effective correction of deformity and decompression of the neural elements. As a result, they are associated with good neurological recovery many cases, especially in trauma with acute neurological deficits, producing neurological improvement in up to 90% of patients [237]. The chief disadvantages of this are an increased rate of post-operative wound infection [238] and C5 palsy [233], though the latter is usually transient and improves within 3 months in most patients.

The two chief questions that must be asked when considering posterior cervical fusion are whether to include the occiput and whether to place pedicle screws or lateral mass screws. Most surgeons elect to place pedicle screws within the axis, due to the relatively large pedicles, and lateral mass screws within the other vertebral levels. The chief advantage of lateral mass screws in the atlas and subaxial spine is that they reduce the risk of vertebral artery injury relative to pedicle screws. Some *in vitro* studies have suggested that the lateral mass screws may have significantly lower pullout strengths, with one study suggesting a pullout strength of 25% of that seen in pedicle screws [239]. But *in vivo* studies examining complications secondary to both instrumentation techniques have suggested similar rates of pseudarthrosis, screw pullout, loss of reduction, screw loosening, and revision surgery [240]. A second alternative to pedicle screws are translaminar screws or transspinous screws, which reduce the risk of vertebral artery injury [241, 242]. These screws have been shown in some studies to have similar pullout strengths to pedicle screws [241] and can be used in patients with small lateral masses or who have previously failed attempts at lateral mass instrumentation. They are contraindicated in any patients with neural arch damage though and may be difficult to incorporate into intermediate construct levels.

The decision to include the occiput in the fusion construct is not one that can be made lightly, as it significantly limits the patient's range of motion in the sagittal plane. Such limitations can have significant impacts on a patient's quality of life, including the elimination of their ability to operate a motor vehicle. Current indications for occipitocervical fusion in the setting of trauma are atlanto-occipital dissociation and type III occipital condyle fractures, both of which are highly unstable lesions [243]. Additionally, patients with irreducible atlantoaxial dislocations may be candidates for occipitocervical fusion. In all cases, the potential benefit of improved stability must be weighed against the inherent surgical morbidity.

The procedure itself is well described in the literature [243–245]. The patient is first placed prone in three-point Mayfield tongs, with 15–20 pounds of traction placed to reduce the fracture or subluxation being addressed by the surgery. A midline incision is then made extending from the inion to the last vertebral level to be instrumented. Subperiosteal dissection is performed over the included vertebral levels, extending out to the lateral masses to provide adequate exposure for instrumentation. Care must be taken during dissection over the atlantoaxial segments in order avoid damaging the prominent C2 nerve roots or V3 segment of the vertebral artery, which runs in the sulcus arteriosus along the superior edge of the atlas. The vertebrae are then instrumented with C2 pedicle screws, C1 lateral mass screws and lateral mass screws at the other included levels. An occipital plate, if required, is applied slightly caudal to the inion using bicortical screws. This placement takes advantage of the thick bone in the region of the inion while decreasing the risk of skin erosion, which is seen in patients with plate placement on the inion itself. Rods are then applied to the screws, reducing the dislocated level or post-traumatic deformity being addressed. Final rod contouring should be based upon thorough pre-operative evaluation of the C2-7 plumb line and cervical lordosis to ensure that a natural head position is achieved in the final construct. After verification of positioning on radiograph, a drain is placed, the wound is closed, and a rigid cervical collar is placed to facilitate healing.

Thoracolumbar Spine

Though less common than symptomatic cervical trauma, myelopathy-associated thoracolumbar trauma is also relatively common, and its operative management has been thoroughly described in the literature, most commonly for thoracolumbar burst fractures. Approaches to the treatment of thoracolumbar trauma can be divided into three main categories – anterior or thoracoscopic approaches, direct lateral approaches, and median or paramedian posterior approaches. Anterior approaches offer the best decompression of the spinal canal in cases of comminuted vertebral fractures, but are relatively morbid in thoracic surgery, owing to the requirement for thoracoscopy. Additionally, they provide correction of sagittal deformity that is inferior to the posterior approach, and in the case of lumbar lesion, require an access surgeon and so may not be feasible options in the emergent setting. Direct lateral approaches are relatively new compared with anterior or posterior approaches, and are most commonly employed for trauma to the lumbar spine or thoracolumbar junction. Unlike anterior surgery of the lumbar spine, direct lateral approaches do not require an access surgeon, but like anterior approaches, they may be infeasible in patients with large body habitus and suboptimal in patients with significant post-traumatic kyphosis. The last and best described approach to thoracolumbar pathology are the posterior approaches, which can be midline posterior, midline paramedian, or costotransverse. All of them offer similar results with respect to risk profile, fusion rates and correction of post-traumatic deformity. However, paramedian and costotransverse approaches allow for better access to the anterior column and so may be preferred in cases requiring corpectomy and anterior column reconstruction.

Extreme or Direct Lateral Approach (Transpsoas Approach)

The direct lateral approach is a minimally invasive technique for the treatment of lumbar pathology that was first presented in 2001 [246]. The patient is placed in a true lateral decubitus position, with the table flexed to increase the space between the twelfth rib and iliac crest; it may help to place a bump or roll underneath the dependent flank to increase the lateral flexion [247]. A K-wire is then used to identify the relevant level, which is marked on the patient's skin. Two small incisions are produced at this level, one in the midaxillary line and one at the border of the erector spinae and abdominal obliques. The surgeon introduces their finger through the posterior incision and uses it to divide the muscles of the abdominal wall. The retroperitoneal space is identified and the peritoneum is swept forward to help create a corridor for the future working channel. The surgeon then palpates the psoas muscles over the surgical and sweeps their finger laterally so that it is in line with the anterior incision. An EMG-equipped dilator (MaXcess™, NuVasive™) is then introduced through the anterior incision and guided to the lateral face of the psoas using the surgeon's finger. The dilator is then used to gently dissect the psoas fibers between the anterior one-third and posterior two-third to minimize damage to the genitofemoral nerve that runs through the psoas, and the lumbosacral plexus, which is intimately related with the medial surface of the muscle. The EMG capability of the dilator allows for periodic stimulation in order to further reduce the risk of nerve injury. Once the psoas has been transverse and the dilator is docked onto the lateral face of the affected level, sequential dilators are introduced to expose a working channel. Corpectomy is performed using a high-speed drill to decompression the spinal canal and the superior and inferior endplates are prepared. A distractible, wide footprint cage is then placed, expanded to reduce kyphosis, and packed with autograft from the corpectomy [191, 248, 249]. A retaining plate may then be applied to maintain cage positioning, though proper compression of the spinal segment following cage replacement can eliminate the need for such a cage. Closure is then performed in a standard fashion, at which time the patient may be flipped for posterior percutaneous pedicle screw instrumentation [248].

Posterior Approach

Posterior approaches to the thoracic and lumbar spine include both midline posterior approaches and paramedian costotransversectomy approaches, both of which allow effective decompression and reconstruction of the damaged segment [250]. One approach described by Sciubba and colleagues for the correction of focal kyphosis secondary to anterior column burst fracture is the bilateral modified costotransversectomy approach, which allows for circumferential decompression of the cord and reconstruction of the vertebral body. Furthermore, this approach can be utilized in patients who are too medically unstable to undergo a combined anterior plus posterior approach.

The procedure begins by placing the patient prone on a Jackson table and acquiring intraoperative SEPs and MEPs. A midline incision is created and subperiosteal dissection is performed in standard fashion over the damaged level and up to 3 segments above and below the level of the lesion, depending upon the length of the construct to be used. The number of levels to be included is somewhat controversial. Some groups prefer instrumentation of 2 or 3 levels above the lesion, especially for trauma to the thoracolumbar junction, but more recent research has suggested that short-segment constructs may be just as stable as longer constructs [251, 252]. After dissecting the paraspinal tissues off the posterior elements, laminectomies are performed over the traumatized vertebrae to decompress the cord. Pedicle screws are placed bilaterally at the levels above and below the lesion and a temporary rod is placed to maintain distraction. Bilateral facetectomies are performed at the lesion levels, with resection of the proximal 1–2 cm of rib in cases of thoracic trauma. A high-speed drill is then used to perform corpectomy of the damaged vertebrae and to prepare the superior and inferior endplates. A distractible cage is then placed in the site of the defect, expanded and packed with bone, including autograft from the site of trauma. In thoracic lesions, ligation of the nerve root may be required to place the cage. Ultrasonography is used to confirm decompression of thecal sac and placement of the cage. The final rods are then contoured and applied to the pedicle screw instrumentation, and reduced down to lock the cage into place. A drain is then placed and the wound is closed in the traditional fashion. Minimally invasive variations of this procedure have since been described and have proven to provide acceptable results in most cases [194, 253, 254].

Case Example

One example of post-traumatic myelopathy that we present here is a 41-year-old female who sustained cervical spine trauma secondary to a fall from height. At the time of injury, the patient was utilizing a 100-foot zip line, from which she fell 15 feet, landing directly on her head and losing consciousness. Emergency services arrived on scene to find the patient responsive, though she complained of numbness and tingling involving the entire distal right upper extremity and pain localized to her neck and upper back. The patient was immediately immobilized using a cervical collar and spinal board, and was then transferred to an outside emergency department. Upon presentation, she was Glasgow Coma Score 15, but had 4/5 strength in the right upper extremity. She was 5/5 strength through the left upper and bilateral lower extremities and had 2+ deep tendon reflexes throughout all extremities, but on head and cervical spine CT and CT angiography was noted to have an occluded right vertebral artery, left anterolateral atlantal arch fracture, right C7 facet fracture, and C2 compound type III odontoid and right-sided Hangman's fracture (Fig. 4.1). MRI was performed to evaluate the cord and soft tissues, which revealed an epidural

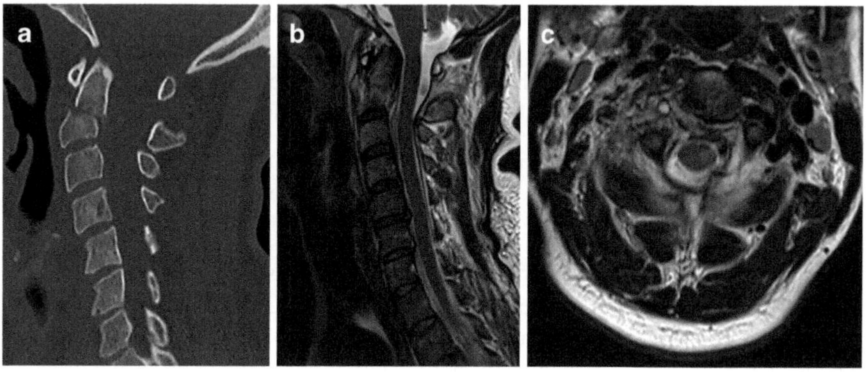

Fig. 4.1 Preoperative imaging demonstrating an acute significantly comminuted, displaced type III Dens fracture with posterior displacement of fracture fragments into the central canal. (**a**) Sagittal CT (**b**) Sagittal T2-weighted MRI (**c**) Axial T2-weighted MRI

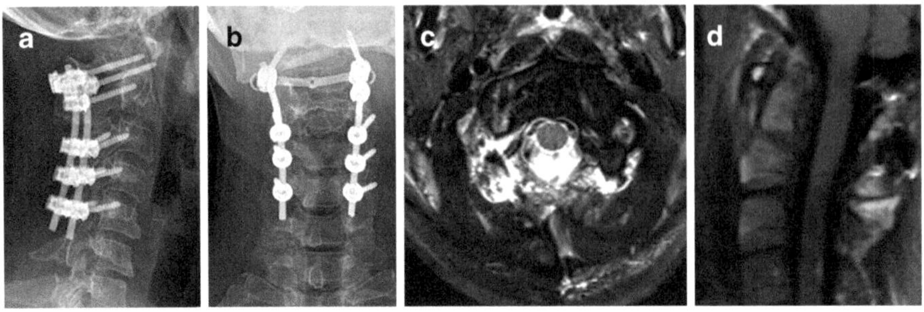

Fig. 4.2 Post-operative imaging demonstrating posterior bilaterally instrumented arthrodesis from C1-C5. (**a**) Lateral plain radiograph (**b**) AP plain radiograph (**c**) Axial T2-weighted MRI (**d**) Sagittal T1-weighted FLAIR

hematoma anterior to the C2 cord without obvious signs of cord compression or signal change.

Following work-up, a recommendation was made to transfer the patient to a facility with comprehensive spine services for operative management of her injury, which she underwent the following morning, less than 24 hours following her injury. Surgery consisted of a posterior instrumented fusion of C1-C5 with placement of a left C2 pedicle screw and bilateral lateral mass screws at the other levels (Fig. 4.2). Open reduction of the C1 and C2 fractures was also performed. Both C2 roots had to be sacrificed to completely access the complex axis fracture. Post-operative DVT and antibiotic prophylaxis were instituted and the patient was placed in a Miami J collar to facilitate fusion of the construct. MRI imaging of the brain was also performed post-operatively to evaluate for possible infarcts secondary to the right vertebral artery dissection, but none were noted. The post-operative course was overall unremarkable, with significant improvement of right upper extremity numbness by post-operative day 3 and discharge home on post-operative day 8. Axial pain was significantly improved by the three-month follow-up visit, at which point the patient had been weaned from the cervical collar. By the sixth month follow-up, full strength had returned to the right upper extremity and radiographic evidence of fusion was present. The patient retained no residual deficits from the accident, though her neck mobility is limited due to inclusion of the atlantoaxial joint in the construct.

Conclusion

Each year 11,000–15,000 Americans suffer traumatic spinal cord injury. Injury most commonly occurs in the cervical segments, but may also occur in either the thoracic or lumbar spine. Current guidelines suggest that initial treatment in most patients be conservative management with external immobilization of the affected spinal segments. However, given that most patients have associated vertebral dislocations or fractures, many patients will require operative management. In such cases, the focus must be placed on both decompressing the neural elements and on correcting the post-traumatic deformity. Our goal in this chapter has been to describe both the sequelae of spinal trauma and summarize current guidelines for the treatment of these injuries. Despite significant work towards the development of guidelines, further work is necessary to obtain higher quality evidence that can be used to guide the care of patients with these injuries.

References

1. McKinley W, Santos K, Meade M, Brooke K. Incidence and outcomes of spinal cord injury clinical syndromes. J Spinal Cord Med. 2007;30(3):215–24.
2. Papadopoulos SM, Selden NR, Quint DJ, Patel N, Gillespie B, Grube S. Immediate spinal cord decompression for cervical spinal cord injury: feasibility and outcome. J Trauma. 2002 Feb;52(2):323–32.
3. Stevens EA, Marsh R, Wilson JA, Sweasey TA, Branch CL Jr, Powers AK. A review of surgical intervention in the setting of traumatic central cord syndrome. Spine J. 2010 Oct;10(10):874–80.
4. Sweis R, Biller J. Systemic complications of spinal cord injury. Curr Neurol Neurosci Rep. 2017 Feb;17(2):8. https://doi.org/10.1007/s11910-017-0715-4.
5. Sekhon LHS, Fehlings MG. Epidemiology, demographics, and pathophysiology of acute spinal cord injury. Spine (Phila Pa 1976). 2001;26(24S):S2–S12.
6. DeVivo MJ. Causes and costs of spinal cord injury in the United States. Spinal Cord. 1997 Dec;35(12):809–13.
7. DeVivo MJ, Krause JS, Lammertse DP. Recent trends in mortality and causes of death among persons with spinal cord injury. Arch Phys Med Rehabil. 1999 Nov;80(11):1411–9.
8. Jain NB, Ayers GD, Peterson EN, Harris MB, Morse L, O'Connor KC, et al. Traumatic spinal cord injury in the United States, 1993–2012. JAMA. 2015 Jun 9;313(22):2236–43.
9. Falci SP, Indeck C, Lammertse DP. Posttraumatic spinal cord tethering and syringomyelia: surgical treatment and long-term outcome. J Neurosurg Spine. 2009 Oct;11(4):445–60.
10. Devivo MJ. Epidemiology of traumatic spinal cord injury: trends and future implications. Spinal Cord. 2012 May;50(5):365–72.
11. LoPachin RM, Lehning EJ. Mechanism of calcium entry during axon injury and degeneration. Toxicol Appl Pharmacol. 1997;143(2):233–44.
12. Hausmann ON. Post-traumatic inflammation following spinal cord injury. Spinal Cord. 2003;41(7):369–78.
13. Popovich PG. Immunological regulation of neuronal degeneration and regeneration in the injured spinal cord. Prog Brain Res. 2000;128:43–58.
14. Cavus G, Altas M, Aras M, Özgür T, Serarslan Y, Yilmaz N, et al. Effects of montelukast and methylprednisolone on experimental spinal cord injury in rats. Eur Rev Med Pharmacol Sci. 2014;18(12):1770–7.
15. Liu D, Li L, Augustus L. Prostaglandin release by spinal cord injury mediates production of hydroxyl radical, malondialdehyde and cell death: a site of the neuroprotective action of methylprednisolone. J Neurochem. 2001;77(4):1036–47.
16. Hurlbert RJ, Hadley MN, Walters BC, Aarabi B, Dhall SS, Gelb DE, et al. Pharmacological therapy for acute spinal cord injury. Neurosurgery. 2013;72(Suppl 3):93–105.
17. Li Y, Lucas-Osma AM, Black S, Bandet MV, Stephens MJ, Vavrek R, et al. Pericytes impair capillary blood flow and motor function after chronic spinal cord injury. Nat Med. 2017;23(6):733–41.
18. Muradov JM, Ewan EE, Hagg T. Dorsal column sensory axons degenerate due to impaired microvascular perfusion after spinal cord injury in rats. Exp Neurol. 2013;249:59–73.

19. Allen BL, Ferguson RL, Lehmann TR, O'Brien RP. A mechanistic classification of closed, indirect fractures and dislocations of the lower cervical spine. Spine (Phila Pa 1976). 1982;7(1):1–27.
20. Harris JH Jr, Edeiken-Monroe B, Kopaniky DR. A practical classification of acute cervical spine injuries. Orthop Clin North Am. 1986;17(1):15–30.
21. Moore T, Vaccaro AR, Anderson PA. Classification of lower cervical spine injuries. Spine (Phila Pa 1976). 2006;31(11S):S37–43.
22. Patel AA, Dailey AT, Brodke DS, Daubs M, Anderson PA, Hurlbert RJ, et al. Subaxial cervical spine trauma classification: the Subaxial Injury Classification system and case examples. Neurosurg Focus. 2008;25(5):E8.
23. Vaccaro AR, Lehman RA Jr, Hurlbert RJ, Anderson PA, Harris MB, Hedlund R, et al. A new classification of thoracolumbar injuries: the importance of injury morphology, the integrity of the posterior ligamentous complex, and neurologic status. Spine (Phila Pa 1976). 2005;30(20):2325–33.
24. Aarabi B, Walters BC, Dhall SS, Gelb DE, Hurlbert RJ, Rozzelle CJ, et al. Subaxial cervical spine injury classification systems. Neurosurgery. 2013;72(Suppl 3):170–86.
25. Chhabra HS, Kaul R, Kanagaraju V. Do we have an ideal classification system for thoracolumbar and subaxial cervical spine injuries: what is the expert's perspective? Spinal Cord. 2015;53(1):42–8.
26. Klekamp J. Treatment of posttraumatic syringomyelia. J Neurosurg Spine. 2012 Sep;17(3):199–211.
27. Ushewokunze SO, Gan YC, Phillips K, Thacker K, Flint G. Surgical treatment of post-traumatic syringomyelia. Spinal Cord. 2010 Sep;48(9):710–3.
28. Fischbein NJ, Dillon WP, Cobbs C, Weinstein PR. The "presyrinx" state: a reversible myelopathic condition that may precede syringomyelia. AJNR Am J Neuroradiol. 1999 Jan;20(1):7–20.
29. Quencer RM, Green BA, Eismont FJ. Posttraumatic spinal cord cysts: clinical features and characterization with metrizamide computed tomography. Radiology. 1983 Feb;146(2):415–23.
30. Bonfield CM, Levi AD, Arnold PM, Okonkwo DO. Surgical management of post-traumatic syringomyelia. Spine (Phila Pa 1976). 2010 Oct 1;35(21 Suppl):S245–58.
31. Hayashi T, Ueta T, Kubo M, Maeda T, Shiba K. Subarachnoid-subarachnoid bypass: a new surgical technique for posttraumatic syringomyelia. J Neurosurg Spine. 2013 Apr;18(4):382–7.
32. Holly LT, Johnson JP, Masciopinto JE, Batzdorf U. Treatment of posttraumatic syringomyelia with extradural decompressive surgery. Neurosurg Focus. 2000 Mar 15;8(3):E8.
33. Ko HY, Kim W, Kim SY, Shin MJ, Cha YS, Chang JH, et al. Factors associated with early onset post-traumatic syringomyelia. Spinal Cord. 2012 Sep;50(9):695–8.
34. Vannemreddy SS, Rowed DW, Bharatwal N. Posttraumatic syringomyelia: predisposing factors. Br J Neurosurg. 2002 Jun;16(3):276–83.
35. Abel R, Gerner HJ, Smit C, Meiners T. Residual deformity of the spinal canal in patients with traumatic paraplegia and secondary changes of the spinal cord. Spinal Cord. 1999 Jan;37(1):14–9.
36. Curati WL, Kingsley DPE, Kendall BE, Moseley IF. MRI in chronic spinal cord trauma. Neuroradiology. 1992;35(1):30–5.
37. Perrouin-Verbe B, Lenne-Aurier K, Robert R, Auffray-Calvier E, Richard I. Mauduyt de la Grève I, et al. Post-traumatic syringomyelia and post-traumatic spinal canal stenosis: a direct relationship: review of 75 patients with a spinal cord injury. Spinal Cord. 1998 Feb;36(2):137–43.
38. Enicker B, Gonya S, Hardcastle TC. Spinal stab injury with retained knife blades: 51 Consecutive patients managed at a regional referral unit. Injury. 2015;46(9):1726–33.
39. Jacobsohn M, Semple P, Dunn R, Candy S. Stab injuries to the spinal cord: a retrospective study on clinical findings and magnetic resonance imaging changes. Neurosurgery. 2007;61(6):1262–7.

40. Peacock WJ, Shrosbree RD, Key AG. A review of 450 stabwounds of the spinal cord. S Afr Med J. 1977;51(26):961–4.
41. Miranda P, Gomez P, Alday R, Kaen A, Ramos A. Brown-Sequard syndrome after blunt cervical spine trauma: clinical and radiological correlations. Eur Spine J. 2007;16(8):1165–70.
42. Roth EJ, Park T, Pang T, Yarkony GM, Lee MY. Traumatic cervical Brown-Sequard and Brown-Sequard-plus syndromes: the spectrum of presentations and outcomes. Paraplegia. 1991;29(9):582–9.
43. Shen C, Wang Y, Yang D, Wang F, Shen BB. Brown-Séquard syndrome associated with Horner's syndrome in cervical epidural hematoma. Spine (Phila Pa 1976). 1995;20(2):244–7.
44. García-Manzanares MD, Belda-Sanchis JI, Giner-Pascual M, Miguel-Leon I, Delgado-Calvo M, Alió y Sanz JL. Brown-Sequard syndrome associated with Horner's syndrome after a penetrating trauma at the cervicomedullary junction. Spinal Cord. 2000;38(11):705–7.
45. Edwards A, Andrews R. A case of Brown-Sequard syndrome with associated Horner's syndrome after blunt injury to the cervical spine. Emerg Med J. 2001;18:512–3.
46. Johnson S, Jones M, Zumsteg J. Brown-Séquard syndrome without vascular injury associated with Horner's syndrome after a stab injury to the neck. J Spinal Cord Med. 2016;39(1):111–4.
47. Russell JH, Joseph SJ, Snell BJ, Jithoo R. Brown-Sequard syndrome associated with Horner's syndrome following a penetrating drill bit injury to the cervical spine. J Clin Neurosci. 2009;16(7):975–7.
48. Meng Y, Zhou L, Liu X, Wang H, Shi J, Guo Y. Brown-Sequard syndrome associated with Horner syndrome following cervical disc herniation. Spinal Cord Ser Cases. 2016;15(2):16037.
49. Caner H, Kilinçoglu BF, Benli S, Altinörs N, Bavbek M. Magnetic resonance image findings and surgical considerations in T1-2 disc herniation. Can J Neurol Sci. 2003;30(2):152–4.
50. Hassan ANA, Ballester J, Slater N. Bilateral first rib fractures associated with Horner's Syndrome. Injury. 2000;31(4):273–4.
51. Paiva WS, De Amorim RLO, Tavares WM, EJL A, Jeng BP, Figueiredo EG. Horner's syndrome after blunt cervical and chest trauma: case report. Arq Neuropsiquiatr. 2007;65(4A):1037–9.
52. Ozel SK, Kazez A. Horner syndrome due to first rib fracture after major thoracic trauma. J Pediatr Surg. 2005;40(10):e17–9.
53. Ahmadi O, Saxena P, Wilson BKJ, Bunton RW. First rib fracture and Horner's syndrome: a rare clinical entity. Ann Thorac Surg. 2013;95(1):355.
54. Ahn UM, Ahn NU, Buchowski JM, Garrett ES, Sieber AN, Kostuik JP. Cauda equina syndrome secondary to lumbar disc herniation: a meta-analysis of surgical outcomes. Spine (Phila Pa 1976). 2000;25(12):1515–22.
55. Dhatt S, Tahasildar N, Tripathy SK, Bahadur R, Dhillon M. Outcome of spinal decompression in cauda equina syndrome presenting late in developing countries: case series of 50 cases. Eur Spine J. 2011;20(12):2235–9.
56. Dinning TAR, Schaeffer HR. Discogenic compression of the cauda equina: a surgical Emergency. Aust NZ J Surg. 1993;63(12):927–34.
57. McCarthy MJ, Aylott CE, Grevitt MP, Hegarty J. Cauda equina syndrome: factors affecting long-term functional and sphincteric outcome. Spine (Phila Pa 1976). 2007;32(2):207–16.
58. O'Laorie SA, Crockard HA, Thomas DG. Prognosis for sphincter recovery after operation for cauda equina compression owing to lumbar disc prolapse. Br Med J (Clin Res Ed). 1981;282(6279):1852–4.
59. Martin ND, Kepler C, Zubair M, Sayadipour A, Cohen M, Weinstein M. Increased mean arterial pressure goals after spinal cord injury and functional outcome. J Emerg Trauma Shock. 2015;8(2):94–8.
60. Quencer RM, Bunge RP, Egnor M, Green BA, Puckett W, Naidich TP, et al. Acute traumatic central cord syndrome: MRI-pathological correlations. Neuroradiology. 1992;34(2):85–94.
61. Aito S, D'Andrea M, Werhagen L, Farsetti L, Cappelli S, Bandini B, et al. Neurological and functional outcome in traumatic central cord syndrome. Spinal Cord. 2007 Apr;45(4):292–7.
62. Brooks NP. Central Cord Syndrome. Neurosurg Clin N Am. 2017 Jan;28(1):41–7.

63. Dvorak MF, Fisher CG, Hoekema J, Boyd M, Noonan V, Wing PC, et al. Factors predicting motor recovery and functional outcome after traumatic central cord syndrome: a long-term follow-up. Spine (Phila Pa 1976). 2005 Oct 15;30(20):2303–11.
64. Aarabi B, Hadley MN, Dhall SS, Gelb DE, Hurlbert RJ, Rozzelle CJ, et al. Management of Acute Traumatic Central Cord Syndrome (ATCCS). Neurosurgery. 2013;72(Suppl 3):195–204.
65. Lenehan B, Fisher CG, Vaccaro A, Fehlings M, Aarabi B, Dvorak MF. The urgency of surgical decompression in acute central cord injuries with spondylosis and without instability. Spine (Phila Pa 1976). 2010 Oct 1;35(21 Suppl):S180–6.
66. Chen L, Yang H, Yang T, Xu Y, Bao Z, Tang T. Effectiveness of surgical treatment for traumatic central cord syndrome. J Neurosurg Spine. 2009 Jan;10(1):3–8.
67. Hagen EM. Acute complications of spinal cord injuries. World J Orthop. 2015 Jan 18;6(1):17–23.
68. Ryken TC, Hurlbert RJ, Hadley MN, Aarabi B, Dhall SS, Gelb DE, et al. The acute cardiopulmonary management of patients with cervical spinal cord injuries. Neurosurgery. 2013;72(Suppl 3):84–92.
69. Krassioukov AV, Furlan JC, Fehlings MG. Autonomic dysreflexia in acute spinal cord injury: an under-recognized clinical entity. J Neurotrauma. 2003 Aug;20(8):707–16.
70. Ropper AE, Ropper AH. Acute spinal cord compression. N Engl J Med. 2017;376(14):1358–69.
71. Belanger E, Picard C, Lacerte D, Lavallee P, Levi AD. Subacute posttraumatic ascending myelopathy after spinal cord injury. Report of three cases. J Neurosurg. 2000 Oct;93(2 Suppl):294–9.
72. Zhang J, Wang H, Liu H, Wang G. Subacute post-traumatic ascending myelopathy after T12 burst fracture in a 32-year-old male: case report and surgical result of cervical durotomy. Spinal Cord Ser Cases. 2016 Jul 7;2:16004.
73. Kovanda TJ, Horn EM. Subacute posttraumatic ascending myelopathy in a 15-year-old boy. J Neurosurg Spine. 2014 Sep;21(3):454–7.
74. Planner AC, Pretorius PM, Graham A, Meagher TM. Subacute progressive ascending myelopathy following spinal cord injury: MRI appearances and clinical presentation. Spinal Cord. 2008 Feb;46(2):140–4.
75. Zhang J, Wang G. Subacute posttraumatic ascending myelopathy: a literature review. Spinal Cord. 2017 Jul;55(7):644–50.
76. Aito S, El Masry WS, Gerner HJ, Lorenzo ND, Pellicano G, D'Andrea M, et al. Ascending myelopathy in the early stage of spinal cord injury. Spinal Cord. 1999 Sep;37(9):617–23.
77. Harrop JS, Sharan AD, Vaccaro AR, Przybylski GJ. The cause of neurologic deterioration after acute cervical spinal cord injury. Spine (Phila Pa 1976). 2001 Feb 15;26(4):340–6.
78. Marshall LF, Knowlton S, Garfin SR, Klauber MR, Eisenberg HM, Kopaniky D, et al. Deterioration following spinal cord injury. A multicenter study. J Neurosurg. 1987 Mar;66(3):400–4.
79. Miller BA, Roy AK, Boucher AB, Pradilla G, Ahmad FU. Subacute posttraumatic ascending myelopathy after an incomplete spinal cord injury from a gunshot wound to the spine: case report and review of the literature. World Neurosurg. 2016 Apr;88:687.e13–7.
80. Bailitz J, Starr F, Beecroft M, Bankoff J, Roberts R, Bokhari F, et al. CT should replace three-view radiographs as the initial screening test in patients at high, moderate, and low risk for blunt cervical spine injury: a prospective comparison. J Trauma. 2009 Jun;66(6):1605–9.
81. Mathen R, Inaba K, Munera F, Teixeira PG, Rivas L, McKenney M, et al. Prospective evaluation of multislice computed tomography versus plain radiographic cervical spine clearance in trauma patients. J Trauma. 2007 Jun;62(6):1427–31.
82. Ryken TC, Hadley MN, Walters BC, Aarabi B, Dhall SS, Gelb DE, et al. Radiographic assessment. Neurosurgery. 2013;72(Suppl 3):54–72.
83. Parizel PM, van der Zijden T, Gaudino S, Spaepen M, Voormolen MHJ, Venstermans C, et al. Trauma of the spine and spinal cord: imaging strategies. Eur Spine J. 2010;19(Suppl 1):8–17.
84. Potter K, Saifuddin A. MRI of chronic spinal cord injury. Br J Radiol. 2003;76(905):347–52.

85. Dundamadappa SK, Cauley KA. MR imaging of acute cervical spinal ligamentous and soft tissue trauma. Emerg Radiol. 2012;19(4):277–86.
86. Kulkarni MV, McArdle CB, Kopanichy D, Miner M, Cotler HB, Lee KF, et al. Acute spinal cord injury: MR imaging at 1.5T. Radiology. 1987;164(3):837–43.
87. Wang D, Bodley R, Sett P, Gardner B, Frankel H. A clinical magnetic resonance imaging study of the traumatised spinal cord more than 20 years following injury. Paraplegia. 1996;34(2):65–81.
88. Kelley BJ, Erickson BJ, Weinshenker BG. Compressive myelopathy mimicking transverse myelitis. Neurologist. 2010;16(2):120–2.
89. Theodore N, Hadley MN, Aarabi B, Dhall SS, Gelb DE, Hurlbert RJ, et al. Prehospital cervical spinal immobilization after trauma. Neurosurgery. 2013;72(Suppl 3):22–34.
90. Theodore N, Aarabi B, Dhall SS, Gelb DE, Hurlbert RJ, Rozzelle CJ, et al. Transportation of patients with acute traumatic cervical spine injuries. Neurosurgery. 2013;72(Suppl 3):35–9.
91. Hadley MN, Walters BC, Aarabi B, Dhall SS, Gelb DE, Hurlbert RJ, et al. Clinical assessment following acute cervical spinal cord injury. Neurosurgery. 2013;72(Suppl 3):40–53.
92. Gelb DE, Hadley MN, Aarabi B, Dhall SS, Hurlbert RJ, Rozzelle CJ, et al. Initial closed reduction of cervical spinal fracture-dislocation injuries. Neurosurgery. 2013;72(Suppl 3):73–83.
93. Theodore N, Aarabi B, Dhall SS, Gelb DE, Hurlbert RJ, Rozzelle CJ, et al. Occipital condyle fractures. Neurosurgery. 2013;72(Suppl 3):106–13.
94. Ryken TC, Aarabi B, Dhall SS, Gelb DE, Hurlbert RJ, Rozzelle CJ, et al. Management of isolated fractures of the atlas in adults. Neurosurgery. 2013;72(Suppl 3):127–31.
95. Ryken TC, Hadley MN, Aarabi B, Dhall SS, Gelb DE, Hurlbert RJ, et al. Management of isolated fractures of the axis in adults. Neurosurgery. 2013;72(Suppl 3):132–50.
96. Ryken TC, Hadley MN, Aarabi B, Dhall SS, Gelb DE, Hurlbert RJ, et al. Management of acute combination fractures of the atlas and axis in adults. Neurosurgery. 2013;72(Suppl 3):151–8.
97. Rozzelle CJ, Aarabi B, Dhall SS, Gelb DE, Hurlbert RJ, Ryken TC, et al. Os Odontoideum. Neurosurgery. 2013;72(Suppl 3):159–69.
98. Gelb DE, Aarabi B, Dhall SS, Hurlbert RJ, Rozzelle CJ, Ryken TC, et al. Treatment of subaxial cervical spinal injuries. Neurosurgery. 2013;72(Suppl 3):187–94.
99. Rozzelle CJ, Aarabi B, Dhall SS, Gelb DE, Hurlbert RJ, Ryken TC, et al. Management of pediatric cervical spine and spinal cord injuries. Neurosurgery. 2013;72(Suppl 3):205–26.
100. Rozzelle CJ, Aarabi B, Dhall SS, Gelb DE, Hurlbert RJ, Ryken TC, et al. Spinal cord Injury Without Radiographic Abnormality (SCIWORA). Neurosurgery. 2013;72(Suppl 3):227–33.
101. Harrigan MR, Hadley MN, Dhall SS, Walters BC, Aarabi B, Gelb DE, et al. Management of vertebral artery injuries following non-penetrating cervical trauma. Neurosurgery. 2013;72(Suppl 3):234–43.
102. Dhall SS, Hadley MN, Aarabi B, Gelb DE, Hurlbert RJ, Rozzelle CJ, et al. Deep venous thrombosis and thromboembolism in patients with cervical spinal cord injuries. Neurosurgery. 2013;72(Suppl 3):244–54.
103. Dhall SS, Hadley MN, Aarabi B, Gelb DE, Hurlbert RJ, Rozzelle CJ, et al. Nutritional support after spinal cord injury. Neurosurgery. 2013;72(Suppl 3):255–9.
104. Gunby I. New focus on spinal cord injury. JAMA. 1981 Mar 27;245(12):1201–6.
105. Waters RL, Meyer PR Jr, Adkins RH, Felton D. Emergency, acute, and surgical management of spine trauma. Arch Phys Med Rehabil. 1999 Nov;80(11):1383–90.
106. Stroh G, Braude D. Can an out-of-hospital cervical spine clearance protocol identify all patients with injuries? An argument for selective immobilization. Ann Emerg Med. 2001 Jun;37(6):609–15.
107. Domeier RM, Evans RW, Swor RA, Rivera-Rivera EJ, Frederiksen SM. Prehospital clinical findings associated with spinal injury. Prehosp Emerg Care. 1997 Jan-Mar;1(1):11–5.
108. Domeier RM, Evans RW, Swor RA, Hancock JB, Fales W, Krohmer J, et al. The reliability of prehospital clinical evaluation for potential spinal injury is not affected by the mechanism of injury. Prehosp Emerg Care. 1999 Oct-Dec;3(4):332–7.

109. Tator CH, Rowed DW, Schwartz ML, Gertzbein SD, Bharatwal N, Barkin M, et al. Management of acute spinal cord injuries. Can J Surg. 1984 May;27(3):289–93.
110. Tator CH, Duncan EG, Edmonds VE, Lapczak LI, Andrews DF. Changes in epidemiology of acute spinal cord injury from 1947 to 1981. Surg Neurol. 1993 Sep;40(3):207–15.
111. Zäch GA, Seiler W, Dollfus P. Treatment results of spinal cord injuries in the Swiss Parplegic Centre of Basle. Paraplegia. 1976 May;14(1):58–65.
112. Burney RE, Waggoner R, Maynard FM. Stabilization of spinal injury for early transfer. J Trauma. 1989 Nov;29(11):1497–9.
113. Graves DE, Frankiewicz RG, Donovan WH. Construct validity and dimensional structure of the ASIA motor scale. J Spinal Cord Med. 2006;29(1):39–45.
114. Marino RJ, Graves DE. Metric properties of the ASIA motor score: subscales improve correlation with functional activities. Arch Phys Med Rehabil. 2004 Nov;85(11):1804–10.
115. Anderson K, Aito S, Atkins M, Biering-Sorensen F, Charlifue S, Curt A, et al. Functional recovery measures for spinal cord injury: an evidence-based review for clinical practice and research. J Spinal Cord Med. 2008;31(2):133–44.
116. Catz A, Itzkovich M, Tesio L, Biering-Sorensen F, Weeks C, Laramee MT, et al. A multicenter international study on the Spinal Cord Independence Measure, version III: rasch psychometric validation. Spinal Cord. 2007 Apr;45(4):275–91.
117. Itzkovich M, Gelernter I, Biering-Sorensen F, Weeks C, Laramee MT, Craven BC, et al. The Spinal Cord Independence Measure (SCIM) version III: reliability and validity in a multicenter international study. Disabil Rehabil. 2007 Dec 30;29(24):1926–33.
118. Horn EM, Lekovic GP, Feiz-Erfan I, Sonntag VK, Theodore N. Cervical magnetic resonance imaging abnormalities not predictive of cervical spine instability in traumatically injured patients. Invited submission from the Joint Section Meeting on Disorders of the Spine and Peripheral Nerves, March 2004. J Neurosurg Spine. 2004 Jul;1(1):39–42.
119. Duane TM, Cross J, Scarcella N, Wolfe LG, Mayglothling J, Aboutanos MB, et al. Flexion-extension cervical spine plain films compared with MRI in the diagnosis of ligamentous injury. Am Surg. 2010 Jun;76(6):595–8.
120. Malham GM, Ackland HM, Jones R, Williamson OD, Varma DK. Occipital condyle fractures: incidence and clinical follow-up at a level 1 trauma centre. Emerg Radiol. 2009 Jul;16(4):291–7.
121. Maddox JJ, Rodriguez-Feo JA 3rd, Maddox GE, Gullung G, McGwin G, Theiss SM. Nonoperative treatment of occipital condyle fractures: an outcomes review of 32 fractures. Spine (Phila Pa 1976). 2012 Jul 15;37(16):E964–8.
122. Jea A, Tatsui C, Farhat H, Vanni S, Levi AD. Vertically unstable type III odontoid fractures: case report. Neurosurgery. 2006;58(4):E797. discussion E797
123. Theodore N, Aarabi B, Dhall SS, Gelb DE, Hurlbert RJ, Rozzelle CJ, et al. The diagnosis and management of traumatic atlanto-occipital dislocation injuries. Neurosurgery. 2013;72(Suppl 3):114–26.
124. Fard SA, Avila MJ, Johnstone CM, Patel AS, Walter CM, Skoch J, et al. Prognostic factors in traumatic atlanto-occipital dislocation. J Clin Neurosci. 2016;33:63–8.
125. Mendenhall SK, Sivaganesan A, Mistry A, Sivasubramaniam P, McGirt MJ, Devin CJ. Traumatic atlantooccipital dislocation: comprehensive assessment of mortality, neurologic improvement, and patient-reported outcomes at a Level 1 trauma center over 15 years. Spine J. 2015;15(11):2385–95.
126. Wholey MH, Bruwer A, Baker HL Jr. The lateral roentgenogram of the neck with comments on the atlanto-odontoid-basion relationship. Radiology. 1958;71(3):350–6.
127. Harris JH Jr, Carson GC, Wagner LK, Kerr N. Radiologic diagnosis of traumatic occipitovertebral dissociation: 2. Comparison of three methods of detecting occipitovertebral relationships on lateral radiographs of supine subjects. AJR Am J Roentgenol. 1994;162(4):887–92.
128. Harris JH Jr, Carson GC, Wagner LK. Radiologic diagnosis of traumatic occipitovertebral dissociation: 1. Normal occipitovertebral relationships on lateral radiographs of supine subjects. AJR Am J Roentgenol. 1994;162(4):881–6.

129. Powers B, Miller MD, Kramer RS, Martinez S, Gehweiler JA Jr. Traumatic anterior atlanto-occipital dislocation. Neurosurgery. 1979;4(1):12–7.
130. Sun PP, Poffenbarger GJ, Durham S, Zimmerman RA. Spectrum of occipitoatlantoaxial injury in young children. J Neurosurg. 2000;93(Spine 1):28–39.
131. Hall GC, Kinsman MJ, Nazar RG, Hruska RT, Mansfield KJ, Boakye M, et al. Atlanto-occipital dislocation. World J Orthop. 2015 Mar 18;6(2):236–43.
132. Clark CR, White AA 3rd. Fractures of the dens. A multicenter study. J Bone Joint Surg Am. 1985 Dec;67(9):1340–8.
133. Polin RS, Szabo T, Bogaev CA, Replogle RE, Jane JA. Nonoperative management of Types II and III odontoid fractures: the Philadelphia collar versus the halo vest. Neurosurgery. 1996;38(3):450–6. discussion 456-7
134. Wang GJ, Mabie KN, Whitehill R, Stamp WG. The nonsurgical management of odontoid fractures in adults. Spine (Phila Pa 1976). 1984 Apr;9(3):229–30.
135. Woods RO, Inceoglu S, Akpolat YT, Cheng WK, Jabo B, Danisa O. C1 lateral mass displacement and transverse atlantal ligament failure in Jefferson's fracture: a biomechanical study of the "Rule of Spence". Neurosurgery. 2017 Apr;20
136. Perez-Orribo L, Snyder LA, Kalb S, Elhadi AM, Hsu F, Newcomb AG, et al. Comparison of CT versus MRI measurements of transverse atlantal ligament integrity in craniovertebral junction injuries. Part 1: a clinical study. J Neurosurg Spine. 2016 Jun;24(6):897–902.
137. Robinson AL, Moller A, Robinson Y, Olerud C. C2 fracture subtypes, incidence, and treatment allocation change with age: a retrospective cohort study of 233 consecutive cases. Biomed Res Int. 2017;2017:8321680.
138. Fielding JW, Francis WR Jr, Hawkins RJ, Pepin J, Hensinger R. Traumatic spondylolisthesis of the axis. Clin Orthop Relat Res. 1989 Feb;(239):47–52.
139. Francis WR, Fielding JW, Hawkins RJ, Pepin J, Hensinger R. Traumatic spondylolisthesis of the axis. J Bone Joint Surg Br. 1981;63-B(3):313–8.
140. Grauer JN, Shafi B, Hilibrand AS, Harrop JS, Kwon BK, Beiner JM, et al. Proposal of a modified, treatment-oriented classification of odontoid fractures. Spine J. 2005 Mar–Apr;5(2):123–9.
141. Greene KA, Dickman CA, Marciano FF, Drabier JB, Hadley MN, Sonntag VK. Acute axis fractures. Analysis of management and outcome in 340 consecutive cases. Spine (Phila Pa 1976). 1997 Aug 15;22(16):1843–52.
142. Julien TD, Frankel B, Traynelis VC, Ryken TC. Evidence-based analysis of odontoid fracture management. Neurosurg Focus. 2000 Jun 15;8(6):e1.
143. Platzer P, Thalhammer G, Ostermann R, Wieland T, Vecsei V, Gaebler C. Anterior screw fixation of odontoid fractures comparing younger and elderly patients. Spine (Phila Pa 1976). 2007 Jul 15;32(16):1714–20.
144. Platzer P, Thalhammer G, Sarahrudi K, Kovar F, Vekszler G, Vecsei V, et al. Nonoperative management of odontoid fractures using a halothoracic vest. Neurosurgery. 2007;61(3):522–9. discussion 529-30
145. Gleizes V, Jacquot FP, Signoret F, Feron JM. Combined injuries in the upper cervical spine: clinical and epidemiological data over a 14-year period. Eur Spine J. 2000 Oct;9(5):386–92.
146. Longo UG, Denaro L, Campi S, Maffulli N, Denaro V. Upper cervical spine injuries: indications and limits of the conservative management in Halo vest. A systematic review of efficacy and safety. Injury. 2010 Nov;41(11):1127–35.
147. Wang S, Wang C, Yan M, Zhou H, Dang G. Novel surgical classification and treatment strategy for atlantoaxial dislocations. Spine (Phila Pa 1976). 2013;38(21):E1348–56.
148. Milhorat TH, Bolognese PA, Nishikawa M, McDonnell NB, Francomano CA. Syndrome of occipitoatlantoaxial hypermobility, cranial settling, and chiari malformation type I in patients with hereditary disorders of connective tissue. J Neurosurg Spine. 2007 Dec;7(6):601–9.
149. Garrett M, Consiglieri G, Kakarla UK, Chang SW, Dickman CA. Occipitoatlantal dislocation. Neurosurgery. 2010;66(Suppl 3):A48–55.
150. Yang SY, Boniello AJ, Poorman CE, Chang AL, Wang S, Passlas PG. A review of the diagnosis and treatment of atlantoaxial dislocations. Global Spine J. 2014;4(3):197–210.

151. Shetty A, Kumar A, Chacko A, Guthe S, Kini AR. Reduction techniques in the management of atlantoaxial subluxation. Indian J Orthop. 2013;47(4):333–9.
152. Fielding JW, Hawkins RJ. Atlanto-axial rotatory fixation. (Fixed rotatory subluxation of the atlanto-axial joint). J Bone Joint Surg Am. 1977;59(1):37–44.
153. Goel A, Desai KI, Muzumdar DP. Atlantoaxial fixation using plate and screw method: a report of 160 treated patients. Neurosurgery. 2002;51(6):1351–7.
154. Dmitriev AE, Lehman RA Jr, Helgeson MD, Sasso RC, Kuhns C, Riew DK. Acute and long-term stability of atlantoaxial fixation methods: a biomechanical comparison of pars, pedicle, and intralaminar fixation in an intact and odontoid fracture model. Spine (Phila Pa 1976). 2009;34(4):365–70.
155. Du JY, Aichmair A, Kueper J, Wright T, Lebl DR. Biomechanical analysis of screw constructs for atlantoaxial fixation in cadavers: a systematic review and meta-analysis. J Neurosurg Spine. 2015;22(2):151–61.
156. Claybrooks R, Kayanja M, Milks R, Benzel E. Atlantoaxial fusion: a biomechanical analysis of two C1–C2 fusion techniques. Spine J. 2007;7(6):682–8.
157. Finn MA, Fassett DR, Mccall TD, Clark R, Dailey AT, Brodke DS. The cervical end of an occipitocervical fusion: a biomechanical evaluation of 3 constructs. J Neurosurg Spine. 2008;9(3):296–300.
158. Lapsiwala SB, Anderson PA, Oza A, Resnick DK. Biomechanical comparison of four C1 to C2 rigid fixative techniques: anterior transarticular, posterior transarticular, C1 to C2 pedicle, and C1 to C2 intralaminar screws. Neurosurgery. 2006;58(3):516–21.
159. Fredø HL, Rizvi SA, Rezai M, Ronning P, Lied B, Helseth E. Complications and long-term outcomes after open surgery for traumatic subaxial cervical spine fractures: a consecutive series of 303 patients. BMC Surg. 2016 Aug 15;16(1):56. https://doi.org/10.1186/s12893-016-0172-z.
160. Quarrington RD, Jones CF, Tcherveniakov P, Clark JM, Sandler SJI, Lee YC, et al. Traumatic subaxial cervical facet subluxation and dislocation: epidemiology, radiographic analyses, and risk factors for spinal cord injury. Spine J. 2017 Jul;21
161. Kotani Y, Abumi K, Ito M, Minami A. Cervical spine injuries associated with lateral mass and facet joint fractures: new classification and surgical treatment with pedicle screw fixation. Eur Spine J. 2005 Feb;14(1):69–77.
162. Pang D. Spinal cord injury without radiographic abnormality in children, 2 decades later. Neurosurgery. 2004;55(6):1325–42. discussion 1342-3
163. Farrell CA, Hannon M, Lee LK. Pediatric spinal cord injury without radiographic abnormality in the era of advanced imaging. Curr Opin Pediatr. 2017;29(3):286–90.
164. Knox J. Epidemiology of spinal cord injury without radiographic abnormality in children: a nationwide perspective. J Child Orthop. 2016;10(3):255–60.
165. Bosch PP, Vogt MT, Ward WT. Pediatric spinal cord injury without radiographic abnormality (SCIWORA): the absence of occult instability and lack of indication for bracing. Spine (Phila Pa 1976). 2002 Dec 15;27(24):2788–800.
166. Pang D, Wilberger JE Jr. Spinal cord injury without radiographic abnormalities in children. J Neurosurg. 1982;57(1):114–29.
167. Bracken MB, Collins WF, Freeman DF, Shepard MJ, Wagner FW, Silten RM, et al. Efficacy of methylprednisolone in acute spinal cord injury. JAMA. 1984 Jan 6;251(1):45–52.
168. Bracken MB, Shepard MJ, Collins WF, Holford TR, Young W, Baskin DS, et al. A randomized, controlled trial of methylprednisolone or naloxone in the treatment of acute spinal-cord injury. Results of the Second National Acute Spinal Cord Injury Study. N Engl J Med. 1990 May 17;322(20):1405–11.
169. Bracken MB, Shepard MJ, Holford TR, Leo-Summers L, Aldrich EF, Fazl M, et al. Administration of methylprednisolone for 24 or 48 hours or tirilazad mesylate for 48 hours in the treatment of acute spinal cord injury. Results of the third national acute spinal cord injury randomized controlled trial. National acute spinal cord injury study. JAMA. 1997 May 28;277(20):1597–604.

170. Bracken MB, Shepard MJ, Holford TR, Leo-Summers L, Aldrich EF, Fazl M, et al. Methylprednisolone or tirilazad mesylate administration after acute spinal cord injury: 1-year follow up. Results of the third national acute spinal cord injury randomized controlled trial. J Neurosurg. 1998 Nov;89(5):699–706.
171. Bracken MB, Holford TR. Neurological and functional status 1 year after acute spinal cord injury: estimates of functional recovery in national acute spinal cord injury study II from results modeled in national acute spinal cord injury study III. J Neurosurg. 2002 Apr;96(3 Suppl):259–66.
172. Inaba K, Nosanov L, Menaker J, Bosarge P, Williams L, Turay D, et al. Prospective derivation of a clinical decision rule for thoracolumbar spine evaluation after blunt trauma: an American association for the surgery of trauma multi-institutional trials group study. J Trauma Acute Care Surg. 2015;78(3):459–65. discussion 465-7
173. Verheyden AP, Holzl A, Ekkerlein H, Gercek E, Hauck S, Josten C, et al. Recommendations for the treatment of thoracolumbar and lumbar spine injuries. Unfallchirurg. 2011 Jan;114(1):9–16.
174. Vaccaro AR, Schroeder GD, Kepler CK, Öner FC, Vialle LR, Kandziora F, et al. The surgical algorithm for the AOSpine thoracolumbar spine injury classification system. Eur Spine J. 2016;25(4):1087–94.
175. Kepler CK, Vaccaro AR, Koerner JD, Dvorak MF, Kandziora F, Rajasekaran S, et al. Reliability analysis of the AOSpine thoracolumbar spine injury classification system by a worldwide group of naïve spinal surgeons. Eur Spine J. 2016;25(4):1082–6.
176. Savage JW, Moore TA, Arnold PM, Thakur N, Hsu WK, Patel AA, et al. The reliability and validity of the thoracolumbar injury classification system in pediatric spine trauma. Spine (Phila Pa 1976). 2015;40(18):E1014–8.
177. Sixta S, Moore FO, Ditillo MF, Fox AD, Garcia AJ, Holena D, et al. Screening for thoracolumbar spinal injuries in blunt trauma: an Eastern Association for the Surgery of Trauma practice management guideline. J Trauma Acute Care Surg. 2012 Nov;73(5 Suppl 4):S326–32.
178. Xu GJ, Li ZJ, Ma JX, Zhang T, Fu X, Ma XL. Anterior versus posterior approach for treatment of thoracolumbar burst fractures: a meta-analysis. Eur Spine J. 2013 Oct;22(10):2176–83.
179. Gnanenthiran SR, Adie S, Harris IA. Nonoperative versus operative treatment for thoracolumbar burst fractures without neurologic deficit: a meta-analysis. Clin Orthop Relat Res. 2012 Feb;470(2):567–77.
180. Wood K, Buttermann G, Mehbod A, Garvey T, Jhanjee R, Sechriest V. Operative compared with nonoperative treatment of a thoracolumbar burst fracture without neurological deficit. A prospective, randomized study. J Bone Joint Surg Am. 2003 May;85-A(5):773–81.
181. Urquhart JC, Alrehaili OA, Fisher CG, Fleming A, Rasoulinejad P, Gurr K, et al. Treatment of thoracolumbar burst fractures: extended follow-up of a randomized clinical trial comparing orthosis versus no orthosis. J Neurosurg Spine. 2017 Jul;27(1):42–7.
182. Bourghli A, Obeid I, Boissiere L, Vital J, Tabboush Z, Al SM. Management of a high thoracic chance fracture. Eur Spine J. 2017; Epub ahead of print
183. Karargyris O, Morassi LG, Zafeiris C, Evangelopoulos DS, Pneumaticos SG. The unusual chance fracture: case report & literature review. Open Orthop J. 2013;7:301–3.
184. Andras LM, Skaggs KF, Badkoobehi H, Choi PD, Skaggs DL. Chance fractures in the pediatric population are often misdiagnosed. J Pediatr Orthop. 2017; Epub ahead of print
185. Damar Ç, Özbayrak M, Süleyman E, Yazol M, Karaarslan E. A chance fracture and accompanying injuries secondary to seat belt trauma in childhood. Spine J. 2016;16(10):e647–8.
186. Sander AL, Laurer H, El Saman A, Ploss C, Mack MG, Maier B, et al. Chance fracture of the upper thoracic spine in a child. Eur J Trauma Emerg Surg. 2009;35(3):318–21.
187. Boham M, O'Connell K. Unusual mechanism of injury resulting in a thoracic chance fracture in a rodeo athlete: a case report. J Athl Train. 2014;49(2):274–9.
188. Okamoto K, Doita M, Yoshikawa M, Manabe M, Sha N, Yoshiya S. Lumbar chance fracture in an adult snowboarder: unusual mechanism of a chance fracture. Spine (Phila Pa 1976). 2005;30(2):E56–9.

189. Bourne JT, Baker ADL, Khatri M. A combined bony and soft tissue, thoracic chance fracture: late displacement following conservative treatment. Case Rep Orthop. 2017;2017:6528673.
190. Sasani M, Ozer AF. Single-stage posterior corpectomy and expandable cage placement for treatment of thoracic or lumbar burst fractures. Spine (Phila Pa 1976). 2009 Jan 1;34(1):E33–40.
191. Smith WD, Dakwar E, Le TV, Christian G, Serrano S, Uribe JS. Minimally invasive surgery for traumatic spinal pathologies: a mini-open, lateral approach in the thoracic and lumbar spine. Spine (Phila Pa 1976). 2010;35(26 Suppl):S338–46.
192. Blondel B, Fuentes S, Pech-Gourg G, Adetchessi T, Tropiano P, Dufour H. Percutaneous management of thoracolumbar burst fractures: Evolution of techniques and strategy. Orthop Traumatol Surg Res. 2011 Sep;97(5):527–32.
193. Korovessis P, Hadjipavlou A, Repantis T. Minimal invasive short posterior instrumentation plus balloon kyphoplasty with calcium phosphate for burst and severe compression lumbar fractures. Spine (Phila Pa 1976). 2008 Mar 15;33(6):658–67.
194. Agarwal N, Choi PA, Sekula RF Jr. Minimally invasive spine surgery for unstable thoracolumbar burst fractures: a case series. Surg J (N Y). 2016;2(4):e131–8.
195. Ni WF, Huang YX, Chi YL, Xu HZ, Lin Y, Wang XY, et al. Percutaneous pedicle screw fixation for neurologic intact thoracolumbar burst fractures. J Spinal Disord Tech. 2010 Dec;23(8):530–7.
196. Palmisani M, Gasbarrini A, Barbanti Brodano G, De lure F, Cappuccio M, Boriani L, et al. Minimally invasive percutaneous fixation in the treatment of thoracic and lumbar spine fractures. Eur Spine J. 2009;18(Suppl 1):71–4.
197. Yang WE, Ng ZX, Koh KM, Low SW, Lwin S, Choy KS, et al. Percutaneous pedicle screw fixation for thoracolumbar burst fracture: a Singapore experience. Singapore Med J. 2012 Sep;53(9):577–81.
198. Wild MH, Glees M, Plieschnegger C, Wenda K. Five-year follow-up examination after purely minimally invasive posterior stabilization of thoracolumbar fractures: a comparison of minimally invasive percutaneously and conventionally open treated patients. Arch Orthop Trauma Surg. 2007 Jul;127(5):335–43.
199. Endo S, Shimamura T, Nakae H, Takakuwa T, Yamada Y, Kasai T, et al. Cervical spinal cord injury associated with ossification of the posterior longitudinal ligament. Arch Orthop Trauma Surg. 1994;113(4):218–21.
200. Epstein NE. Laminectomy for cervical myelopathy. Spinal Cord. 2003;41(6):317–27.
201. Chikuda H, Seichi A, Takeshita K, Matsunaga S, Watanabe M, Nakagawa Y, et al. Acute cervical spinal cord injury complicated by preexisting ossification of the posterior longitudinal ligament: a multicenter study. Spine (Phila Pa 1976). 2011;36(18):1453–8.
202. Choi B, Song K, Chang H. Ossification of the posterior longitudinal ligament: a review of literature. Asian Spine J. 2011;5(4):267–76.
203. Jung J, Chung CK, Kim CH, Choi Y. Risk factors and prognosis for acute progression of myelopathic symptoms in patients with ossification of the posterior longitudinal ligament after minor trauma. Spine (Phila Pa 1976). 2017; Epub ahead of print
204. Benglis DM, Sandberg DI. Acute neurological deficit after minor trauma in an infant with achondroplasia and cervicomedullary compression Case report and review of the literature. J Neurosurg Pediatr. 2007;107(2):152–5.
205. Torg JS, Naranja RJ Jr, Pavlov H, Galinat BJ, Warren R, Stine RA. The relationship of developmental narrowing of the cervical spinal canal to reversible and irreversible injury of the cervical spinal cord in football players. An epidemiological study. J Bone Joint Surg Am. 1996;78(9):1308–14.
206. Nouri A, Montejo J, Sun X, Virojanapa J, Kolb LE, Abbed KM, et al. Cervical cord-canal mismatch: a new method for identifying predisposition to spinal cord injury. World Neurosurg. 2017;108(12):112–7.
207. Freedman BA, Hoffler CE II, Cameron BM, Rhee JM, Bawa M, Malone DG, et al. A comparison of computed tomography measures for diagnosing cervical spinal stenosis associated with myelopathy: a case-control study. Asian Spine J. 2015;9(1):22–9.

208. Harmatz P, Mengel KE, Giugliani R, Valayannopoulos V, Lin S, Parini R, et al. The Morquio A clinical assessment program: baseline results illustrating progressive, multisystemic clinical impairments in Morquio A subjects. Mol Genet Metab. 2013;109(1):54–61.
209. Hendriksz CJ, Harmatz P, Beck M, Jones S, Wood T, Lachman R, et al. Review of clinical presentation and diagnosis of mucopolysaccharidosis IVA. Mol Genet Metab. 2013 Sep-Oct;110(1-2):54–64.
210. Kopits SE. Orthopedic complications of dwarfism. Clin Orthop Relat Res. 1976;114(1):153–79.
211. Meikle PJ, Hopwood JJ, Clague AE, Carey WF. Prevalence of lysosomal storage disorders. JAMA. 1999 Jan 20;281(3):249–54.
212. Montaño AM, Tomatsu S, Gottesman GS, Smith M, Orii T. International Morquio A registry: clinical manifestation and natural course of Morquio A disease. J Inherit Metab Dis. 2007;30(2):165–74.
213. Muenzer J. Overview of the mucopolysaccharidoses. Rheumatology (Oxford). 2011 Dec;50(Suppl 5):v4–12.
214. Northover H, Cowie RA, Wraith JE. Mucopolysaccharidosis type IVA (Morquio syndrome): a clinical review. J Inherit Metab Dis. 1996;19(3):357–65.
215. Dempster AG, Heap SW. Fatal high cervical spinal cord injury in an automobile accident complicating Os Odontoideum. Am J Forensic Med Pathol. 1990;11(3):252–6.
216. McGoldrick JM, Marx JA. Traumatic central cord syndrome in a patient with Os Odontoideum. Ann Emerg Med. 1989;18(12):1358–61.
217. Zhang Z, Zhou Y, Wang J, Chu T, Li C, Ren X, et al. Acute traumatic cervical cord injury in patients with os odontoideum. J Clin Neurosci. 2010;17(10):1289–93.
218. Bethem D, Winter RB, Lutter L, Moe JH, Bradford DS, Lonstein JE, et al. Spinal disorders of dwarfism. Review of the literature and report of eighty cases. J Bone Joint Surg Am. 1981;63(9):1412–25.
219. Cheung MS, Arponen H, Roughley P, Azouz ME, Glorieux FH, Waltimo-Sirén J, et al. Cranial base abnormalities in osteogenesis imperfecta: phenotypic and genotypic determinants. J Bone Miner Res. 2011;26(2):405–13.
220. Janus GJM, Engelbert RHH, Beek E, Gooskens RHJM, Prujis JEH. Osteogenesis imperfecta in childhood: MR imaging of basilar impression. Eur J Radiol. 2003;47(1):19–24.
221. Han MH, Ryu JI, Kim CH, Kim JM, Cheong JH, Bak KH, et al. Influence of systemic bone mineral density on atlantoaxial subluxation in patients with rheumatoid arthritis. Osteoporos Int. 2017 Jun;28(6):1931–8.
222. Han MH, Ryu JI, Kim CH, Kim JM, Cheong JH, Bak KH, et al. Factors that predict risk of cervical instability in rheumatoid arthritis patients. Spine (Phila Pa 1976). 2017 Jul 1;42(13):966–73.
223. Naranjo A, Carmona L, Gavrila D, Balsa A, Belmonte MA, Tena X, et al. Prevalence and associated factors of anterior atlantoaxial luxation in a nation-wide sample of rheumatoid arthritis patients. Clin Exp Rheumatol. 2004 Jul-Aug;22(4):427–32.
224. Smith PH, Benn RT, Sharp J. Natural history of rheumatoid cervical luxations. Ann Rheum Dis. 1972 Nov;31(6):431–9.
225. Hobbs WR, Sponseller PD, Weiss AP, Pyeritz RE. The cervical spine in Marfan syndrome. Spine (Phila Pa 1976). 1997 May 1;22(9):983–9.
226. Nader-Sepahi A, Casey ATH, Hayward R, Crockard HA, Thompson D. Symptomatic atlantoaxial instability in Down syndrome. J Neurosurg Pediatr. 2005;103(3):231–7.
227. Nakamura N, Inaba Y, Aota Y, Oba M, Machida J, Aida N, et al. New radiological parameters for the assessment of atlantoaxial instability in children with Down syndrome: the normal values and the risk of spinal cord injury. Bone Joint J. 2016;98-B(12):1704–10.
228. Henderson FCS, Austin C, Benzel E, Bolognese P, Ellenbogen R, Francomano CA, et al. Neurological and spinal manifestations of the Ehlers-Danlos syndromes. Am J Med Genet C Semin Med Genet. 2017 Mar;175(1):195–211.
229. Kim TY, Ratnayake K. Os Odontoideum discovered after minor cervical trauma. Pediatr Emerg Care. 2017;33(2):104–6.

230. Satar A, Wazir Z, Saeed M, Arif M, Inam M. Early outcome of surgical intervention in subaxial cervical spine injuries. J Pak Med Assoc. 2014 Dec;64(12 Suppl 2):S83–6.
231. Wang T, Tian XM, Liu SK, Wang H, Zhang YZ, Ding WY. Prevalence of complications after surgery in treatment for cervical compressive myelopathy: a meta-analysis for last decade. Medicine (Baltimore). 2017 Mar;96(12):e6421.
232. Huang D, Du X, Liang H, Hu W, Hu H, Cheng X. Anterior corpectomy versus posterior laminoplasty for the treatment of multilevel cervical myelopathy: a meta-analysis. Int J Surg. 2016 Nov;35:21–7.
233. Shou F, Li Z, Wang H, Yan C, Liu Q, Xiao C. Prevalence of C5 nerve root palsy after cervical decompressive surgery: a meta-analysis. Eur Spine J. 2015 Dec;24(12):2724–34.
234. Rieger A, Holz C, Marx T, Sanchin L, Menzel M. Vertebral autograft used as bone transplant for anterior cervical corpectomy: technical note. Neurosurgery. 2003;52(2):449–53. discussion 453-4
235. Schulz C, Mauer UM, Mathieu R. Clinical and radiological results after anterior cervical corpectomy with cage fusion – a retrospective comparison of PEEK vs. titanium cages. Z Orthop Unfall. 2017 Apr;155(2):201–8.
236. Yeh KT, Lee RP, Chen IH, Yu TC, Liu KL, Peng CH, et al. Fresh frozen cortical strut allograft in two-level anterior cervical corpectomy and fusion. PLoS One. 2017 Aug 25;12(8):e0183112.
237. Klimo P Jr, Kan P, Rao G, Apfelbaum R, Brockmeyer D. Os odontoideum: presentation, diagnosis, and treatment in a series of 78 patients. J Neurosurg Spine. 2008 Oct;9(4):332–42.
238. Kato S, Nouri A, Wu D, Nori S, Tetreault L, Fehlings MG. Comparison of anterior and posterior surgery for degenerative cervical myelopathy: an MRI-based propensity-score-matched analysis using data from the prospective multicenter AOSpine CSM North America and international studies. J Bone Joint Surg Am. 2017 Jun 21;99(12):1013–21.
239. Ito Z, Higashino K, Kato S, Kim SS, Wong E, Yoshioka K, et al. Pedicle screws can be 4 times stronger than lateral mass screws for insertion in the midcervical spine: a biomechanical study on strength of fixation. J Spinal Disord Tech. 2014 Apr;27(2):80–5.
240. Yoshihara H, Passias PG, Errico TJ. Screw-related complications in the subaxial cervical spine with the use of lateral mass versus cervical pedicle screws: a systematic review. J Neurosurg Spine. 2013 Nov;19(5):614–23.
241. Liu GY, Mao L, Xu RM, Ma WH. Biomechanical comparison of pedicle screws versus spinous process screws in C2 vertebra: a cadaveric study. Indian J Orthop. 2014 Nov;48(6):550–4.
242. Saetia K, Phankhongsab A. C2 anatomy for translaminar screw placement based on computerized tomographic measurements. Asian Spine J. 2015 Apr;9(2):205–9.
243. Vaccaro AR, Lim MR, Lee JY. Indications for surgery and stabilization techniques of the occipito-cervical junction. Injury. 2005 Jul;36(Suppl 2):B44–53.
244. Kukreja S, Ambekar S, Sin AH, Nanda A. Occipitocervical fusion surgery: review of operative techniques and results. J Neurol Surg B Skull Base. 2015 Sep;76(5):331–9.
245. Wertheim SB, Bohlman HH. Occipitocervical fusion. Indications, technique, and long-term results in thirteen patients. J Bone Joint Surg Am. 1987 Jul;69(6):833–6.
246. Arnold PM, Anderson KK, McGuire RA Jr. The lateral transpsoas approach to the lumbar and thoracic spine: A review. Surg Neurol Int. 2012;3(Suppl 3):S198–215.
247. Ozgur BM, Aryan HE, Pimenta L, Taylor W. Extreme Lateral Interbody Fusion (XLIF): a novel surgical technique for anterior lumbar interbody fusion. Spine J. 2006;6(4):435–43.
248. Amaral R, Marchi L, Oliveira L, Coutinho T, Pimenta L. Acute lumbar burst fracture treated by minimally invasive lateral corpectomy. Case Rep Orthop. 2013;2013:953897.
249. Theologis AA, Tabaraee E, Toogood P, Kennedy A, Birk H, McClellan RT, et al. Anterior corpectomy via the mini-open, extreme lateral, transpsoas approach combined with short-segment posterior fixation for single-level traumatic lumbar burst fractures: analysis of health-related quality of life outcomes and patient satisfaction. J Neurosurg Spine. 2016;24(1):60–8.
250. Sciubba DM, Gallia GL, McGirt MJ, Woodworth GF, Garonzik IM, Witham T, et al. Thoracic kyphotic deformity reduction with a distractible titanium cage via an entirely posterior approach. Oper Neurosurg (Hagerstown). 2007;60(Suppl_4):ONS-223-ONS-231.

251. Elmasry S, Asfour S, Travascio F. Effectiveness of pedicle screw inclusion at the fracture level in short-segment fixation constructs for the treatment of thoracolumbar burst fractures: a computational biomechanics analysis. Comput Methods Biomech Biomed Engin. 2017 Aug;17:1–9.
252. Ozbek Z, Ozkara E, Onner H, Bas G, Erman IC, Ozen H, et al. Treatment of unstable thoracolumbar fractures: does fracture level fixation accelerate the bone healing? World Neurosurg. 2017;107:362–70.
253. Kalra RR, Schmidt MH. The role of a miniopen thoracoscopic-assisted approach in the management of burst fractures involving the thoracolumbar junction. Neurosurg Clin N Am. 2017 Jan;28(1):139–45.
254. Li C, Pan J, Gu Y, Dong J. Minimally invasive pedicle screw fixation combined with percutaneous vertebroplasty for the treatment of thoracolumbar burst fracture. Int J Surg. 2016 Dec;36(Pt A):255–60.
255. Daniels AH, Arthur M, Hart RA. Variability in rates of arthrodesis for patients with thoracolumbar spine fractures with and without associated neurologic injury. Spine (Phila Pa 1976). 2007;32(21):2334–8.
256. Falci SP, Lammertse DP, Best L, Starnes CA, Prenger EC, Stavros AT, et al. Surgical treatment of posttraumatic cystic and tethered spinal cords. J Spinal Cord Med. 1999 Fall;22(3):173–81.
257. Guest J, Eleraky MA, Apostolides PJ, Dickman CA, Sonntag VK. Traumatic central cord syndrome: results of surgical management. J Neurosurg. 2002 Jul;97(1 Suppl):25–32.
258. Klekamp J, Batzdorf U, Samii M, Bothe HW. Treatment of syringomyelia associated with arachnoid scarring caused by arachnoiditis or trauma. J Neurosurg. 1997 Feb;86(2):233–40.
259. Krebs J, Koch HG, Hartmann K, Frotzler A. The characteristics of posttraumatic syringomyelia. Spinal Cord. 2016 Jun;54(6):463–6.
260. Rahimi-Movaghar V, Vaccaro AR, Mohammadi M. Efficacy of surgical decompression in regard to motor recovery in the setting of conus medullaris injury. J Spinal Cord Med. 2006;29(1):32–8.
261. Sgouros S, Williams B. Management and outcome of posttraumatic syringomyelia. J Neurosurg. 1996 Aug;85(2):197–205.

The Spinal Cord Arterial Supply

5

Philippe Gailloud

Contents

Introduction

The configuration of the spinal arterial vascularization dictates the distribution of parenchymal damage during ischemia. This chapter describes features of the cord supply relevant to the diagnosis of spinal stroke.

The Spinal Arterial Vasculature

Three main longitudinal arteries supply the spinal cord, the anterior spinal artery (ASA) and the paired posterior spinal arteries (PSA) . The ASA extends from the vertebrobasilar junction to the tip of the conus medullaris; it is generally uninterrupted but varies in caliber. The left and right PSAs are plexiform; each includes a posterolateral (primary) and a posteromedial (secondary) component, respectively located in front of or behind the dorsal nerve roots. A superficial arterial

P. Gailloud (✉)
Division of Interventional Neuroradiology, The Johns Hopkins Hospital, Baltimore, MD, USA
e-mail: phg@jhmi.edu

B. Greenberg (ed.), *Myelopathy*, https://doi.org/10.1007/978-3-030-99906-3_5

network—the *vasocorona*—interconnects the ASA and PSAs. Despite its plexiform appearance, the *vasocorona* is not a significant source of collateral supply (Fig. 5.1).

From a developmental standpoint, the ASA and PSAs are longitudinal anastomotic chains derived from the radiculomedullary branches of the primitive intersegmental arteries (ISA) [1]. Only a few of these primitive contributions remain functionally significant at the adult stage, including the anterior vertebrospinal trunks (C0-C1), the superior and inferior arteries of the cervical enlargement (C4-C6, C7-T1), the artery of von Haller (T4-T5), and the artery of the lumbosacral

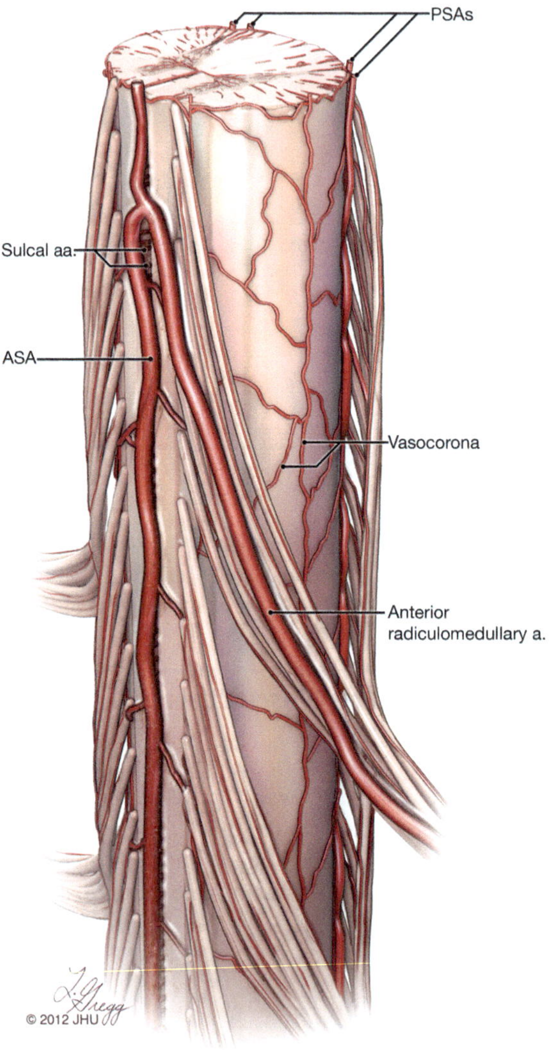

Fig. 5.1 Extrinsic arterial vascularization of the spinal cord

The extrinsic spinal arterial system consists of longitudinal arteries (principally the anterior spinal artery (ASA) and the paired posterior spinal arteries (PSAs)) supplied by a limited number of radiculomedullary arteries and interconnected by a delicate mesh, the *vasocorona* enlargement (T6-L4) [2, 3]. There are more posterior than anterior radiculomedullary arteries (RMA), including a dominant branch in the thoracolumbar region [4].

Sulcal arteries arise from the ASA's concealed surface and penetrate the spinal cord in the depth of the anteromedian fissure (Fig. 5.1); their territory is typically unilateral [4], but trunks with multiple ipsilateral or bilateral branches exist [5, 6]. Therefore, damage to a single sulcal artery can lead to a limited homolateral infarct (sulcal syndrome) or be longitudinally and transversally more extensive. Sulcal syndromes tend to occur in the cervical region, where the ASA is frequently duplicated [7]; occlusion of a duplicated ASA segment thus seems a likelier "sulcal syndrome" mechanism than occlusion of a single sulcal branch. The variability in the density of sulcal arteries (number of vessels per length unit) derives from regional differences in spinal cord elongation during fetal life; the thoracic cord has the lowest sulcal artery density [8, 9], a factor believed to increase its sensitivity to ischemia.

The intrinsic arterial system consists of two converging circulations: the sulcal arteries principally supply the central gray matter (centrifugal system), the PSAs and the *vasocorona* vascularize most of the surrounding white matter (centripetal system) (Fig. 5.2a) [10]. Although both circulations interconnect at the capillary level, there is limited potential for collateral supply: spinal perforators are, from a functional standpoint, end-arteries.

Spinal Collateral Pathways

Collateral supply to the spinal cord depends primarily on extradural osseous and muscular anastomoses, on the recruitment of alternate RMAs, and on the periconal arterial anastomotic circle, the only functionally significant connection between the anterior and posterior spinal circulations. Collateral pathways influence the extent and severity of ischemic damages; their availability varies with age and the arterial injury's timing and location. The principles proposed by Lazorthes in 1971 remain valid [9]:

(i) "The nearer the arterial obstruction is to the aortal origin and the farther it is removed from the spinal cord, the greater the possibilities of anastomotic substitution",

(ii) "The slower the obstruction is in establishing itself, the greater the chances of effective intervention by the substitution pathways, whereas a sudden obstruction takes the substitution pathways by surprise."

Postmortem observations of occluded dominant anterior RMAs without clinical or histopathological consequences confirm that collateral pathways can, at least in the context of a slowly evolving process, take over the cord supply [11]. The greater availability of collateral channels in young individuals has a protective role, for example, during aortic or spine surgery [12].

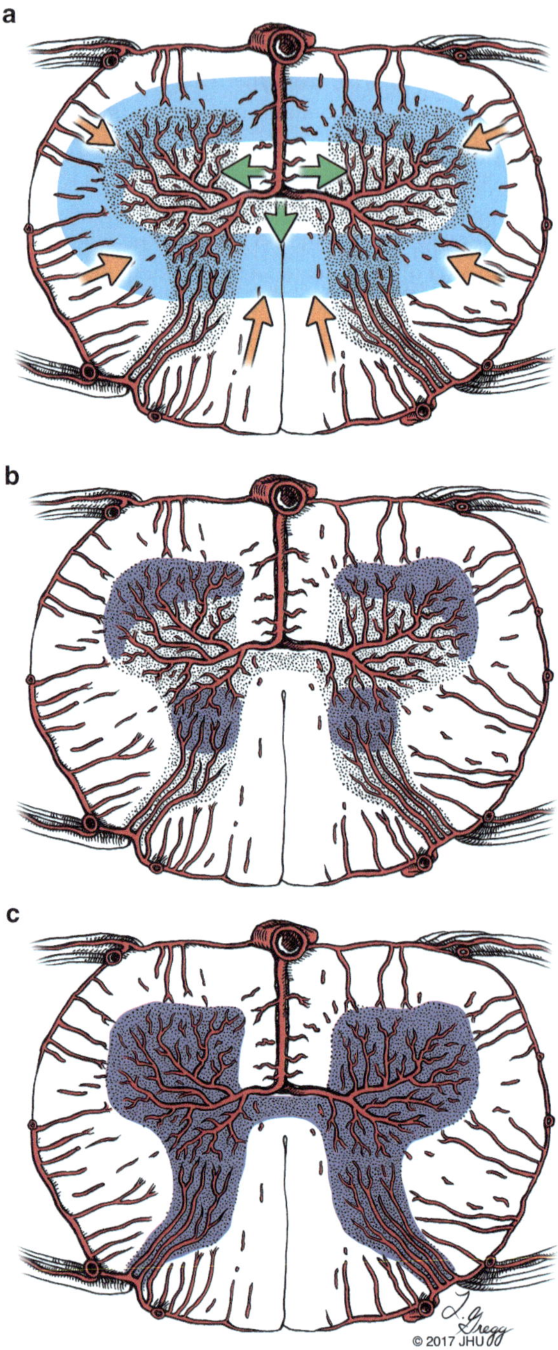

Fig. 5.2 Intrinsic arterial circulation and axial watershed zones. (**a**) Adamkiewicz divided the intrinsic arterial system into central (or centrifugal, green arrows) and peripheral (or centripetal, orange arrows) systems. Their interface constitutes a ring-like anatomical zone at risk for ischemia (blue ring). (**b**) The combination of the ring-like anatomical watershed area with the increased gray matter sensitivity to ischemia defines focal zones at risk in the anterior and posterior horns ("snake eyes" pattern). (**c**) When ischemia involves the entire gray matter but spares the white matter, the injury adopts a "butterfly" pattern

Spinal Blood Flow

The spinal supply is peculiar for its apparent frailty and the lack of readily available reserve under normal conditions. As Feeney and Watterson noted in 1946 [13]:

> [...] there exists a very close relationship between the metabolic requirements of the nervous tissue and the final distribution of intraneural vessels in the adult, a relationship which functions in such a way as to provide the nervous system with a blood supply just adequate for its minimal needs.

Animal studies have shown higher blood flow in the cervical and lumbosacral cord and a positive gray matter to white matter ratio at all levels (up to 5:1 in primates) [14, 15]. These findings are consistent with the higher gray matter's sensitivity to ischemia observed both experimentally [16] and clinically [17].

The spinal circulation is protected from pressure variations by an autoregulation process similar to the mechanism adjusting the cerebral circulation [18]. Spinal flow is also sensitive to chemical mediation (increased by hypoxia and hypercapnia, decreased by hypocapnia), while metabolic stimulation only increases flow to the gray matter [14]. Spinal autoregulation does not depend on cerebral centers since hypercapnia increases flow in transected cords [19]. Systemic blood pressure directly influences blood flow within the superficial spinal circulation [20].

Sensitivity to ischemia varies among and within cell groups: for example, neurons are, as a group, more sensitive than the microglia, but certain types of neurons are more vulnerable than others. This relative sensitivity seems to play a role early in the ischemic process, while the injury pattern resulting from severe and prolonged ischemia depends more on local angioarchitectural factors [21, 22].

Spinal Watershed Zones

Watershed zones are ischemia-prone areas located at the interface between convergent arterial circulations [23, 24]. Watershed zones are involved early in the ischemic process and therefore represent essential clinical and histopathological markers.

Axial Watershed Zone

The axial watershed zone lies at the interface between the centripetal and centrifugal intrinsic circulations [10]. While the zone at risk is in theory ring-shaped [9], its combination with increased gray matter vulnerability—due in part to the neurons higher metabolic needs [25, 26]—results in a "snake eyes" appearance typical of minimal or early injuries [27] (Fig. 5.2b). More severe lesions—for example, in the setting of systemic hypotension [28] or aortic dissection [29]—can involve the whole gray matter yet still spare the white matter [17] (Fig. 5.2c). Finally, profound ischemia leads to extensive lesions that involve the deep white matter before the peripheral white matter [30, 31]. However, even severe ischemia may spare the peripheral white matter or the lateral edge of the anterior horns, or both [32].

A single lesion can combine various ischemic patterns, either in a topographical distribution corresponding to variable locoregional degrees of injury or in successive imaging studies indicating damage progression over time. A watershed pattern is typically found at the edge of a lesion, where collateral flow limits the severity of ischemia [29] (Fig. 5.3).

Longitudinal Watershed Zones

As Lazorthes and colleagues pointed out, the value of the anterior and posterior longitudinal spinal arteries as collateral pathways is limited:

> [...] there is no continuous perimedullary longitudinal substitution pathway. The three areas that we have described are functionally isolated: the upper cervicothoracic and lower thoracolumbar areas are separated by the midthoracic area, whose poor vascularization we know, and where anastomoses are more or less nonexistent. [9]

Mettler [33], Zülch [23], and Di Chiro [34] reported the existence of longitudinal watershed zones at the junction between adjacent arterial territories. Since the plexiform nature of the PSAs offers better protection against ischemia, longitudinal watershed zones predominantly involve the ASA territory; their topography depends on the number, size, and location of anterior RMAs, and the mechanism leading to ischemia (*e.g.*, single branch occlusion *versus* hypotensive episode).

The classic description of a midthoracic zone of "ischemic vulnerability" is not confirmed by modern anatomical and clinical data, notably the constant presence of an upper thoracic anterior RMA [35] and the sparing of the midthoracic cord during severe systemic hypotension [28, 36, 37].

Posterior Lumbosacral Watershed Zone

The periconal arterial anastomotic circle—the only functionally significant anastomosis between the ASA and PSAs—is the spinal counterpart of the circle of Willis. Through this anastomotic circle, the ASA supplies the caudal end of the PSAs, in which the flow is ascending [38]. This configuration creates a longitudinal junctional territory along the posterior aspect of the conus medullaris, the posterior lumbosacral watershed zone (Fig. 5.4) [39]. Flow impairment in the caudal portion of the ASA—after occlusion of the artery of Adamkiewicz, for example—can thus simultaneously impact the anterior and posterior circulations, explaining why transverse lesions are more common in the lumbosacral region.

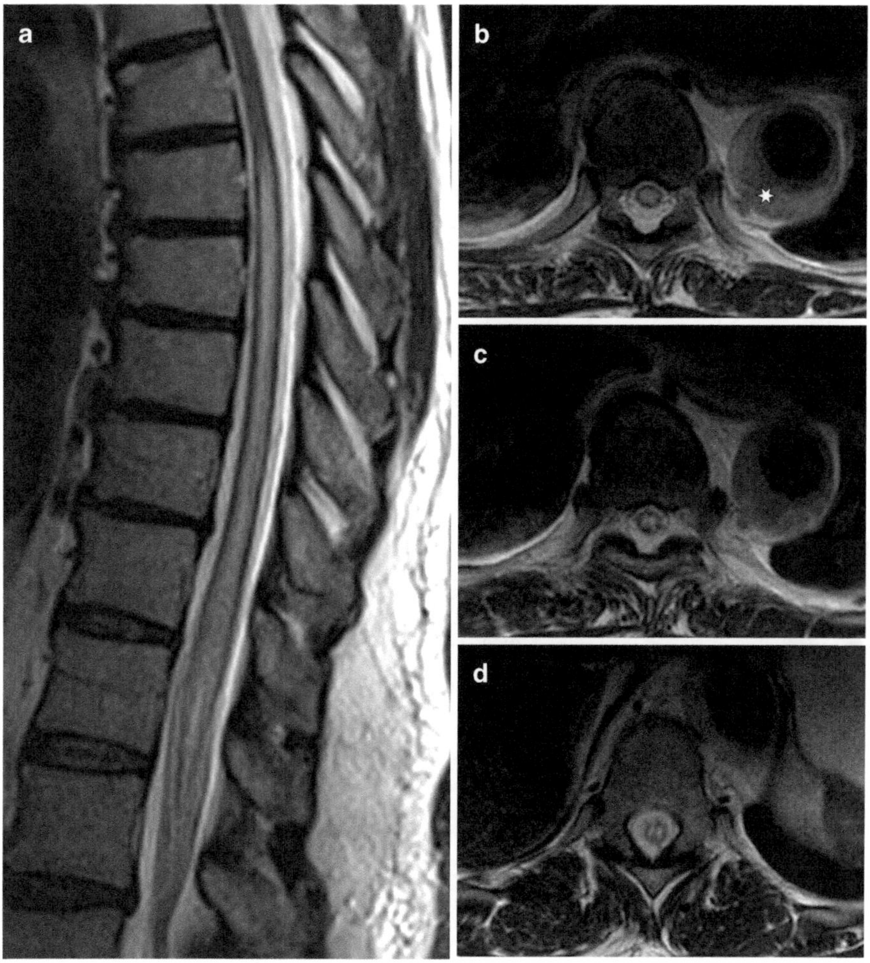

Fig. 5.3 Spinal stroke following occlusion of the artery of Adamkiewicz by an acute aortic dissection. (**a**) MRI, T2-weighted sagittal image, documenting signal hyperintensity and cord swelling from the midthoracic region to the tip of the conus medullaris. (**b**) MRI, T2-weighted axial images at T12, showing near-complete transverse infarction with a peripheral rim of spared tissue. Parietal thrombus is visible within the aortic dissection (star). (**c**) MRI, T2-weighted axial images at T8; closer to the upper limit of the lesion—and sources of collateral supply—the damage only involves the gray matter ("butterfly" pattern). (**d**) MRI, T2-weighted axial images at T7; the damage is minimal at the edge of the lesion, taking a "snake-eye" appearance

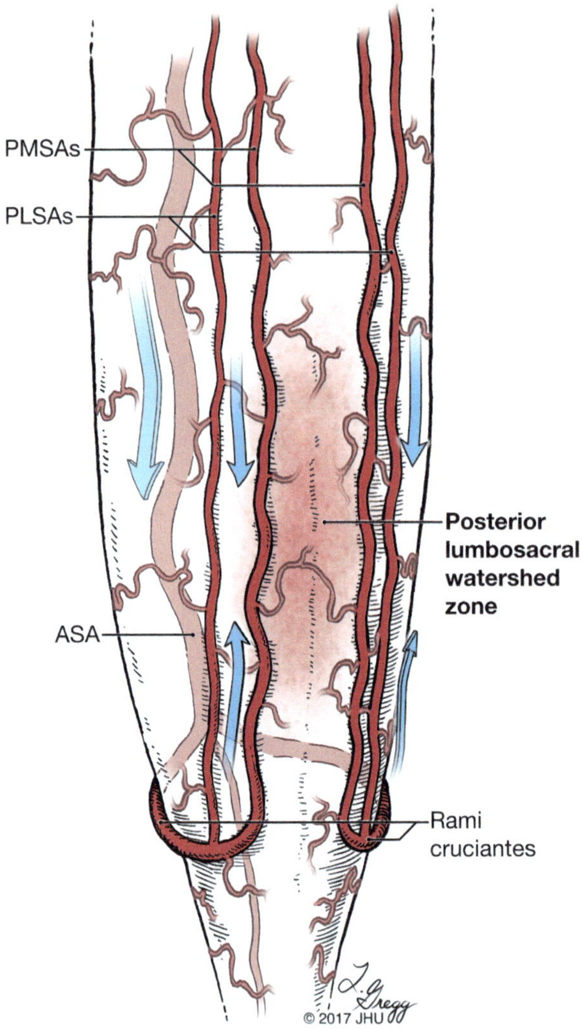

Fig. 5.4 The posterior lumbosacral watershed zone

The anterior spinal artery (ASA) connects around the tip of the conus medullaris with the posterior-medial and posterior-lateral spinal arteries (PMSAs, PLSAs) via the *rami cruciantes*. Both the anterior and posterior arterial systems participate in the supply of the caudal portion of the posterior spinal territory, creating a watershed zone at their interface, the posterior lumbosacral watershed zone

References

1. Evans HM. The development of the vascular system. In: Keibel F, Mall FP, editors. Manual of human embryology, vol. 2. Philadelphia/London: J.B. Lippincott; 1912. p. 570–708.
2. Adamkiewicz A. Die Blutgefässe des menschlichen Rückenmarkes. II. Theil. Die Gefässe der Rückenmarks-Oberfläche. Sitzungsberichten der Kaiserlichen Akademie der Wissenschaften, Mathematisch-naturwissenschaftliche Classe. 1882;85:101–30.
3. Von Haller A. Iconum anatomicarum quibus aliquae partes corporis humani delineatae traduntur. Fasciculus VII - Arteriae cerebri Medullae spinalis Oculi. Widow of Abram Vandenhoeck: Göttingen; 1754.

4. Kadyi H. Über die Blutgefässe des Menschlichen Rückenmarkes. Gubrynowicz & Schmidt: Lemberg; 1889.
5. Hassler O. Blood supply to human spinal cord: a microangiographic study. Arch Neurol. 1966;15(3):302.
6. Zhang Z-A, Nonaka H, Hatori T. The microvasculature of the spinal cord in the human adult. Neuropathology. 1997;17(1):32–42.
7. Weidauer S, Nichtweiss M, Hattingen E, Berkefeld J. Spinal cord ischemia: aetiology, clinical syndromes and imaging features. Neuroradiology. 2015;57(3):241–57.
8. Hassler O. The arteries of the spinal chord. Differences in morphology at various levels. Anat Anz. 1963;112:19–24.
9. Lazorthes G, Gouaze A, Zadeh JO, Santini JJ, Lazorthes Y, Burdin P. Arterial vascularization of the spinal cord. Recent studies of the anastomotic substitution pathways. J Neurosurg. 1971;35(3):253–62.
10. Adamkiewicz A. Die Blutgefässe des menschlichen Rückenmarkes. I. Theil. Die Gefässe der Rückenmarkssubstanz. Sitzungsberichten der Kaiserlichen Akademie der Wissenschaften, Mathematisch-naturwissenschaftliche Classe. 1881;84:469–502.
11. Maliszewski M, Ladzinski P, Aleksandrowicz R, Majchrzak H, Bierzynska-Macyszyn G, Wolanska-Karut J. Occlusion of radicular arteries – reasons, consequences and anastomotic substitution pathways. Spinal Cord. 1999;37(10):710–6.
12. Adams HD, Van Geertruyden HH. Neurologic complications of aortic surgery. Ann Surg. 1956;144(4):574–610.
13. Feeney JF Jr, Watterson RL. The development of the vascular pattern within the walls of the central nervous system of the chick embryo. J Morphol. 1946;78:231–303.
14. Marcus ML, Heistad DD, Ehrhardt JC, Abboud FM. Regulation of total and regional spinal cord blood flow. Circ Res. 1977;41(1):128–34.
15. Sandler AN, Tator CH. Regional spinal cord blood flow in primates. J Neurosurg. 1976;45(6):647–59.
16. DeGirolami U, Zivin JA. Neuropathology of experimental spinal cord ischemia in the rabbit. J Neuropathol Exp Neurol. 1982;41(2):129–49.
17. Kepes JJ. Selective necrosis of spinal cord gray matter. A complication of dissecting aneurysm of the aorta. Acta Neuropathol. 1965;4(3):293–8.
18. Hickey R, Albin MS, Bunegin L, Gelineau J. Autoregulation of spinal cord blood flow: is the cord a microcosm of the brain? Stroke. 1986;17(6):1183–9.
19. Kindt GW. Autoregulation of spinal cord blood flow. Eur Neurol. 1971;6(1):19–23.
20. Otomo E, Wolbarsht ML, Van Buskirk C, Davidson M. A comparison of spinal cord, cortical and superficial circulation. J Nerv Ment Dis. 1960;131:418–27.
21. Scholz W. Selective neuronal necrosis and its topistic patterns in hypoxemia and oligemia. J Neuropathol Exp Neurol. 1953;12(3):249–61.
22. Spronck C-H-H. Contribution à l'étude expérimentale des lésions de la moelle épinière déterminées par l'anémie passagère de cet organe. Archives de Physiologie Normale et Pathologique. 1888;20:1–31.
23. Zülch KJ. Mangeldurchblutung als Ursache ungeklärter Rückenmarksschädigungen. Deutsche Zeitschrift fur Nervenheilkunde. 1954;172(1):81–101.
24. Schneider M. Durchblutung und Sauerstoffversorgung des Gehirns. In: Thauer R, editor. Verhandlungen der Deutschen Gesellschaft für Kreislaufforschung. Darmstadt: Verlag von Dr. Dietrich Steinkopff; 1953. p. 3–25.
25. Craigie EH. On the relative vascularity of various parts of the central nervous system of the albino rat. J Comp Neurol. 1920;31(5):429–64.
26. Gelfan S, Tarlov IM. Differential vulnerability of spinal cord structures to anoxia. J Neurophysiol. 1955;18(2):170–88.
27. Hundsberger T, Thomke F, Hopf HC, Fitzek C. Symmetrical infarction of the cervical spinal cord due to spontaneous bilateral vertebral artery dissection. Stroke. 1998;29(8):1742.

28. Blumbergs PC, Byrne E. Hypotensive central infarction of the spinal cord. J Neurol Neurosurg Psychiatry. 1980;43(8):751–3.
29. Kalisher O. Demonstration eines Präparat (Aneurysma dissecans der Aorta mit Paraplegie). Berliner Klinische Wochenschrift. 1914;115:1286–7.
30. Thompson GB. Dissecting aortic aneurysm with infarction of the spinal cord. Brain. 1956;79(1):111–8.
31. Fried LC, Aparicio O. Experimental ischemia of the spinal cord. Histologic studies after anterior spinal artery occlusion. Neurology. 1973;23(3):289–93.
32. Ishizawa K, Komori T, Shimada T, Arai E, Imanaka K, Kyo S, et al. Hemodynamic infarction of the spinal cord: involvement of the gray matter plus the border-zone between the central and peripheral arteries. Spinal Cord. 2005;43(5):306–10.
33. Mettler FA. Neuroanatomy. 2nd ed. The C.V. Mosby Company: St. Louis; 1948.
34. Di Chiro G, Fried LC. Blood flow currents in spinal cord arteries. Neurology. 1971;21(11):1088–96.
35. Gailloud P. The artery of von Haller: a constant anterior radiculomedullary artery at the upper thoracic level. Neurosurgery. 2013;73(6):1034–43.
36. Duggal N, Lach B. Selective vulnerability of the lumbosacral spinal cord after cardiac arrest and hypotension. Stroke. 2002;33(1):116–21.
37. Gilles FH, Nag D. Vulnerability of human spinal cord in transient cardiac arrest. Neurology. 1971;21(8):833–9.
38. Bolton B. The blood supply of the human spinal cord. J Neurol Psychiatry. 1939;2(2):137–48.
39. Gailloud P, Gregg L, Galan P, Becker D, Pardo C. Periconal arterial anastomotic circle and posterior lumbosacral watershed zone of the spinal cord. J Neurointervention Surg. 2014;7(11):848–53.

Venous Hypertensive Myelopathies

6

Philippe Gailloud

Contents

Introduction

Aminoff and colleagues realized that some spinal vascular malformations become symptomatic by elevating the perimedullary venous pressure in 1974 [1]. Although most spinal shunts can induce venous hypertension, this chapter focuses on a group of radiologically inconspicuous anomalies that frequently belong in the differential diagnosis of myelopathies of unclear etiology, the low-flow spinal arteriovenous fistulas (SAVFs).

P. Gailloud (✉)
Division of Interventional Neuroradiology, The Johns Hopkins Hospital,
Baltimore, MD, USA
e-mail: phg@jhmi.edu

B. Greenberg (ed.), *Myelopathy*, https://doi.org/10.1007/978-3-030-99906-3_6

Low-Flow Spinal Arteriovenous Fistulas

Spinal vascular malformations are divided into three categories based on flow characteristics [2]:

1. Anomalies with a high-flow shunt
2. Anomalies with a low-flow shunt
3. Anomalies without a shunt

Anomalies without shunt (e.g., a cavernous malformation) or with a high-flow shunt (e.g., a spinal cord arteriovenous malformation) are generally conspicuous on MRI and rarely overlooked [3]. Low-flow spinal SAVFs, on the other hand, have insidious clinical and radiological features. They are commonly misdiagnosed, generally as an inflammatory myelopathy [4]. Low-flow spinal SAVFs represent about 80% of all spinal vascular anomalies; three types are identified based on the shunt location (Fig. 6.1):

A. Low-flow perimedullary arteriovenous fistulas (PmAVF)
B. Low-flow dural arteriovenous fistulas (SDAVF)
C. Low-flow spinal extradural arteriovenous fistulas (SEAVF)

Historical Background

Spinal vascular anomalies were hard to characterize before the advent of spinal angiography in the 1960s [5, 6]. Kendall and Logue described SDAVFs in 1977; they identified the existence of a focal shunt along the spinal nerve root and recognized the secondary nature of the accompanying perimedullary venous engorgement [7]. Merland and colleagues reported the first cases of low-flow SEAVFs and PmAVFs in 1980 [8].

Physiopathology

The progressive myelopathy caused by low-flow SAVFs results from an elevation of the perimedullary venous pressure. The discrepancy between these seemingly benign low-output shunts and the devastating spinal cord damages they induce is perplexing at first. Logue suggested the role of concomitant venous deficiency in 1979 [9]; drainage impairment is due to a reduction in the number of functional radiculomedullary veins (RMV), notably in older men. Thrombosis is the probable cause of this progressive loss of RMVs. The antireflux mechanism—a valve-like configuration of the RMV at its point of passage through the dural sac [10–12] (Fig. 6.1)—likely contributes both to RMV thrombosis and the development of SDAVFs [13].

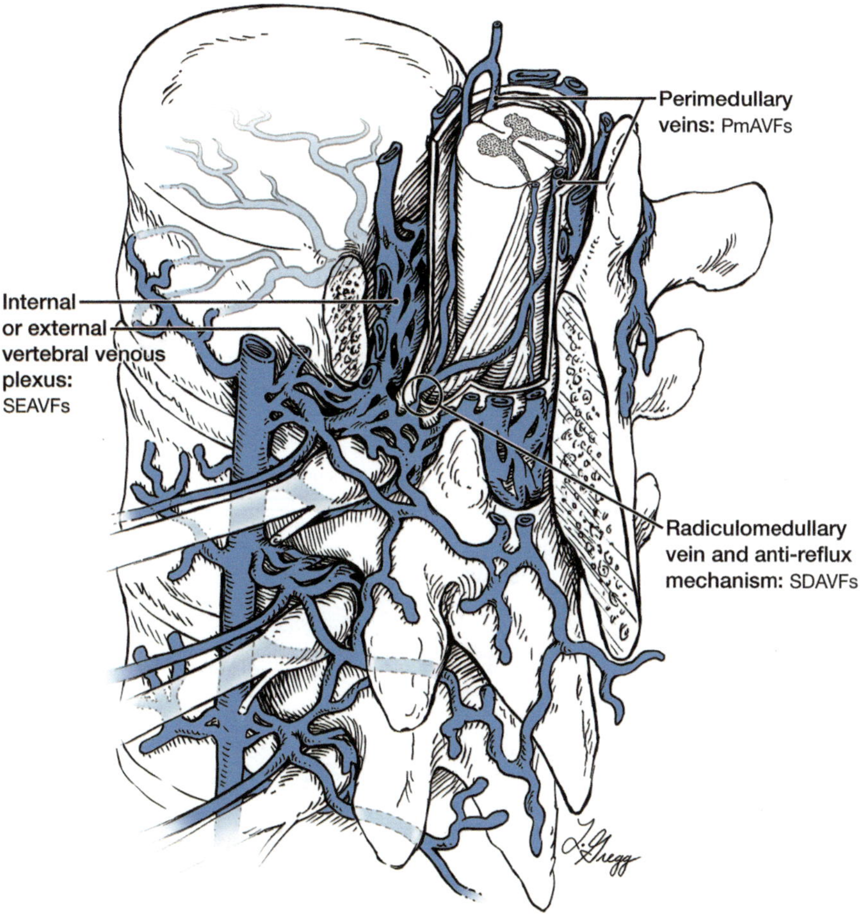

Fig. 6.1 Topographical classification of spinal arteriovenous fistulas

Low-flow perimedullary arteriovenous fistulas (PmAVF) are found on the pial surface of the spinal cord, spinal dural arteriovenous fistulas (SDAVF) along the inner surface of the thecal sac, and low-flow spinal extradural arteriovenous fistulas (SEAVF) in the epidural or paravertebral spaces

Etiology and Morphology

Low-flow SAVFs probably form in a context of venous thrombosis followed by recanalization and arterialization, a mechanism similar to the development of cranial dural arteriovenous fistulas [14]. The thrombotic process participates in the shunt formation and influences its clinical expression by limiting the availability of drainage pathways. The thrombosed venous structure predisposing to shunt formation is specific to each type of SAVF:

(i) SDAVFs: the shunt involves an RMV immediately before its passage through the thecal sac, on the intradural versant of the antireflux mechanism [15] (Fig. 6.2A). The venous drainage is typically intradural [16].

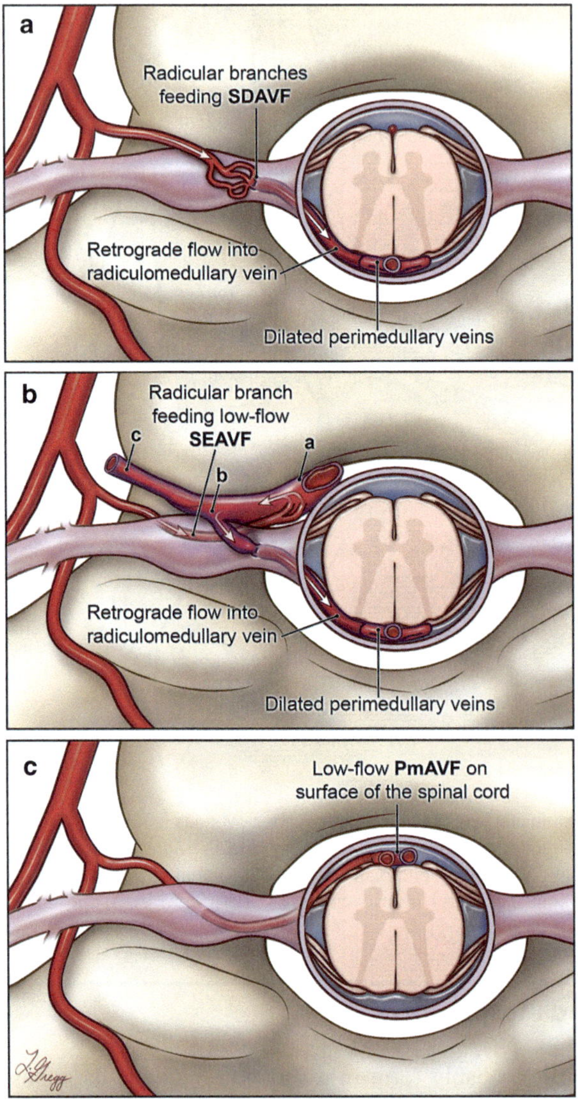

Fig. 6.2 Angioarchitecture of symptomatic low-flow spinal arteriovenous fistulas
(**A**) **SDAVF**—the shunt is located on the inner surface of the thecal sac and drains intradurally
(**B**) **SEAVF**—the shunt involves a pouch of epidural plexus (**a**) and drains into one or more radiculomedullary vein(s). Shunts involving foraminal (**b**) or paravertebral (**c**) veins have similar presentations
(**C**) **PmAVF**—the shunt lies over the pial surface and drains into the perimedullary venous system

(ii) Low-flow SEAVFs: the shunt involves an epidural venous pouch partially or completely isolated from the rest of the epidural plexus (Fig. 6.2B). The perimedullary venous pressure only increases when the arterialized pouch is connected to the intradural venous system by one or more RMVs, and the antireflux mechanism fails to prevent retrograde drainage.

(iii) Low-flow PmAVFs: The shunt most often interconnects the anterior spinal artery and vein on the anterior surface of the cord (Fig. 6.2C).

Clinical Presentation

Low-flow SAVFs tend to occur in older men (50 and above); they are less common in women and exceptional under the age of 30 [17]. They typically present with a progressive venous hypertensive myelopathy (VHM), a remote and non-localizing consequence of the arteriovenous shunt. SDAVFs can cause a radicular pain predating the onset of other symptoms by months or years [18].

The combination of spinal venous hypertension with cofactors reducing the systemic arterial pressure (*e.g.*, aortic atheroma, dehydration, antihypertensive therapy) participates in the proteiform clinical picture of low-flow SAVFs. Patients not infrequently present with acute or subacute worsening of a previously slowly evolving myelopathy or even with an inaugural "stroke-like" acute episode. Cervical lesions can cause acute hemiplegia simulating cerebral ischemia [19]. Intermittent spinal cord claudication is frequent. The sudden pejoration of a progressive myelopathy following steroid administration—intravenously [20], percutaneously [21, 22], or even per os (personal observation)—must raise concern for the diagnosis of low-flow SAVF.

Maximum disability is reached within a year in about half the cases, the evolution being possibly more severe in women [23]. This rapid progression leads to the notion of a "narrow therapeutic window," i.e., a limited interval during which therapy can provide meaningful functional improvement. Unfortunately, the diagnosis frequently remains elusive for months or years [24].

Noninvasive Imaging

Conventional MRI

MRI is the technique of choice for the screening of myelopathies, although patients with vascular malformations may undergo CT myelography when MRI is contraindicated. Low-flow SAVFs have a nonspecific appearance on conventional MRI, including longitudinally extensive T2 hypersignal with a central distribution and variable degree of enhancement after gadolinium administration (Fig. 6.3). "Flow voids" on T2-weighted images strongly suggest a vascular malformation, but their absence does not exclude a SAVF: flow voids are most often subtle or absent [3]. Signs of superimposed arterial ischemia (*i.e.*, partial of complete gray matter

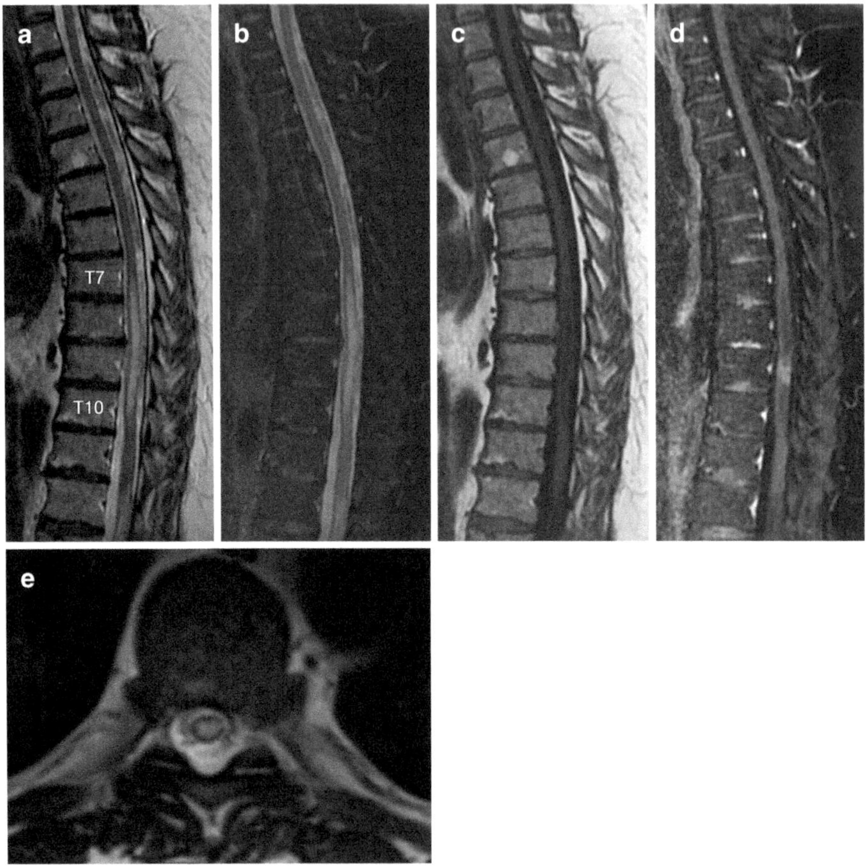

Fig. 6.3 Typical MRI features of spinal venous hypertension. (**a**), MRI, sagittal T2-weighted image, documenting spinal cord edema as an area of increased T2 signal between T7 to T10. (**b**), MRI, sagittal STIR image, confirming the extent of the edematous area. While both the T2-weighted and STIR sequences show dorsal CSF flow artifacts, neither documents conspicuous "flow-voids." (**c**), MRI, sagittal T1-weighted image; the spinal cord edema appears as a central area of hyposignal. (**d**), MRI, sagittal T1-weighted image after gadolinium administration; there is a focal area of parenchymal enhancement at T10, without clear evidence of dilated perimedullary vessels. (**e**), MRI, axial T2-weighted image showing the central pattern of T2 hypersignal typical of venous hypertension

hypersignal in a "snake-eye" or 'butterfly" pattern) are not uncommon. Focal lesions are infrequent, and the absence of cord anomaly in symptomatic patients is exceptional.

Advanced MRI Techniques

While the sensitivity and specificity of conventional MRI for low-flow SAVFs are poor, advanced techniques—such as time-resolved contrast-enhanced MRA

(CE-MRA)—carry high expectations, notably as an adjunct modality guiding subsequent conventional angiography (Fig. 6.4). These new modalities show promise for the detection of spinal vascular anomalies in general [25–27], with sensitivity rates between 81% [27] and 100% [26]. However, most published series are small and fail to distinguish between low-flow and high-flow SAVFs, which offer drastically different challenges since MRI exceptionally overlooks high-flow lesions [3]. One study specifically evaluating CE-MRA's efficacy for diagnosing SDAVFs reported a detection rate of 81%, with flow voids noted on conventional MRI in all cases [27]. It thus appears that CE-MRA, in that instance, merely confirmed the presence of low-flow lesions already detected by conventional MRI [3]. The yield of CE-MRA for the detection of low-flow SAVFs without flow voids is, to our knowledge, undetermined. High-resolution three-dimensional MRI sequences (e.g.,

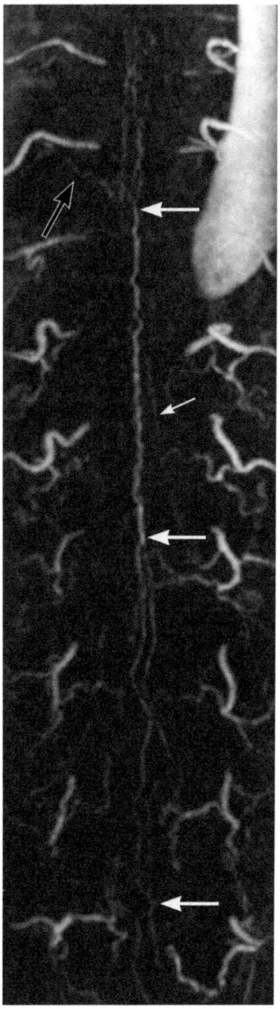

Fig. 6.4 Contrast-enhanced MRA (coronal reconstruction) in a 68-year-old patient with progressive myelopathy documenting dilated perimedullary veins (large white arrows). The artery of Adamkiewicz is visible (small white arrow). Based on this study, the patient was referred for the treatment of a right T7 spinal dural arteriovenous fistula (black arrow). Instead, spinal angiography revealed a pelvic arteriovenous fistula, while the suspicious structure shown by MRA was a draining vein. Conventional angiography during endovascular therapy can easily correct misleading MRA findings, but a misguided surgical approach based on inaccurate MRA data could prove catastrophic

CISS) are useful in studying the relationship between a vascular anomaly and its surroundings, for example, to distinguish between intra- and extramedullary lesions.

The impact of advanced MRI techniques for the evaluation of myelopathic patients remains unclear at this time: a study dividing 154 patients with low-flow SAVFs into early (1986–1999) and recent (2000–2008) cohorts showed no diagnostic delay reduction despite the advent of modern imaging [28]. Broader use of advanced MRI techniques in suspected vascular myelopathies should nonetheless improve the detection rate of low-flow lesions and allow earlier treatment. A normal MRI, or MRA, however, should not discourage a clinician from obtaining a conventional spinal angiogram in patients with high pretest probabilities of having a low-flow SAVF.

Computed Tomography (CT) and Computed Tomography Angiography (CTA)

The role of CTA for the screening of low-flow SAVFs is currently limited. CTA is associated with narrow longitudinal coverage, low spatial and temporal resolutions, and high radiation doses. Studies recommending extensive CTA evaluations (*e.g.*, T1 to L4) rarely include radiation exposure information [29]. However, a recent article suggested that CTA should be restricted to "difficult-to-find AVFs" because of high doses (over 40 mSv in the thoracolumbar region) [30].

On the other hand, thoracic and abdominal contrast-enhanced CT routinely obtained during the workup of suspected inflammatory myelopathies could play a significant but currently unexploited role in the early diagnosis of low-flow SAVFs: the observation of enhancing intracanalar structures can, in many cases, suggest the presence of a low-flow SAVF [31] (Fig. 6.5).

Digital Subtraction Angiography

Spinal digital subtraction angiography (DSA) is safe in experienced hands: the occurrence of neurological complications is extremely low nowadays [32], thanks in part to the introduction of nonionic contrast agents in the 1980s [33] (Fig. 6.6). Sophisticated techniques such as three-dimensional spinal DSA [34] or flat panel catheter angiotomography [35] increase the yield of conventional angiography by offering high-resolution multiplanar reconstructions [36, 37] (Fig. 6.7).

Complete spinal DSA must investigate each pair of intersegmental arteries (ISA) of aortic origin, the subclavian artery and its branches, and the pelvic vasculature (median and lateral sacral arteries). Carotid artery injections are necessary to exclude cranial anomalies with perimedullary venous drainage [38]. Angiographers must remember that VHM has no localizing value [39]: a cervical SDAVF can, for example, induce devastating lumbosacral changes but spare the thoracic cord (a C1 SDAVF caused the myelopathy shown in Fig. 6.3).

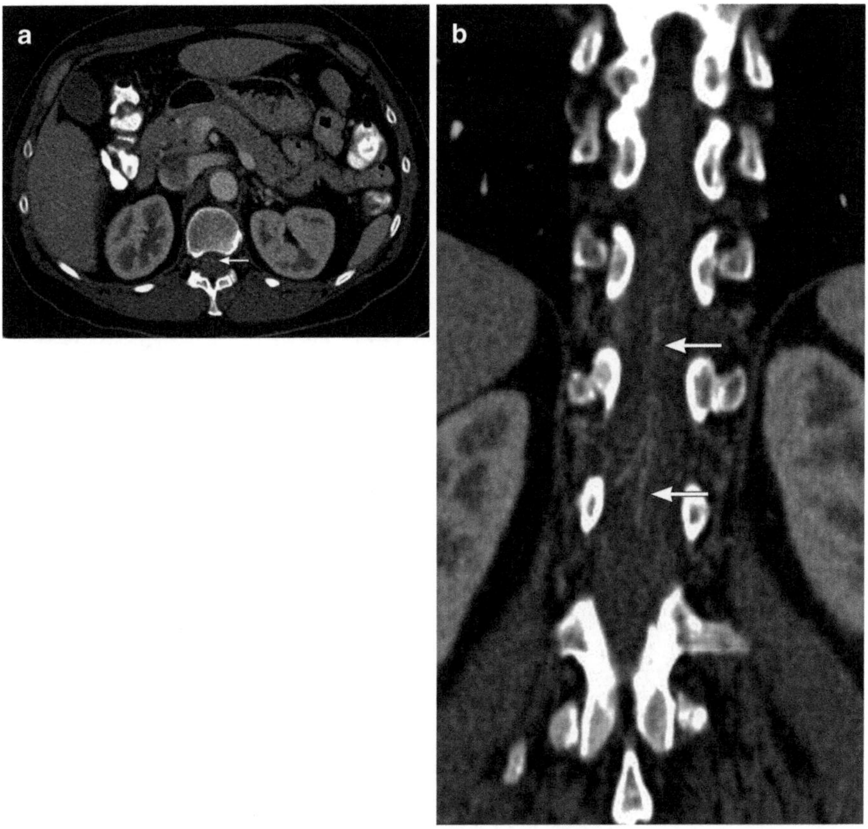

Fig. 6.5 A 56-year-old woman with a progressive myelopathy worsened after intravenous steroid administration. Angiography diagnosed a right L3 dural arteriovenous fistula. The detection of enhancing intracanalar structures in a thoracoabdominal CT obtained during her initial workup could have led to earlier diagnosis (arrows in axial images (**a**) and coronal reconstructions (**b**))

Treatment Options

Until the 1970s, treatment generally consisted of excision of the congested perimedullary veins associated with low-flow SAVFs, worsening venous hypertension, and leading to infarction. Kendall and Logue's identification of the focal nature of SDAVFs in 1977 led the way to modern therapy focusing on the shunt itself and the adjoining segments of the feeding artery and draining vein [40, 41]. Surgical treatment of a low-flow SAVF can be achieved by merely interrupting its draining vein [41].

Endovascular techniques for spinal vascular lesions appeared in the early 1970s [42, 43]. With the introduction of liquid embolic agents able to cross the arteriovenous shunt and seal the draining vein's proximal portion [44, 45], embolization has become a valid alternative to surgical treatment for low-flow SAVFs [2, 8, 46].

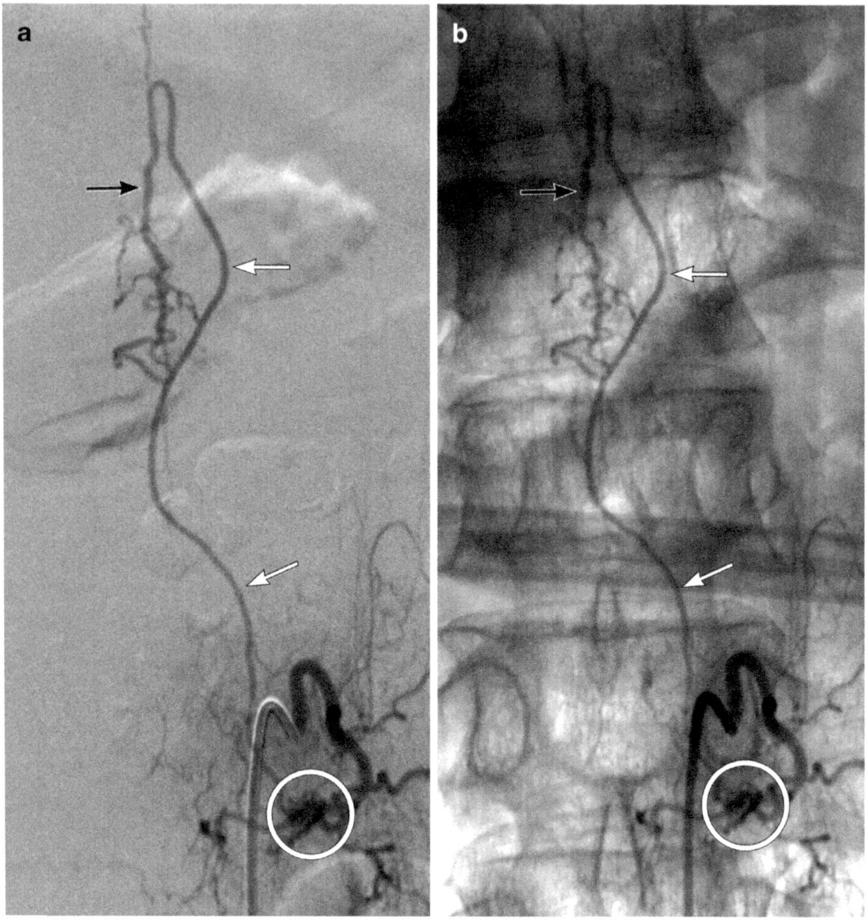

Fig. 6.6 Typical angiographic appearance of a left L1 spinal dural arteriovenous fistula. (**a**), DSA, left L1 injection, subtracted view, posteroanterior projection. The circle indicates the location of the shunt in the vicinity of the vertebral pedicle. The shunt drains into a dilated perimedullary venous system (black arrow) via a left L1 radiculomedullary vein (white arrows). (**b**), DSA, Same injection, non-subtracted image, shown for topographic orientation

Treatment Outcomes

Most if not all low-flow SAVFs are curable, but the functional outcome depends on the extent of spinal cord damage at the time of diagnosis. Prolonged delays and severe neurological deficits before treatment considerably impact the potential for recovery [47]. MRI findings have, in our experience, a limited predictive value, except maybe when showing signs of concomitant arterial ischemia. Untreated spinal venous hypertension leads to infarction with hemorrhagic transformation

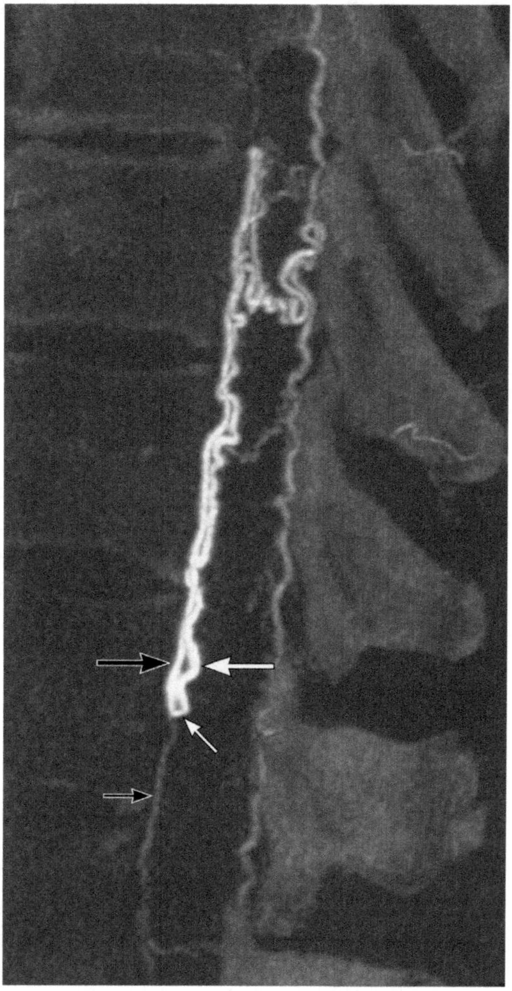

Fig. 6.7 Flat-panel catheter angiotomography in a 43-year-old woman with a low-flow perimedullary arteriovenous fistula at the conus medullaris level (sagittal reconstruction). The caliber of the ASA (large black arrow) drops abruptly (small black arrow) past the site of the arteriovenous shunt (small white arrow). The anterior-median spinal vein (large white arrow), deep to the ASA, drains cranially

(Foix-Alajouanine syndrome) [48, 49]. Although outcomes are at this stage generally bleak, therapy remains warranted since significant clinical improvement can still be observed [50]. Spinal venous thrombosis or a second vascular malformation must be suspected when the myelopathy fails to improve or worsens after therapy. Patients managed endovascularly are heparinized during and after treatment to limit the risk of perimedullary venous thrombosis. Antiplatelet or anticoagulation can also be started before or immediately after treatment.

In summary, therapy's primary goal for patients with VHM is to stop the disease's progression. While functional recovery—ranging from minimal to complete—is generally observed, individual treatment benefits are difficult to predict. Diagnostic delays represent a significant obstacle to favorable outcomes.

Diagnostic Errors and Low-Flow Spinal Arteriovenous Fistulas

The clinical diagnosis of spinal vascular malformations is challenging. Before the advent of modern neuroimaging, identification relied on surgical exploration or necropsy, sometimes after years of evolution. Diagnostic errors remain an issue nowadays: the author believes that a majority of low-flow SAVFs elude detection. Patients presenting with intermittent claudication are often treated for suspected narrow lumbar canal or peripheral arteriopathy, while older men complaining of bladder dysfunction generally get prostate surgery first. The predominant misdiagnosis is, in our experience, transverse myelitis, primarily because of the lack of specificity of conventional MRI: a recent survey of the yield of initial MRI in patients with low-flow SAVFs showed a false-negative rate of more than 60% [3]. The assumptions that a lack of flow-voids rules out a vascular malformation and that cord enhancement after gadolinium administration points towards an inflammatory myelopathy are critical factors in that dismal sensitivity rate [3].

Conventional angiography also suffers from pitfalls. Studies are frequently incomplete, technically inadequate, or performed by inexperienced physicians. A recent analysis of 30 spinal angiograms falsely reported as normal discovered cognitive errors in most cases: the SAVF was documented but not recognized (55.6%), or the angiogram was incomplete (29.6%). Therefore, a "negative angiogram" should not rule out the diagnostic of SAVF until the study quality is confirmed.

Conclusions

The diagnosis of low-flow SAVFs is challenging. A majority of low-flow SAVFs remain undetected despite the recent progress of noninvasive neuroimaging. Most if not all are amenable to endovascular or surgical therapy, often with significant functional improvement when addressed within a reasonable timeframe. Logue's 1979 observation on low-flow SAVFs remains pertinent [9]: "Any improvement in results can only come from greater awareness of the condition leading to earlier diagnosis and operation."

References

1. Aminoff MJ, Barnard RO, Logue V. The pathophysiology of spinal vascular malformations. J Neurol Sci. 1974;23(2):255–63.
2. Gailloud P. Spinal vascular malformations: angiographic evaluation and endovascular management. In: Hetts S, Cooke D, editors. Handbook of clinical neurology, vol. 176. Elsevier; 2021. p. in press.
3. El Mekabaty A, Pardo CA, Gailloud P. The yield of initial conventional MRI in 115 cases of angiographically confirmed spinal vascular malformations. J Neurol. 2017;264(4):733–9.
4. Murphy OC, Hedjoudje A, Salazar-Camelo A, Pardo CA, Gailloud P. Clinical characteristics, misdiagnosis and outcomes of patients with low-flow spinal arteriovenous fistulas. J Neurol Sci. 2020;413:116863.

5. Di Chiro G, Doppman J, Ommaya AK. Selective arteriography of arteriovenous aneurysms of spinal cord. Radiology. 1967;88(6):1065–77.
6. Djindjian R, Houdart R, Hurth M. Acquisitions récentes en angiographie médullaire. Rev Neurol (Paris). 1966;115(6):1068–9.
7. Kendall BE, Logue V. Spinal epidural angiomatous malformations draining into intrathecal veins. Neuroradiology. 1977;13(876450):181–9.
8. Merland JJ, Riche MC, Chiras J. Intraspinal extramedullary arteriovenous fistulae draining into the medullary veins. J Neuroradiol. 1980;7:271–320.
9. Logue V. Angiomas of the spinal cord: review of the pathogenesis, clinical features, and results of surgery. J Neurol Neurosurg Psychiatry. 1979;42(1):1–11.
10. Tadié M, Hemet J, Aaron C, Bianco C, Huard P. Les veines radiculaires de drainage de la moelle ont-elles un dispositif de sécurité anti-reflux ? Bull Acad Natl Med. 1978;162(6):550–4.
11. Tadié M, Hemet J, Aaron C, Bianco C, Creissard P, Huard P. Le dispositif protecteur anti-reflux des veines de la moelle. Neuro-Chirurgie. 1979;25:28–30.
12. van der Kuip M, Hoogland PV, Groen RJ. Human radicular veins: regulation of venous reflux in the absence of valves. Anat Rec. 1999;254(2):173–80.
13. Gailloud P. The antireflux mechanism – angiographic anatomy and clinical implications. Interv Neuroradiol. 2020;26(6):691–702.
14. Chaudhary MY, Sachdev VP, Cho SH, Weitzner I Jr, Puljic S, Huang YP. Dural arteriovenous malformation of the major venous sinuses: an acquired lesion. AJNR Am J Neuroradiol. 1982;3(1):13–9.
15. Takai K, Komori T, Taniguchi M. Microvascular anatomy of spinal dural arteriovenous fistulas: arteriovenous connections and their relationships with the dura mater. J Neurosurg Spine. 2015;23(4):526–33.
16. Gailloud P. Spinal dural arteriovenous fistula (SDAVF) variant with dual perimedullary and epidural drainage. Eur Spine J. 2017;27(Suppl 3):375–9.
17. Jellema K, Tijssen CC, van Gijn J. Spinal dural arteriovenous fistulas: a congestive myelopathy that initially mimics a peripheral nerve disorder. Brain. 2006;129(Pt 12):3150–64.
18. Aminoff MJ, Logue V. Clinical features of spinal vascular malformations. Brain J Neurol. 1974;97(4373119):197–210.
19. Moisset X, Taithe F, Cotte V, Jean B, Ferrier A, Clavelou P. Une hémiplégie brutale, révélant une malformation artério-veineuse médullaire cervicale. Rev Neurol (Paris). 2012;168(S2):A93–A4.
20. Soderlund ME, Benisty S, Gaston A, Djindjian M, Cesaro P, Creange A. Can myelopathies secondary to arterio-venous dural fistulae be aggravated by intravenous corticosteroid therapy? Rev Neurol (Paris). 2007;163(2):235–7.
21. Kim S, Choi Y, Park J, Sung DH. Acute paraplegia after lumbar steroid injection in patients with spinal Dural arteriovenous fistulas: case reports. Ann Rehabil Med. 2016;40(5):949–54.
22. Hetts SW, Narvid J, Singh T, Meagher S, Corcoran K, Higashida RT, et al. Association between lumbar epidural injection and development of acute paraparesis in patients with spinal dural arteriovenous fistulas. AJNR Am J Neuroradiol. 2007;28(3):581–3.
23. Aminoff MJ, Logue V. The prognosis of patients with spinal vascular malformations. Brain. 1974;97(1):211–8.
24. Jellema K, Canta LR, Tijssen CC, van Rooij WJ, Koudstaal PJ, van Gijn J. Spinal dural arteriovenous fistulas: clinical features in 80 patients. J Neurol Neurosurg Psychiatry. 2003;74(10):1438–40.
25. Amarouche M, Hart JL, Siddiqui A, Hampton T, Walsh DC. Time-resolved contrast-enhanced MR angiography of spinal vascular malformations. AJNR Am J Neuroradiol. 2015;36(2):417–22.
26. Unsrisong K, Taphey S, Oranratanachai K. Spinal arteriovenous shunts: accuracy of shunt detection, localization, and subtype discrimination using spinal magnetic resonance angiography and manual contrast injection using a syringe. J Neurosurg Spine. 2016;24(4):664–70.

27. Lindenholz A, TerBrugge KG, van Dijk JM, Farb RI. The accuracy and utility of contrast-enhanced MR angiography for localization of spinal dural arteriovenous fistulas: the Toronto experience. Eur Radiol. 2014;24(11):2885–94.
28. Saladino A, Atkinson JL, Rabinstein AA, Piepgras DG, Marsh WR, Krauss WE, et al. Surgical treatment of spinal dural arteriovenous fistulae: a consecutive series of 154 patients. Neurosurgery. 2010;67(5):1350–7. discussion 7-8
29. Si-jia G, Meng-wei Z, Xi-ping L, Yu-shen Z, Jing-hong L, Zhong-hui W, et al. The clinical application studies of CT spinal angiography with 64-detector row spiral CT in diagnosing spinal vascular malformations. Eur J Radiol. 2009;71(1):22–8.
30. Yamaguchi S, Takemoto K, Takeda M, Kajihara Y, Mitsuhara T, Kolakshyapati M, et al. The position and role of four-dimensional computed tomography angiography in the diagnosis and treatment of spinal arteriovenous fistulas. World Neurosurg. 2017;103:611–9.
31. Hedjoudje A, Murphy OC, Gregg L, Pardo CA, Gailloud P. Spinal fistulas documented by contrast enhanced computed tomography during myelopathy workup: a lost opportunity. Neuroradiology. 2021;63(2):201–7.
32. Chen J, Gailloud P. Safety of spinal angiography: complication rate analysis in 302 diagnostic angiograms. Neurology. 2011;77(13):1235–40.
33. Kendall B. Spinal angiography with iohexol. Neuroradiology. 1986;28(1):72–3.
34. Prestigiacomo CJ, Niimi Y, Setton A, Berenstein A. Three-dimensional rotational spinal angiography in the evaluation and treatment of vascular malformations. AJNR Am J Neuroradiol. 2003;24(7):1429–35.
35. Aadland TD, Thielen KR, Kaufmann TJ, Morris JM, Lanzino G, Kallmes DF, et al. 3D C-arm conebeam CT angiography as an adjunct in the precise anatomic characterization of spinal dural arteriovenous fistulas. AJNR Am J Neuroradiol. 2010;31(3):476–80.
36. Chen J, Ethiati T, Gailloud P. Flat panel catheter angiotomography of the spinal venous system: an enhanced venous phase for spinal digital subtraction angiography. AJNR Am J Neuroradiol. 2012;33(10):1875–81.
37. Pearl MS, Chen JX, Gregg L, San Millan D, Belzberg A, Jallo G, et al. Angiographic detection and characterization of "cryptic venous anomalies" associated with spinal cord cavernous malformations using flat-panel catheter angiotomography. Neurosurgery. 2012;71(1 Suppl Operative):125–32.
38. Gobin YP, Rogopoulos A, Aymard A, Khayata M, Reizine D, Chiras J, et al. Endovascular treatment of intracranial dural arteriovenous fistulas with spinal perimedullary venous drainage. J Neurosurg. 1992;77(5):718–23.
39. Martinez M, Hedjoudje A, Pardo C, Tamargo RJ, Gailloud P. Cervical spinal dural fistulas leading to remote thoracolumbar myelopathy: a diagnostic pitfall. Neurol Clin Pract. 2020;10(4):340–3.
40. Oldfield EH, Di Chiro G, Quindlen EA, Rieth KG, Doppman JL. Successful treatment of a group of spinal cord arteriovenous malformations by interruption of dural fistula. J Neurosurg. 1983;59(6):1019–30.
41. Afshar JK, Doppman JL, Oldfield EH. Surgical interruption of intradural draining vein as curative treatment of spinal dural arteriovenous fistulas. J Neurosurg. 1995;82(2):196–200.
42. Newton TH, Adams JE. Angiographic demonstration and nonsurgical embolization of spinal cord angioma. Radiology. 1968;91(5):873-6 passim.
43. Djindjian R, Cophignon J, Hurth M, Comoy J, Houdart R. 1st attempts of fragmentary muscle embolization via the femoral route in a case of medullary and craniocerebral angioma. Presse Med. 1971;79(40):1757.
44. Margolis MT, Freeny PC, Kendrick MM. Cyanoacrylate occlusion of a spinal cord arteriovenous malformation. Case Rep J Neurosurg. 1979;51(1):107–10.
45. Kerber CW, Cromwell LD, Sheptak PE. Intraarterial cyanoacrylate: an adjunct in the treatment of spinal/paraspinal arteriovenous malformations. AJR Am J Roentgenol. 1978;130(1):99–103.
46. Gokhale S, Khan SA, McDonagh DL, Britz G. Comparison of surgical and endovascular approach in management of spinal dural arteriovenous fistulas: a single center experience of 27 patients. Surg Neurol Int. 2014;5:7.

47. Van Dijk JM, TerBrugge KG, Willinsky RA, Farb RI, Wallace MC. Multidisciplinary management of spinal dural arteriovenous fistulas: clinical presentation and long-term follow-up in 49 patients. Stroke. 2002;33(6):1578–83.
48. Foix C, Alajouanine T. La myélite nécrotique subaiguë. Rev Neurol (Paris). 1926;11:1–42.
49. Jellinger K, Minauf M, Garzuly F, Neumayer E. Angiodysgenetic necrotizing myelopathy (report on 7 cases). Arch Psychiatr Nervenkr (1970). 1968;211(4):377–404.
50. Aghakhani N, Parker F, David P, Lasjaunias P, Tadie M. Curable cause of paraplegia: spinal dural arteriovenous fistulae. Stroke. 2008;39(10):2756–9.

Transverse Myelitis

7

Ram N. Narayan and Benjamin Greenberg

Contents

Nomenclature

The term "myelopathy" refers to spinal cord dysfunction. The term transverse myelitis (TM) commonly refers to an acquired inflammatory disorder of the spinal cord resulting in various degrees of motor, sensory and autonomic impairment [1]. The word "myelitis" refers to inflammation of the spinal cord and the word "transverse" refers to inflammation that spreads across the transverse section on the spinal

R. N. Narayan (✉)
Barrow Neurological Institute, Phoenix, AZ, USA
e-mail: ram.narayan@commonspirit.org

B. Greenberg
Department of Neurology, University of Texas Southwestern, Dallas, TX, USA

B. Greenberg (ed.), *Myelopathy*, https://doi.org/10.1007/978-3-030-99906-3_7

cord at any particular level. Since not all forms of TM involve the entire transverse section of the spinal cord, a more appropriate term would be "inflammatory myelopathy" or simply "myelitis". TM can occur as an independent entity (idiopathic TM) where the presumed etiology is a post-infectious immune-mediated pathology. It can also occur as a manifestation of neuro-immunological disorders (disease associated TM) like multiple sclerosis (MS), neuromyelitis optica spectrum disorders (NMOSD) or acute disseminated encephalomyelitis (ADEM). While evaluating patients with TM, it is important to rule out compressive and non-inflammatory causes of myelopathy and to delineate the various underlying etiologies since the treatment, risk of recurrence and prognosis varies according to the type of TM.

History of Transverse Myelitis

In 1882 Bastian et al. described several cases of "acute myelitis" and pathological analysis revealed vascular lesions in some of them and acute inflammation in others. In the early 1920s about 200 cases of "post-vaccinal encephalomyelitis" characterized by inflammation of the spinal cord was described as a rare complication of smallpox vaccination in the United Kingdom. These cases revealed inflammatory cells and demyelination on autopsy. In 1928, Ford et al. first postulated a "post-infectious" rather than an "infectious" cause for acute myelitis because the rash and fever was noted to have resolved when the symptoms of myelitis began. Therefore, it was proposed that an "allergic" response to the virus rather than the virus itself caused spinal cord injury. Suchett-Kaye Al et al. used the term "acute transverse myelitis" in 1948 while describing a case of inflammatory myelopathy complicating pneumonia [2].

Pathophysiology

Understanding the pathophysiology of TM has direct clinical implications. The three key elements in the development of TM irrespective of the underlying effector mechanisms are (1) Inflammation (2) Demyelination and (3) Axonal degeneration (except in cases of acute flaccid myelitis, which by definition has predominant anterior horn cell damage). It is important to recognize that these three elements tend to evolve sequentially in most cases (Fig. 7.1) and so early recognition and treatment can potentially delay and minimize progression to the process of axonal degeneration at which stage, the disease process is irreversible and causes significant morbidity.

The inflammatory phase of TM is characterized by perivascular infiltration by monocytes and lymphocytes in the lesion. The white and gray matter areas of the spinal cord are involved to varying degrees suggesting that TM is not a pure demyelinating disorder (confined to the white matter) but rather is a heterogenous inflammatory disorder that affects neurons, axons, oligodendrocytes and myelin. Axonal degeneration occurs in the final phase and is likely responsible for most lingering deficits. In recent years, a subtype of myelitis, known as Acute Flaccid Myelitis

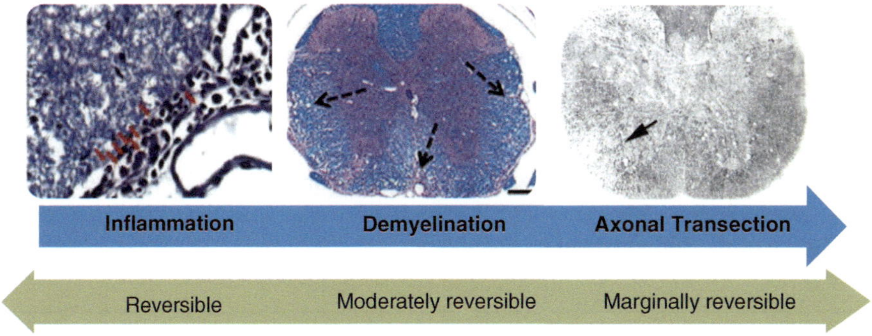

Fig. 7.1 Stages of inflammatory myelopathy

(AFM) has been recognized in the US and throughout the world. This phenotype is characterized by a preponderance of gray matter damage and is most associated with acute viral infections. Some patients will have concomitant white matter involvement that likely represents parainfectious inflammatory damage to spinal cord. Thus, while most myelitis is purely immune mediated, some rare cases have evidence of a cord infection causing an immune response that independently causes damage [3].

Epidemiology

The incidence of TM is probably underestimated. A database from Israel reported an incidence of 1.34 per million population. Large population-based studies in the United States are currently lacking. A US based study based on 33 cases of TM reported an annual incidence of 4.6 per million. Hence TM still remains a rare condition when compared to a disease like multiple sclerosis whose estimated prevalence is about 1000 per million populations. The incidence of pediatric TM is similar to that in the adult population and is estimated at 1.7–2 per million children per year. Based on these numbers about 1500 cases are expected in the US every year and about 34,000 individuals are expected to be left with chronic morbidity from TM at any time. TM affects men and women equally although with MS-associated TM, females tend to be more frequently affected; both in adult and pediatric populations. A bimodal age distribution is noted between 10 to 19 years and between 30 to 39 years [4, 5]. Children account for about 20% of cases of TM. Amongst children there is another bimodal pattern with the under 5 years and above 10 years groups being the most affected [6]. The AFM variant of myelitis disproportionately effects children [7].

With regards to the etiology of TM, 64% of cases were noted to be idiopathic and 36% were found to be disease-associated in one study. In another study, idiopathic TM accounted for about 21% of the cases while 45% were reported as para infectious, 21% as MS-associated and 12% as vascular. A preceding infection was identified in about 47% of the children prior to the onset of TM symptoms. The wide variations in the frequency of various types of TM differs based on the geographical area, ethnicity and more importantly based on improvement in diagnostics and characterization of newer disease entities [8]. For instance, with the advent of the myelin oligodendrocyte glycoprotein (MOG) antibody associated syndromes, the incidence of isolated TM is estimated to be 12% and it is more than likely that these cases were categorized as "idiopathic TM" rather than "disease associated TM" before the discovery of the antibody and its phenotype.

Clinical Presentation

The classic clinical presentation in TM is an acute or subacute onset of neurological symptoms characteristic of a myelopathy; motor, sensory and/or autonomic dysfunction. Depending on the acuity of the disease process and the tracts affected the clinical picture tends to vary at presentation. An important question to ask patients at presentation is how much time it took from onset of symptoms to nadir. An ischemic event of the spinal cord typically evolves over a few minutes to a few hours whereas idiopathic TM typically hits nadir anywhere between several hours to days. Progression over several weeks or months argues significantly against a diagnosis of myelitis [9]. The AFM variant can progress over a few hours or as long as many days.

Motor symptoms in TM can include weakness in the extremities, gait instability or inability to walk, imbalance, stiffness, spasms of affected muscle groups and/or cramping of leg muscles. Sensory symptoms can include numbness, paresthesias and less frequently pain of the affected extremities. These symptoms can be the initial presentation in some cases and patients or health-care providers can be dismissive of these symptoms. A sensory level can be reported by patients and can be described as a loss of sensation below a level, with or without a tight or squeezing band-like sensation at the top of the sensory level (described as MS-hug in patients with multiple sclerosis). A subjective sensory level as reported by the patient indicates spinal cord dysfunction unless proven otherwise and the lesion is likely localized to that dermatomal level or above. This is due to the fact that spinal cord cross section is laminated and so eccentrically located lesions in the cervical spine for example, can cause a subjective sensory level in the thoracic segments and below. Another presentation to recognize is that a stocking-glove sensory distribution does not always indicate a length dependent neuropathy and in an acute setting warrants a search for myelopathic causes. Sometimes myelitis can cause back pain preceding the symptoms of myelopathy. Pain in the trunk and extremities is often a late feature in many cases of TM; especially in TM associated with NMOSD. Autonomic dysfunction is characterized by urinary retention (most common form of autonomic disturbance in the acute phase), increased urinary/fecal urgency, bladder and bowel incontinence, incomplete evacuation and constipation and sexual dysfunction. Urinary retention can be one of the first signs of myelopathy and can bring a patient to the ER before the onset of motor or sensory symptoms. It should be noted in this context that acute urinary retention should cause concern for myelopathy and not be dismissed. Acute urinary retention in an otherwise healthy adult should cause consideration of a neurogenic etiology [10].

Physical examination findings of patients with TM varies according to the timing of the exam with respect to the onset of symptoms. The goals of performing a careful neurological examination in patients with a suspected myelopathic event include (1) To confirm a diagnosis of myelopathy (2) To localize the level of the lesion and (3) To identify patterns of spinal cord involvement and specific clinical syndromes which are sometimes suggestive of the underlying cause (Table 7.1). During the initial acute phase of TM (phase of spinal shock), examination can reveal flaccid

Table 7.1 Clinical syndromes based on anatomic location of lesion in myelitis

	Patterns	Salient clinical features	Common conditions
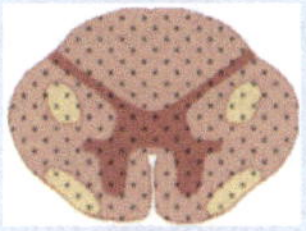	Complete transection	If truly complete transection, complete loss of all motor, sensory, autonomic functions below the level of the lesion. Most often, transection is incomplete; clinical deficits may also be variable/asymmetric. Lower motor neuron signs may be observed at the level of lesion. Urinary urgency is seen early on followed by retention and then incontinence (a late finding). Cervical and thoracic lesions can cause ipsilateral Horner syndrome and autonomic dysreflexia.	Trauma, idiopathic TM
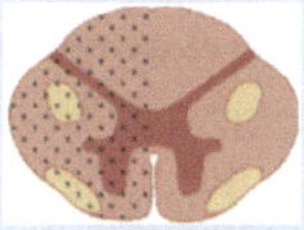	Hemisection	Contralateral loss of pain & temperature, ipsilateral loss of prop and vibrations, ipsilateral UMN pattern weakness, segmental LMN signs and autonomic impairment ipsilaterally.	Extradural lesions like tumor (esp. metastasis), epidural abscess, penetrating trauma, multiple sclerosis.
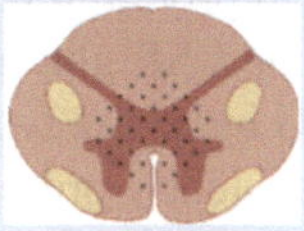	Central	"Dissociated" sensory loss early on followed by segmental LMN weakness and then UMN signs below the level of lesion followed by dorsal column involvement. Sacral sensory sparing until very late.	Syringomyelia, intramedually tumor, hyperextension injury
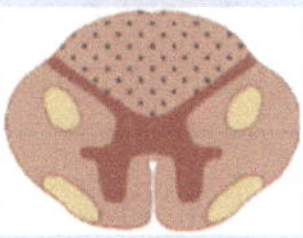	Posterolateral	Early loss of vibrations and proprioception, positive Romberg sign, positive pyramidal signs, Intact spinothalamic tract sensation.	B12 deficiency , HIV, HTLV (TSP), Copper deficiency, spondylotic myelopathy,, MS
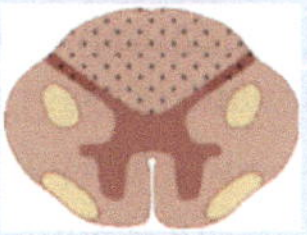	Posterior only	Early and marked loss of vibrations and proprioception with positive Romberg sign and sensory ataxia. Typically, well preserved strength.	Tabes dorsalis, spondylotic myelopathy
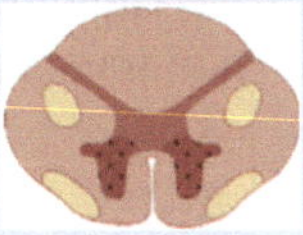	Anterior horn cell	Pure motor involvement, LMN pattern. No sensory or autonomic involvement	Polio, SMA, ALS, Hirayama,

paralysis (with hypotonia, hyporeflexia and absent pathological reflexes) which evolves over days or weeks to a more well-recognizable pyramidal pattern of spastic weakness (of upper motor neuron type) with increased tone, hyperreflexia and the appearance of pathological reflexes like Babinski and Hoffman signs. Another sign described in patients with TM is the Beevor sign which refers to the upward displacement of the umbilicus when a patient attempts to contract the abdominal recti (as while raising the head from an inclined position against resistance). This results from the relative weakness of the muscles below the level of the lesion than those above the lesion. This sign has been historically associated with a thoracic spine lesion between the T10 and T12 segments. The Beevor sign is not specific for myelopathy can be seen in certain conditions like facioscapulohumeral muscular dystrophy or amyotrophic lateral sclerosis which cause lower abdominal weakness. Superficial reflexes like the abdominal, cremasteric and the ano-cutaneous wink reflexes are absent below the level of the spinal cord injury. A patulous rectum and reduced/absent rectal tone on anal examination in another finding in the acute phase of TM [10].

In the AFM variant of TM, patients can present with acute flaccid paralysis/weakness of one or more limbs. Most patients have a cervical cord lesion causing asymmetric upper limb flaccid weakness. Involvement of the cervical corticospinal tracts would lead to upper motor neuron patterns of weakness in the lower limbs. Thus, some patients present with mixed upper and lower motor neuron patterns of weakness [11].

Table 7.1 depicts the various acute spinal cord syndromes with information on specific tracts involved, associated clinical signs and specific conditions as examples.

Cerebrospinal Fluid (CSF)

CSF is abnormal in about 50% of patients with idiopathic TM. Lymphocytic pleocytosis (usually less than 100/mm^3) and elevated protein level (usually 100–120 mg/dL) are common findings. Higher cell counts (mean – 136/mm^3) and protein levels (mean – 173 mg/dL) have been described in a pediatric case series. CSF glucose levels are typically normal. CSF oligoclonal bands and elevated IgG index are typically absent or transiently present in idiopathic TM and when persistently present (especially 2 or more unrestricted bands) suggest a higher risk of subsequent development of MS [9].

Imaging

One of the initial goals of obtaining imaging in the acute phase of a patient with suspected TM is to rule out compressive etiologies. Magnetic resonance imaging (MRI) is the preferred modality of imaging for the spinal cord. This said, there is a role for computerized tomography (CT) scans in select circumstances. For instance, in patients with implantable MRI-incompatible devices such as pacemakers and stimulators, CT myelography is useful in the evaluation of compressive etiologies. Plain films/xrays are generally not useful in patients with non-traumatic myelopathies.

While obtaining a MRI in a suspected case of TM two important decisions have to be made; (1) Timing of imaging and (2) Segment of the spinal cord to be imaged. With regards to timing, in a suspected case of spinal cord compression which is indistinguishable from TM at initial presentation, a stat MRI is recommended to appropriately triage a patient for surgical intervention, particularly if symptoms have evolved in the prior 24 hours. In cases where a compressive etiology is not suspected, imaging can be obtained on an urgent basis. As described above in the section on pathophysiology, since "time is spinal cord tissue", we recommend empiric treatment with high dose steroids in suspected TM cases after a compressive etiology is ruled out with initial imaging even when a clear inflammatory etiology has not been established. In centers where obtaining an MRI might be delayed, an empiric dose of high dose methylprednisolone (1000 mg for adults, administered intravenously) is recommended. With regards to the segment to image, we recommend to first clinically localize the lesion and image the entire neuroaxis proximal to it (at least during the initial phase of evaluation) before embarking on to a more comprehensive evaluation. Standard T1 and T2 sequences including short tau inversion recovery (STIR) sequences are obtained. Gadolinium-based contrast enhanced T1 weighted sequences are also obtained in patients with no contraindications to gadolinium contrast agents. While sagittal cuts give information on the extent of involvement, the axial cuts are critical for identifying the patterns of involvement and the tracts involved in order to generate a differential diagnosis.

The classical MRI finding in TM is a T2 signal abnormality of the spinal cord with post contrast enhancement, of varying lengths and patterns of involvement with or without associated cord edema. When a cord lesion extends to three or more vertebral segments it is termed longitudinally extensive transverse myelitis (LETM). Some common causes of LETM are NMOSD, neurosarcoidosis, systemic lupus erythematosus (SLE) spinal ependymoma, arteriovenous malformations (AVM), infectious causes like varicella zoster and syphilis, B12 and copper deficiency states to name some. Conditions like MS typically cause short-segment discrete lesions which are eccentrically (laterally or dorsally) located on axial sections although there are exemptions to this rule [12].

Another useful approach in classifying TM based on the pattern of MRI involvement is as follows:

- White matter predominant
- Gray matter predominant
- Mixed gray and white matter predominant
- Central cord syndrome
- Anterior cord syndrome

We recommend obtaining a brain MRI with contrast even in the absence of clinical signs of cerebral involvement at presentation. Up to 87% of MS patients that initially presented with myelitis were noted to have brain abnormalities in one series. Asymptomatic brain lesions are not specific to MS and can be seen in conditions like NMOSD, anti-MOG associated disorder and adrenoleukodystrophy. TM associated with neurosarcoidosis commonly exhibits the following clinical features; (1) LETM, (2) Persistent enhancement at 2 months or more and (3) A nodular dorsal sub-pial enhancement pattern although many times it is non-specific.

A summary of MRI findings in some common myelopathic conditions is mentioned in Fig. 7.2.

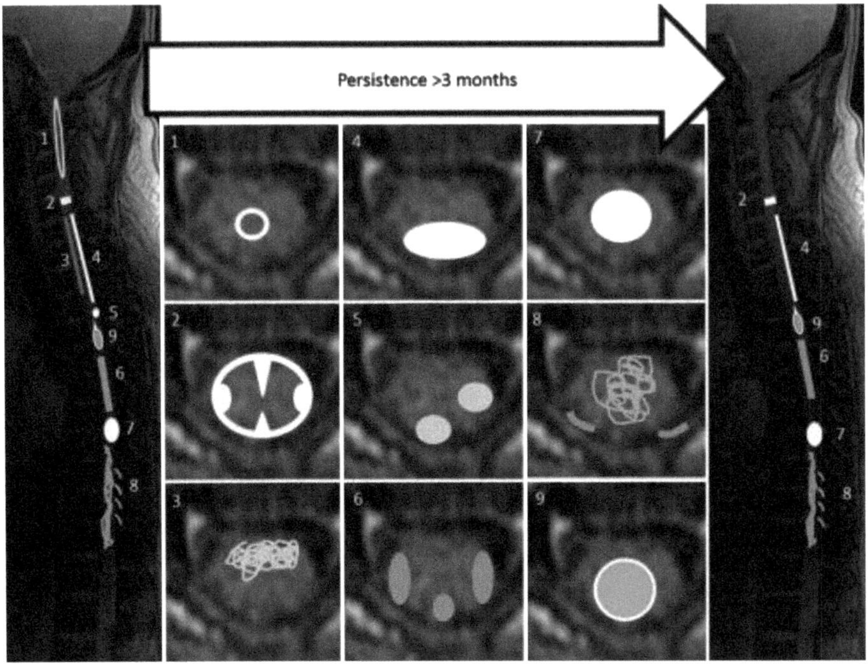

Fig. 7.2 Summary of intramedullary gadolinium enhancement patterns by etiology and their evolution in acute and subacutemyelitis. Sagittal (left, images at initial presentation shown, and right panel, persistently enhancing lesions on follow-up images shown) and axial (middle panels) patterns of gadolinium enhancement. Brighter regions represent higher intensity of enhancement. (1) neuromyelitis optica spectrum (elongated ring appearance in approximately one-third – the remainder usually patchy); (2) cervical spondylotic myelopathy ("pancake-like" or "transverse band" on sagittal images – width of enhancement greater than or equal height – at middle of T2 hyperintensity and associated with moderate or severe stenosis and demonstrating circumferential white-matter enhancement sparing gray matter on axial images; enhancement only present in 7% of spondylotic myelopathies, but when present often mimics tumor or inflammation); (3) anterior spinal artery infarct (patchy in anterior spinal cord; owl eyes or snake eyes may be seen particularly on follow-up MRI); (4) spinal cord sarcoidosis (dorsal subpial linear enhancement extending over multiple segments); (5) multiple sclerosis (dorsal cord or lateral cord; may be nonenhancing; often asymmetric); (6) paraneoplastic symmetric tract-specific enhancement; (7) primary intramedullary spinal cord lymphoma (bright homogeneous enhancement; may be multiple); (8) dural arteriovenous fistula (patchy enhancement; enhancing veins dorsal to spinal cord may be seen; may or may not be associated with gadolinium enhancement); (9) intramedullary spinal cord metastases (thin rim of more intense enhancement surrounding enhancing lesion with a flame-like appearance superiorly – can also be inferior to lesion). (Ref. [13])

MRI Negative TM

In very rare instances, patients with TM have been reported to have normal/negative spinal cord MRI. This is thought to occur due to imaging timing (too early in the disease course before the lesion evolves or too late in the disease course such that the lesion resolves) or due to spinal meningitis without parenchymal involvement (can be missed if a gadolinium sequence is not obtained), but can also be seen in the setting of a functional neurological disorder. A few conditions where this condition has been reported are the early phase of spinal cord ischemia, nutritional myelopathies (B12 and copper deficiency myelopathy) and myelin oligodendrocyte glycoprotein associated disorder (MOGAD). However, in routine clinical practice issues pertaining to radiologic protocols (e.g. lack of good quality axial cuts, unavailability of DWI sequences in suspected cord ischemia), movement and implant-related artefacts are more common causes for an "MRI negative TM" [14].

Classification

Subtypes of TM are differentiated based on the extent of clinical and radiological involvement [15]. These include acute partial TM, acute complete TM and LETM.

1. Acute partial TM refers to spinal cord dysfunction that is asymmetric and incomplete with an MRI involvement of less than three segments.
2. Acute complete TM refers to spinal cord dysfunction that is symmetric, complete or near-complete neurological deficits (paraplegia, quadriplegia, sensory loss and autonomic dysfunction) below the level of the lesion with an MRI involvement of less than three segments.
3. LETM refers to complete or incomplete, symmetric or asymmetric spinal cord dysfunction but extending to three or more vertebral segments.

Diagnosis

TM is suspected when there is an acute or subacute onset of spinal cord dysfunction (motor, sensory and autonomic dysfunction) in patients with no evidence of a compressive cord lesion on imaging. Thus, the diagnosis of idiopathic TM is made when a patient has signs or symptoms of myelopathy, evidence of inflammation on MRI and/or CSF testing, with exclusion of other causes [15].

Clinical Approach and Work Up

The four main steps in the care of a patient with suspected TM include:

1. Acute therapy: This is discussed below in the treatment section, BUT treatment should not be delayed pending work up. Prompt initiation of therapy is recommended once the diagnosis of TM is confirmed on clinical grounds.
2. Determination of the etiology
3. Prevention of future attacks
4. Rehabilitation/Symptom management

Acute Therapy

High dose intravenous glucocorticoid therapy is considered to be the standard first—line therapy. IV methylprednisolone at 30 mg/kg per day (up to a maximum 1000 mg daily dose) given over three to 5 days is a recommended regimen. It is crucial to institute steroid therapy as early as possible in the disease course; typically, within a few hours of admission since it is the most effective measure against edema and worsening inflammation which is the main offender in the initial phases of the TM disease process and is largely reversible (Fig. 7.1). Plasma exchange is effective in cases where high dose steroid therapy has failed or if there is incomplete response. We also recommend plasma exchange as initial therapy in patients who have motor involvement concomitantly with steroid therapy. The recommended regimen for plasma exchange is five to seven treatments; each with 1.1–1.5 plasma volumes every other day for 10–14 days. IV cyclophosphamide (at a dose of 800–1200 mg/m^2 body surface area administered as a single pulse dose) has been used successfully in the acute phase on an anecdotal basis, but is most effective in patients with myelitis related to mixed connective tissue disorders like lupus [16–18].

Determination of the Etiology

The clinical approach to a patient with suspected TM is proposed in Figs. 7.3 and 7.4. The main aim of this work up is to rule out other potentially recurring causes of inflammatory myelitis (which tend to occur as part of an autoimmune disease state) and other types of myelopathy (nutritional, vascular, infectious, etc).

The following investigations are recommended in patients with suspected TM.

(i) MRI of the entire spinal with and without gadolinium contrast (Fig. 7.5)
(ii) Brain MRI with and without gadolinium (to rule out multiple sclerosis).
(iii) Cerebrospinal fluid analysis including cell count, protein, glucose, oligoclonal bands, IgG index, cytology and flow cytometry (in select cases), infectious work-up (in select cases with a high index of suspicion)
(iv) Serum anti-AQP-4 antibodies, anti-MOG antibodies, ANA, SSA/SSB antibodies, TSH, B12 and methylmalonic acid, homocysteine, copper, ceruloplasmin, zinc.

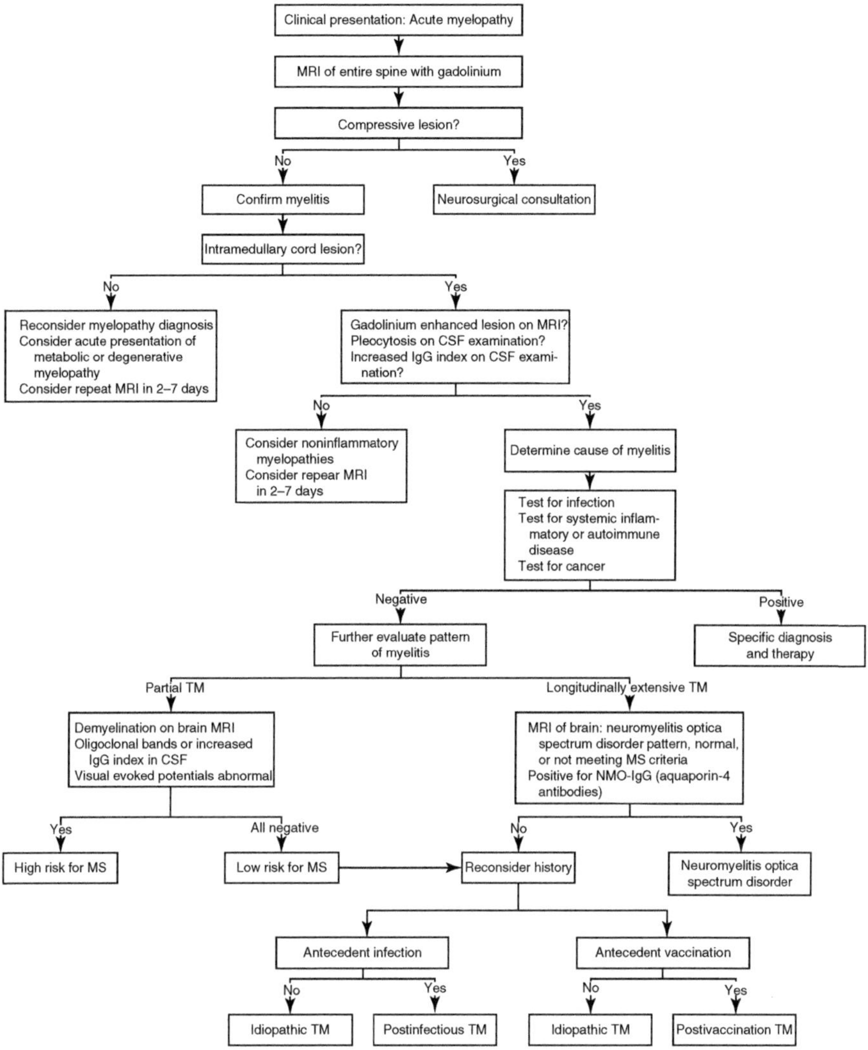

Fig. 7.3 ALGORITHM: Approach to a patient with an acute myelopathy presentation. (Ref. [19])

(v) Infectious studies: CSF gram staining, bacterial and viral culture (in select cases), CSF testing for enterovirus PCR, cytomegalovirus PCR, Epstein-Barr virus PCR, herpes virus PCR (HSV-1, HSV-2, HHV-6 PCR), varicella-zoster virus PCR, West Nile Virus PCR and serology, HTLV-1 antibody and PCR, lyme serology (if epidemiologically relevant), syphilis serology. Serum testing for HIV serology, WNV serology, lyme and syphilis serology.

(vi) In the cases of suspected AFM: nasopharyngeal swabs for viral testing (eg, enterovirus polymerase chain reaction [PCR]), fecal samples (rectal swab) for viral testing (eg, enterovirus PCR).

Potential medical work-up for suspected acute transverse myelitis

Indicative signs and symptoms	Suggested evaluation
Infectious etiology	
Fever	CSF Gram stain and bacterial culture
Meningismus	CSF PCR: HSV-1, HSV-2, HHV-6, VZV, CMV, EBV, enteroviruses D68 and EV71
Rash	CSF viral culture
Concurrent systemic infection	CSF acid fast bacilli smear and tuberculous culture
Immunocompromised state	CSF HSV, VZV, and HTLV-1 antibodies
Recurrent genital infection	CSF anti-*Borrelia burgdorferi* antibodies
Symptoms of zoster radiculopathy	CSF VDRL
Adenopathy	CSF India ink and fungal culture
Residence in area endemic for parasitic infections	Chest radiograph and cranial CT scan
Lymphadenopathy	Serology for antibodies to HIV, HSV, VZV, HTLV-1, *B. burgdorferi*
	Serology for hepatitis A, B, C, and *Mycoplasma*
	Consider serology for parasites
	Blood cultures
Systemic inflammatory disease (vasculitis, collagen vascular diseases, mixed connective tissue disease)	
Rash	Serum ACE
Oral or genital ulcers	Autoantibodies: ANA, ds-DNA, Ro/SSA, La/SSB, Sm, RNP
Adenopathy	Complement levels
Livedo reticularis	Urinalysis with microscopic analysis for hematuria
Serositis	Lip/salivary gland biopsy
Photosensitivity	Chest CT with intravenous contrast
Inflammatory arthritis	Schirmer test
Erythema nodosum	Chest radiograph
Xerostomia	Gallium scan
Keratitis	Antiphospholipid antibodies (anticardiolipin antibodies, Russel viper venom time, partial thromboplastin time)
Conjunctivitis	
Contractures or thickening of skin	
Anemia/leukopenia/thrombocytopenia	
Raynaud phenomenon	
History of arterial and venous thrombosis	
Multiple sclerosis	
Previous demyelination event	Brain MRI
Incomplete deficit clinically with MRI abnormality ≤2 spinal segments and <50 percent of cord diameter	CSF oligoclonal bands and IgG index
Neuromyelitis optica spectrum disorders (NMOSD)	
Optic neuritis	Brain MRI (usually negative)
Clinical deficit with MRI abnormality ≥3 spinal segments	Serum anti-AQP4 IgG and anti-MOG IgG autoantibodies
Paraneoplastic myelopathies	
Spastic paresis with or without bowel and bladder dysfunction, usually with involvement of other areas of the nervous system	Paraneoplastic antibody panel
Longitudinally extensive transverse myelitis on spine MRI	Cancer screening
Idiopathic transverse myelitis	
No clinical or paraclinical features suggestive of another diagnostic category	Rule out infectious etiologies, systemic inflammatory disease, CNS inflammatory disorders, and paraneoplastic myelopathies

ACE: angiotensin-converting enzyme; ANA: antinuclear antibodies; AQP4: aquaporin 4; CMV: cytomegalovirus; CNS: central nervous system; CSF: cerebrospinal fluid; CT: computed tomography; ds-DNA: double stranded DNA; EBV: Epstein-Barr virus; HHV: human herpes virus; HSV: herpes simplex virus; HTLV-1: human T-cell lymphotropic virus 1; IgG: immunoglobulin G; MRI: magnetic resonance imaging; MOG: myelin oligodendrocyte glycoprotein; PCR: polymerase chain reaction; RNP: ribonucleoprotein; VDRL: Venereal Disease Research Laboratory; VZV: varicella zoster virus

Modified with permission from: Transverse Myelitis Consortium Working Group. Proposed diagnostic criteria and nosology of acute transverse myelitis. Neurology 2002; 59:499. Copyright © 2002 Lippincott Williams & Wilkins.

Fig. 7.4 Evaluation of a case of suspected acute non-compressive myelopathy. Modified with permission from Ref. [15]. © 2002 Lippincott Williams & Wilkins. Adoped from Uptodate: Chitra Krishnan, Benjamin Greenberg, et al. Transverse myelitis

Suggestive MRI findings of acute myelopathies

MRI findings	Potential diagnosis
Blood within the spinal cord (bright and dark T1 and T2 signal)	Vascular malformation such as cavernous angioma or dural arteriovenous fistula
Flow voids within spinal cord	Dural arteriovenous fistula or arteriovenous malformation
Central T2 signal abnormality	Venous hypertension
Ring-enhancing lesion	Infection or tumor (but consider course of intravenous glucocorticoids to rule out inflammatory process before progressing to biopsy)
Acute loss of vertical intervertebral disc height and corresponding T2 signal abnormality	Consider fibrocartilaginous embolism
Fusiform lesion extending over >3 spinal cord segments	Consider neuromyelitis optica spectrum disorders (NMOSD) or disease-associated transverse myelitis
T2 bright lesion in white matter occupying less than 2 spinal cord segments in rostral-caudal extent and less than 50 percent of the cord diameter	Consider multiple sclerosis
T2 spinal cord lesion adjacent to disk herniation or spondylitic ridge, but lack of spinal cord compression	Consider dynamic spinal cord compression only during flexion or extension (flexion-extension x-ray to determine the presence of abnormal spinal column mobility; MRI in flexion or extended position instead of in neutral position)

Fig. 7.5 Suggestive MRI findings in TM. Adopted from Uptodate: Chitra Krishnan, Benjamin Greenberg, et al. Transverse myelitis

For patients with LETM we recommend adding.

(vii) Chest CT to evaluate for the presence of hilar adenopathy, FDG-PET scan or gallium nucleotide uptake scan to evaluate for evidence of systemic sarcoidosis.

In rarer instances the following labs are recommended to complete work up (especially if the initial work up is non-contributory);

(viii) Vitamin E, paraneoplastic panel (especially CRMP antibodies), spinal angiogram, CT aorta and prothrombotic workup (in cases of spinal artery stroke), neuroophthalmological evaluation (including an optical coherence tomogram) to look for evidence of optic neuritis, salivary gland biopsy (for suspected Sjogren's myelopathy).

Differential Diagnosis of TM

The differential diagnoses of idiopathic TM can be grouped into three main categories:

(i) Other types of myelopathies – Compressive and other non-inflammatory myelopathies.

(a) Compressive myelopathies include those caused by disc herniation, epidural bleed/abscess, vertebral body compression fracture and spondylosis. An overt evidence of trauma may not always be present. Imaging of the entire spine (screening) is indicated even if the lesion clinically localizes to a particular level. For instance in the case of traumatic paraplegia, even if the lesion localizes to the thoracic spine, an entire cord MRI is obtained to identify concomitant cervical spine lesions. In most instances cord imaging is obtained on an emergent basis (CT or MRI) to plan surgical intervention or make decisions on immobilization.

(b) Non-compressive and non-inflammatory myelopathies include conditions like vascular myelopathies (spinal artery stroke, spinal dural arteriovenous fistula, fibrocartilaginous embolism), metabolic and nutritional myelopathies (Vit B12 and Copper deficiency, nitrous oxide toxicity, neurolathyrism, neurocassavism, Vit E deficiency), neoplasms (intramedullary cord tumor, primary CNS lymphoma, intravascular lymphoma) and radiation myelopathy [20].

(ii) Secondary transverse myelitis (TM) refers to immune mediated myelopathies that occur as part of autoimmune diseases like MS, NMOSD, neurosarcoidosis, etc. It is very important to distinguish idiopathic TM from secondary TM (as mentioned below) since this has implications on determination and prevention of recurrence and long term prognosis [20].

(iii) Acute flaccid myelitis (AFM) – AFM refers to a polio-like myelopathy phenotype that occurs in biennial outbreaks in the United States and Europe associated with enterovirus D68 and D71. This condition occurs mostly in children; adults are rarely affected. Although the clinical presentation in the acute phase is similar to idiopathic TM, the occurrence of fever or a respiratory illness either prior to or concomitantly with neurological symptoms, acute flaccid weakness (mostly asymmetric) evolving over hours to a few days with predominant gray matter involvement on MRI and relevant endemic/epidemiological cues favor AFM over idiopathic TM. A positive EV-PCR from a stool or nasopharyngeal sample confirms the diagnosis [11].

(iv) Guillian-Barre syndrome (GBS) – Acute inflammatory demyelinating polyneuropathy (AIDP) or GBS can have a clinical presentation similar to TM. Distinguishing features (despite some overlap)
Include:

(a) AIDP tends to present with more severe or isolated lower extremity symptoms (usually symmetric) whereas a cervical TM presents with equivalent upper and lower extremity symptoms and a thoracic TM presents with isolated lower extremity involvement.

(b) With regards to autonomic involvement, urinary and/or bowel involvement is more common in TM whereas cardiovascular instability is more common with AIDP.
(c) A sensory level is often definable in TM whereas this is never present in AIDP.
(d) CSF analysis in TM may reveal inflammatory cells and elevated proteins whereas in AIDP, the characteristic finding is cytoalbuminologic dissociation.
(e) Spinal MRI imaging often shows a distinct cord lesion in TM whereas the cord itself is typically normal in AIDP (cauda equina enhancement is often noted).
(f) Electrodiagnostic testing is normal in TM whereas this can be abnormal to varying degrees in AIDP (depending on the timing of the testing).

Determination and Prevention of Recurrence

More than two-thirds of patients experience a monophasic disease course. Recurrence has been reported in about 25%–33% of idiopathic TM cases but these statistics are from studies conducted before the testing of MOG and AQP4 antibodies and so the actual rate of recurrence in idiopathic TM is considered to be lower. When TM occurs secondary to an immune-mediated disease (like MS), the recurrence rate is much higher (as high as 70%). Features that predict recurrence of TM at the time of initial presentation include [21–26]:

- Seropositivity for AQP4 or MOG antibodies
- Presence of unmatched oligoclonal bands in the CSF
- Lesions on brain MRI
- Multifocal lesions or longitudinally extensive involvement on cord MRI
- Presence of autoantibodies indicative of systemic autoimmunity (ANA, ds DNA, phospholipid, c-ANCA)
- Known diagnosis of connective tissue disease(lupus, MCTD)

Prevention of Recurrence

In patients with recurrent disease or indicators of a chronic/recurrent disease course (as with the presence of AQP4 or MOG antibodies) chronic immunosuppressive therapy should be considered. Commonly used agents are azathioprine (150–250 mg/day), methotrexate (15–20 mg per week oral or subcutaneous with folate rescue), mycophenolate (2–3 gm per day) or rituximab (intravenous, 1000 mg single dose or with a second 1000 mg dose at 2 weeks). Newer therapies indicated for anti-AQP4 NMOSD include inebilizumab (CD19 targeted antibody causing B cell depletion), eculizumab (complement C5 inhibitor), tocilizumab (IL6 Receptor inhibitor) and sataralizumab (humanized IL6 inhibitor). In patients with TM who fit criteria for high risk CIS at onset, standard MS disease modifying therapies can be considered.

Prognosis/Recovery

Long term follow-up data on patients with idiopathic TM suggest that about one-third of patients recover with little or no sequelae, one-third are left with a moderate degree of disability (eg: mild spasticity but independent ambulation, sphincter disturbances or disabling sensory impairments) and one-third have severe disabilities (eg: inability to walk, absence of sphincter control, etc). This data was generated prior to more aggressive treatment regimens for acute TM and probably overestimates rates of disability. The disability varies according to the specific setting in which TM has occurred and the age at onset. At the onset of the condition, it is hard to predict which patient will fall into each of these outcome categories although a few prognostic markers have been identified in this regard. A rapid onset with complete paraplegia and spinal shock at onset, prolonged stay in the intensive care unit (ICU), requiring ventilator assistance, the number of white blood cells in the CSF, age of onset less than 3 years, high CSF levels of Il-6 (not routinely checked) are some poor prognostic markers. This said, all patients with acute TM require acute rehabilitation and about 66% of patients might require long-term rehabilitation [27].

Rehabilitation in TM

Two classical approaches to rehabilitation in TM are [28]:

1. Traditional approach which is aimed at maximizing physical indepdence, capabilities and potential.
2. Activity-based restorative approach which addresses the specific impairment and is based on activity-dependent neural plasticity in which changes in the nervous system are driven by repetitive activation of the neuromuscular system above and below the level of lesion.

Traditional Rehabilitation

In this approach, the physical and occupational therapists train patients to increase their strength and joint range of motion (ROM), improve tone, mitigate pain and maximize functional mobility. Equipment evaluation is performed in a systematic and regular manner to augment and optimize functional performance. A thorough home rehabilitation program is designed to sustain the patient's functional gains which are acquired at the therapy site. Some of the specific components of this approach are:

1. Adequate ROM is achieved through stretching exercises, use of appropriate orthoses and strengthening exercises. Daily stretching of muscle with terminal sustained stretch is highly recommended for ROM limitation due to spasticity. The most common sites where contractures limit ROM are shoulder external

rotation, shoulder elevation, scapular depression, shoulder retraction, elbow extension and supination, hip extension, ankle dorsiflexion and great toe flexion. Some muscle tightness may be desirable in certain locations like the finger flexors (to facilitate a stronger grasp) resulting in good wrist extension. Another example is tightness of the back extensors to assist triceps weakness and regain upright sitting. Mild overstretching is permissible can help with adequate hip external rotation required to put on shoes and socks. Aggressive ROM exercises in the absence of supervision by a PT or OT should be avoided especially in the presence of fractures, active heterotopic ossification, deep venous thrombosis and osteoporosis.

2. Muscle strengthening is achieved by exercise training through the maximum range in all spared muscle groups. Exercise training results in increase in type II fibers, increased metabolic capacity and increased levels of myofibrillar proteins. Strength training can be achieved by static or dynamic training performed through isometric, isotonic and isokinetic techniques according to targeted goals and the degree of neurological deficit. Training programs using the DeLorme or Oxford methods are used specifically in patients with paralysis.
3. Activity training progresses from the easiest to the most difficult; i.e. from bed mobility to rolling, prone lying, long sitting, short sitting and sitting up from a lying position. Siting up from a supine position is the first step towards independent dressing and transfers. An appropriate transfer technique has to be identified in patients with paraplegia or tetraplegia. Dependent transfers include sliding transfers, standing pivot technique or the use of Hoyer lifts. Transfers that require some active patient participation include two-man lift and the assisted standing pivot transfer techniques. The goal of assisted transfer techniques is to gradually enable independent transfer. Floor-to-chair transfer technique is important to patients who are prone to falling from wheel chair.
4. Ambulation is a commonly expressed goal of most patients with TM. Patients with injury of myotomes T2 or above are less likely to achieve ambulation whereas those from injury of myotomes between T3 and T11 levels are able to use braces for physiological standing and therapeutic ambulation. The goal for individuals with injury to myotomes between T12 and L2 levels is to achieve ambulation within a household and for the goal for those with injury to myotomes at L3 and lower is to optimize ambulation in the community (i.e a distance of more than 150 feet at a time). It should be noted that these goals vary according to the age and the motivation levels of an individual patient.
5. Bracing is based on the how much muscle function is attained in the back and lower extremity muscles. For example, patients with intact quadriceps and tibialis anterior and tibialis posterior function can walk full time with short leg braces like ankle-foot prosthesis (AFOs) or even supramalleolar orthoses or no braces at all whereas those with weakness of muscles crossing the hip joint (iliopsoas, sartorius, gluteus maximus) but with good control of pelvic muscles and abdominal muscles may require long leg braces (knee-ankle-foot orthoses or KAFOs).
6. Gait training exercises are focused on strengthening the core trunk and abdominal muscles, shoulder depressors and scapula stabilizing muscles besides triceps

and wrist extensors. a structured progressive resistive exercise program for the latissimus dorsi, pectoralis, lower trapezius, and serratus anterior muscles is very important to achieve good trunk and hip stability. During gait training, control of the pelvic musculature is critical for successful ambulation. Gait training includes practicing standing between parallel bars, practicing the gait pattern inside and outside the bars with assistive devices (ie, canes, bilateral forearm or axillary crutches, walkers), walking on an uneven ground, on ramps, walking through doorways and practicing getting into a car for example.

7. Training on safe falling techniques and getting up from a floor is very important in this patient population because of the increased risk of falls.
8. Wheelchair prescription commensurate with the level of deficit and appropriate for an individual's needs and comfort is very essential.

Activity-Based Restorative Therapy

In this approach, motor activation and sensory stimulation are performed with the ultimate goal of neural restoration not mere functional restoration. The tools employed are similar to that in traditional rehabilitation but the underlying principle is that the nervous system is dependent on activity for everything; from myelination to remyelination to new cell and synapse formation leading ultimately to function.

1. Motor activation

   Patterned motor activation can be achieved through task-specific and nonspecific training. Locomotor training (i.e gait training) is an example of patterned task-specific training. It is offered through partially weight-supported environments using treadmill systems, automatic gait robots, aquatic therapy etc. These techniques are based on two main principles; (1) Maximization of load bearing in the lower extremities thereby minimizing shared load-bearing between the upper and lower extremities and (2) Optimizing sensory cues, ensuring normal walking speed and optimizing kinematics (stance/swing phases and arm swing).

   Patterned nontask-specific training is based on the principle of activation of the central pattern generator (CPG) which is thought to be located in the lumbar myotomes of the spinal cord (L2-L5). This is mainly accomplished using functional electrical stimulation (FES). FES is postulated to promote peripheral and central nervous system repair following injury. Following complete spinal cord transection in rats, lower extremity FES induced an 82% to 86% increase in cell birth in the lumbar spinal cord. Hence activation of the CNS influences regenerative cellular mechanisms; activity-dependent gene expression, modification of synapse strength, synapse elimination, myelination and maintenance of myelination and axonal growth. In addition, FES activation increases neurotrophin production below the injury level which forms the biological basis for neural reorganization and functional improvement.

   One of the important prerequisites for the success of FES in TM patients is intact lower motor neuron function. In TM, the lower motor neuron is generally affected at the level of the inflammation. For that reason, muscle contractions in response to FES from levels at the injury site are usually limited or absent in the acute phase but returns in a few weeks or months after the injury. During that period, it is important to try to avoid muscle atrophy and its sequelae at that level. This may be attempted by using other electrical stimulation devices in addition to using traditional rehabilitation approaches (eg, bracing, taping, splinting).

2. Sensory activation

   Sensory stimulation can be used to activate afferent pathways with the goal of providing information that can subsequently be used to perform a motor task with the direct effect being improved motor and sensory function. Focal sensory activation or stimulation and nonfocal activation (eg, epidural stimulation or intrathecal delivery of neurotrophin-3 or brain-derived neurotrophic factor) can also produce complex lower limb cycling-like movements. In a doubleblind, randomized controlled clinical trial using whole-body vibration in patients with MS, Schuhfried and colleagues demonstrated improved postural control and walking speed.

Conclusions

1. The term TM refers to an acquired inflammatory disorder of the spinal cord. Idiopathic TM is an independent entity with no identifiable etiology. Secondary TM is an entity that occurs as part of an autoimmune disease state (like MS or NMOSD).
2. The time course of evolution of symptoms is key to understanding the etiological process.
3. AFM is a variant of TM that presents as a polio like flaccid weakness of one more extremities and is associated with enterovirus D68 infection.
4. In patient with TM, when a cord lesion extends to three or more vertebral segments it is termed longitudinally extensive transverse myelitis (LETM) and this entity has unique diagnostic and prognostic indications.
5. Acute therapy of TM consists of steroids, plasmapheresis and IVIG.
6. The diagnostic work up for TM consists of search for autoimmune, nutritional, neoplastic and vascular causes of spinal cord injury.
7. The presence of brain MRI lesions, positive serology for AQP4 or MOG antibody are among the top features that predict recurrence in TM.
8. The prognosis of TM suggests that a majority of patients recur from their initial attack and the extent of recovery depends on rehabilitation approaches.

References

1. Power H, Sedgwick LW. The new Sydenham Society's lexicon of medicine and the allied sciences, vol. 4. The New Sydenham Society: London; 1892.
2. Kerr D. The history of TM: the origins of the name and the identification of the disease. The Transverse Myelitis Association; 2018. Retrieved 22 July 2018
3. Adams RD, Kubik CS. The morbid anatomy of the demyelinative diseases. Amer J Med. 1952;12:510–46.
4. Berman M, Feldman S, Alter M, et al. Acute transverse myelitis: incidence and etiologic considerations. Neurology. 1981;31:966.

5. Bhat A, Naguwa S, Cheema G, Gershwin ME. The epidemiology of transverse myelitis. Autoimmun Rev. 2010;9:A395.
6. Pidcock FS, Krishnan C, Crawford TO, et al. Acute transverse myelitis in childhood: center-based analysis of 47 cases. Neurology. 2007;68:1474.
7. Theroux LM, Brenton JN. Acute transverse and flaccid myelitis in children. Curr Treat Options Neurol. 2019;21:64.
8. Beh SC, Greenberg BM, Frohman T, Frohman EM. Transverse myelitis. Neurol Clin. 2013;31:79.
9. de Seze J, Stojkovic T, Breteau G, et al. Acute myelopathies: clinical, laboratory and outcome profiles in 79 cases. Brain. 2001;124:1509.
10. Krishnan C, Kaplin AI, Calabresi P, Kerr DA. Clinical characteristics and prognostic factors in 170 patients with idiopathic transverse myelitis. Neurology. 2004;62(Suppl 5):A231.
11. Murphy OC, et al. AFM working group. Acute flaccid myelitis: cause, diagnosis, and management. Lancet. 2021 Jan 23;397(10271):334–46. https://doi.org/10.1016/S0140-6736(20)32723-9.
12. Choi KH, Lee KS, Chung SO, et al. Idiopathic transverse myelitis: MR characteristics. AJNR Am J Neuroradiol. 1996;17:1151.
13. Flanagan EP. Chapter 19: Autoimmune myelopathies. In: Pittock SJ, Vincent A, editors. Handbook of clinical neurology, vol. 133. Amsterdam: Elsevier; 2016. p. 327–51.
14. Sechi E, Krecke KN, Pittock SJ, et al. Frequency and characteristics of MRI-negative myelitis associated with MOG autoantibodies. Mult Scler. 2021;27(2):303–8.
15. Transverse Myelitis Consortium Working Group. Proposed diagnostic criteria and nosology of acute transverse myelitis. Neurology. 2002;59:499.
16. Weinshenker BG, O'Brien PC, Petterson TM, et al. A randomized trial of plasma exchange in acute central nervous system inflammatory demyelinating disease. Ann Neurol. 1999;46:878.
17. Greenberg BM. Treatment of acute transverse myelitis and its early complications. Continuum (Minneap Minn). 2011;17:733.
18. Greenberg BM, Thomas KP, Krishnan C, et al. Idiopathic transverse myelitis: corticosteroids, plasma exchange, or cyclophosphamide. Neurology. 2007;68:1614.
19. Frohman EM, Wingerchuk DM. Clinical practice. Transverse myelitis. N. Engl. J. Med. 2010;363:564–72.
20. Berger JR, Cambi F, Di Rocco A, Farace J. Overview to approach to the patient with noncompressive myelopathy. Continuum (Minneap Minn). 2005;11:13.
21. Bruna J, Martínez-Yélamos S, Martínez-Yélamos A, et al. Idiopathic acute transverse myelitis: a clinical study and prognostic markers in 45 cases. Mult Scler. 2006;12:169.
22. Ganelin-Cohen E, Konen O, Nevo Y, et al. Prognostic parameters of acute transverse myelitis in children. J Child Neurol. 2020;35:999.
23. Seifert T, Enzinger C, Ropele S, et al. Relapsing acute transverse myelitis: a specific entity. Eur J Neurol. 2005;12:681.
24. Kim KK. Idiopathic recurrent transverse myelitis. Arch Neurol. 2003;60:1290.
25. Chen L, Li J, Guo Z, et al. Prognostic indicators of acute transverse myelitis in 39 children. Pediatr Neurol. 2013;49:397.
26. Gajofatto A, Monaco S, Fiorini M, et al. Assessment of outcome predictors in first-episode acute myelitis: a retrospective study of 53 cases. Arch Neurol. 2010;67:724.
27. Ford B, Tampieri D, Francis G. Long-term follow-up of acute partial transverse myelopathy. Neurology. 1992;42:250.
28. Sadowsky CL, et al. Rehabilitation in transverse myelitis. Continuum (Minneap Minn). 2011 Aug;17(4):816–30.

Infectious Myelopathies

8

Olwen C. Murphy and Arun Venkatesan

Contents

Introduction

Infections are an important cause of myelopathy globally. Causative organisms vary by population and region (Tables 8.1 and 8.2). Clinical presentations of infections affecting the spinal cord vary according to the micro-organism involved and the pathological process and can include acute flaccid myelitis, acute myelitis, radiculomyelitis and chronic progressive paraparesis. Certain populations are at increased risk of infectious myelopathies, such as immunocompromised patients. Establishing the correct diagnosis is essential in infectious myelopathies, as many of these diseases are amenable to treatment with specific anti-microbials. The clinical, diagnostic and management considerations for the most common and most important causes of micro-organism associated myelopathy will be presented in this chapter.

O. C. Murphy · A. Venkatesan (✉)
Division of Neuroimmunology and Neuroinfectious Diseases, Department of Neurology, Johns Hopkins University School of Medicine, Baltimore, MD, USA
e-mail: avenkat2@jhmi.edu

B. Greenberg (ed.), *Myelopathy*, https://doi.org/10.1007/978-3-030-99906-3_8

Table 8.1 Important micro-organisms causing infectious or parainfectious myelopathy

Viruses	**Bacteria**
HIV	*Pyogenic abscesses*
HTLV-1	*Mycobacterium tuberculosis*
HSV-2	*Borrelia burgdorferi*
VZV	*Treponema pallidum*
CMV	**Fungi**
Rabies virus	*Cryptococcus neoformans*
West Nile virus	*Aspergillus species*
Zika virus	**Parasites**
Dengue virus	*Schistosoma species*
Japanese encephalitis	*Taenia solium*
Tick-borne encephalitis	

Table 8.2 Infectious myelopathies with regions of endemicity

Micro-organism	Areas of highest incidence	Clinical spinal cord presentation(s)
HIV	Global disease burden with highest frequency in sub-saharan Africa	Chronic progressive spastic paraparesis
HTLV-1	Japan, South America, Caribbean, Africa (west, central and south)	Chronic progressive spastic paraparesis
Rabies virus	Africa, Asia	Flaccid areflexic paralysis evolving to quadriplegia and respiratory failure
West Nile virus	United States, North Africa, Eastern Europe, France	Infectious prodrome followed by acute flaccid paralysis
Zika virus	South America, Central America, Caribbean, Pacific regions	Acute myelitis
Japanese encephalitis	South and East Asia	Acute flaccid paralysis
Tick-borne encephalitis	Europe, Russia, East Asia	Acute flaccid paralysis
Borrelia burgdorferi (Lyme disease)	North America, Europe, Asia	Painful polyradiculitis +/− segmental myelitis Longitudinally extensive myelitis
Schistosoma species	Sub-Saharan Africa, South America (Brazil & Venezuela), Asia (China, Japan & South-East Asia)	Acute painful myelitis and/or polyradiculitis
Taenia solium (cysticercosis)	Sub-Saharan Africa, South & Central America, China, India, South-East Asia	Subacute or chronic myelopathic syndrome

Viral Myelopathies

Retroviruses

HIV

Myelopathy in HIV can result from a number of underlying pathologic processes. The most common form is HIV-associated vacuolar myelopathy, named after the distinct histopathological features described below [1]. HIV-associated vacuolar myelopathy typically occurs in longstanding HIV infection with low CD4 cell counts or in the context of AIDS. However, it has been reported as an early or presenting feature of HIV on rare occasions [2]. Autopsy series in the pre-antiretroviral era demonstrated pathological changes of HIV-associated vacuolar myelopathy in 22% of spinal cords of AIDS-patients, some of whom did not have spinal cord symptoms, suggesting that the clinical syndrome is subtle or asymptomatic in some patients [1].

Early symptoms can include paresthesias, leg discomfort and erectile dysfunction [3, 4]. These are followed by progressive spastic paraparesis which is typically symmetric and may involve gait ataxia [3]. Bowel and bladder dysfunction with incontinence occurs in over half of patients [1]. Sensory deficits predominantly reflect dorsal column involvement with impaired vibration and proprioception [3]. The clinical syndrome may plateau after many years. A caveat in interpreting sensory findings and reflexes in HIV patients is the possibility of a co-existing HIV-associated peripheral neuropathy which has been reported in approximately 40% of patients with HIV [5].

HIV-associated vacuolar myelopathy is considered a clinical diagnosis and one of exclusion in HIV patients, as there are no specific diagnostic investigations other than pathological examination. MRI of the spinal cord is usually unremarkable, although high T2 signal in the posterior and lateral cord may be seen in some cases [6]. CSF analysis is often undertaken to rule out opportunistic infection which can occur in HIV and serological studies for HTLV should be sent, since co-infection with human T-cell lymphotropic virus-1 (HTLV-1) and HIV is associated with increased risk of myelopathy [7].

Anti-retroviral therapy is not thought to alter the natural history of HIV-associated vacuolar myelopathy in individuals [4], although the incidence of this syndrome in the HIV population has reduced since the introduction of highly active anti-retroviral therapy [8].

Characteristic pathological findings at autopsy are vacuolation of the white matter with infiltrate of lipid-laden macrophages, most prominent in the lateral and posterior regions of the mid to lower thoracic spinal cord [1]. As the pathological changes are very similar to those seen in subacute combined degeneration of the cord due to B12 deficiency, it has been suggested that metabolic pathways may be involved in the pathogenesis of this disorder [9]. However, the clinical syndrome does not respond to B12 supplementation [8].

Other causes of myelopathy related to HIV are also possible. Acute transverse myelitis has been reported as a complication of seroconversion and has been successfully treated with corticosteroids and anti-retroviral therapy [10]. Co-infection or opportunistic infection with mycobacterium tuberculosis, HTLV-1, cytomegalovirus, herpes simplex virus, varicella zoster virus, syphilis or cryptococcus neoformans should also be considered as causes of myelopathy, while epidural abscess from a variety of bacteria resulting in compressive myelopathy is also more frequent in HIV patients [4].

Human T-cell Lymphotropic Virus (HTLV)

HTLV is transmitted through exchange of bodily fluids, typically in the setting of sexual intercourse, blood product transfusions, or shared needles. HTLV-1 is endemic in South America, the Caribbean, Japan and western, central and southern Africa [11], while HTLV-2 is found in certain populations in the Americas, such as American Indians [4, 12]. HTLV-1 seropositivity in the United States is very rare, with the exception being intravenous drug users and commercial sex workers in whom sero-prevalence may be as high as 18% [13]. Of the two subtypes, HTLV-1 causes myelopathy much more frequently than HTLV-2, although cases have been reported in association with HTLV-2 [14].

Most individuals with HTLV-1 seropositivity are asymptomatic carriers, with less than 4% of infected persons developing 'HTLV-associated myelopathy' (HAM) or 'tropical spastic paraparesis' (TSP) [15, 16]. Risk of progression from carrier to symptomatic state is thought to be modified by proviral load, host HLA genotype and immune response [11]. Pathological findings seen in the spinal cord at autopsy are perivascular inflammatory infiltrates in the grey and white matter and hyaloid thickening of the media and adventitia of blood vessels, with demyelination and axonal degeneration of the anterior and lateral columns of the spinal cord, most marked in the thoracic region [17].

Clinical presentation is similar to that of HIV-associated myelopathy. Patients develop a slowly progressive myelopathy with prominent spasticity and early bladder dysfunction. Pain and sensory symptoms are less prominent but can occur [18]. Symptoms and signs are typically limited to the lower extremities which results in progressive gait disturbance, without remission or plateau. Patients may become wheelchair-bound around 20 years after symptom onset [11].

Laboratory testing for HTLV-1 antigen and antibody can be performed on both serum and CSF, with newer assays providing high sensitivity and specificity [19]. Proviral load can be tested in peripheral blood [11]. Routine CSF analysis may be normal [20] or may demonstrate mild non-specific abnormalities suggestive of inflammation i.e. mild lymphocytosis, elevated protein or positive oligoclonal bands [8]. MRI of the spinal cord may be normal or show atrophy, with a minority of patients demonstrating focal or diffuse spinal cord lesions [20–22]. It has been suggested that patients with HTLV-1 (both symptomatic and asymptomatic patients) may frequently have non-specific white matter lesions seen on MRI brain [20, 21].

Treatment with corticosteroids may be beneficial in the early inflammatory stage of the disease [11]. Various antivirals and immunomodulatory treatments such as interferon-alpha, cyclosporine A and diazole have also been reported to be of benefit in small numbers of patients [11, 23].

Herpesviruses

Herpesviruses are a family of DNA viruses with high prevalence worldwide. Herpes simplex virus (HSV), varicella zoster virus (VZV), Epstein-Barr virus (EBV) and cytomegalovirus (CMV) can cause a myelitis during primary infection or after remaining latent in sensory ganglia or the immune system for years.

Herpes Simplex Virus (HSV)

HSV-1 is a common infection transmitted via oral contact, while HSV-2 is typically transmitted during sexual contact with active genital lesions. HSV-2 can cause a myeloradiculitis of the lower spinal cord during primary infection or reactivation (Elsberg Syndrome), with symptoms of lower extremity weakness, bladder dysfunction, radicular pain, numbness or paresthesia in a lumbosacral distribution [24]. Attacks are usually self-limiting but can be recurrent. MRI may be normal, or show edema/hyperintensity/enhancement of the lower cord and nerve roots [24].

A more severe presentation of HSV-2 is acute necrotizing myelitis beginning in the lumbo-sacral region and ascending to the thoracic and cervical regions [25]. This presentation is most frequent in the immunocompromised (particularly with HIV), though cases have also been reported in immunocompetent patients [24, 26, 27]. Paraplegia can be severe and in early stages is often flaccid with absent reflexes [8]. CSF usually shows elevated protein and a mild-to-moderate pleocytosis (lymphocyte-predominant, although polymorphs can be seen with necrotizing lesions) [8].

For both presentations of HSV-2 myelitis, viral DNA can usually be detected from CSF using PCR [25, 28]. Patients can be treated with aciclovir, although the benefit of this medication is unproven in this setting. Outcome varies from complete recovery with Elsberg syndrome to severe residual spastic paraparesis with acute necrotizing lesions.

While encephalitis is the recognized manifestation of HSV-1 in the CNS, rare cases of myelitis have been reported with this viral subtype [29].

Varicella Zoster Virus (VZV)

After primary infection, VZV remains latent in the dorsal root ganglion. Reactivation is more common in the immunocompromised and results in a characteristic vesicular painful dermatomal rash commonly known as shingles, with associated neuropathic pain. Rarely, during an episode of zoster, the virus may spread retrogradely to the spinal cord and cause a myelitis, days to weeks after the dermatomal rash [30]. In immunocompetent patients, myelitis symptoms are often mild and self-limiting [31]. By contrast, in immunocompromised individuals, the presentation is more insidious, severe or potentially fatal, and can even occur without preceding zoster rash (zoster sine herpete) [30, 32].

MRI in VZV myelitis demonstrates T2 hyperintensity at the spinal level corresponding to the involved dermatome, with lesions appearing asymmetric in axial sequences [8]. CSF findings are similar to those seen in HSV myelitis. CSF VZV PCR, VZV IgM and IgG should be tested, with antibody tests reported to demonstrate higher sensitivity than PCR tests in diagnosing CNS complications of VZV [33]. However, physicians should remember that a clinical diagnosis of VZV myelitis can often be made in the appropriate context, allowing early treatment with intravenous acyclovir. The addition of corticosteroids has also been reported to be helpful in some patients [34].

VZV vasculopathy is another well-recognized CNS complication of VZV infection, and it is important to remember that this vasculopathy can cause ischemic myelopathy as well as cerebral stroke [30].

Cytomegalovirus (CMV) & Epstein-Barr Virus (EBV)

CMV is a global infection. Population seroprevalence is between 50% and 60% in highly developed countries [35, 36] while developing countries demonstrate higher seroprevalence, even approaching 100% in some populations [37, 38]. CMV can cause a subacute polyradiculomyelitis in immunocompromised patients, particularly in individuals with advanced HIV (CD4 count <50 cells/mm^3) or organ transplant recipients. Clinical presentation is usually ascending weakness and sensory impairment, loss of reflexes and sphincter dysfunction [39]. MRI shows inflammation of the spinal cord and/or nerve roots. Pleocytosis is expected in CSF, and hypoglycorrhachia can also be observed in some cases [39]. CMV DNA can be identified in the CSF with PCR, and serum antibody studies can confirm the presence of CMV IgG antibody. Patients should be treated with intravenous ganciclovir and/or intravenous foscarnet, however, the outcome is often poor [40].

Transverse myelitis occurring in association with primary CMV infection in immunocompetent hosts is likely an immune-mediated phenomenon rather than direct viral infection of the spinal cord, supported by the absence of CMV DNA in CSF of these patients [41], although rare case reports have suggested that direct infection may be possible even in immunocompetent hosts [42]. A similar clinical picture of immune-mediated para-infectious transverse myelitis can occur in association with primary EBV infection, another global infection with high population prevalence [43]. The clinical features of para-infectious transverse myelitis will be discussed later in this chapter.

Rabies Virus

Clinical presentations of rabies virus have become exceedingly rare in developed countries such as the United States, due to effective disease control at an animal level and the availability of rabies vaccine and immunoglobulin for exposed individuals [44]. However, the disease still causes morbidity and mortality in Africa and Asia, with annual human deaths worldwide estimated at almost 60,000 [45]. Rabies virus is transmitted through animal bites (typically dog or bat bites) and spreads to the CNS via peripheral nerves during an incubation period of 20–90 days [44]. Clinical manifestation can be with encephalitic 'furious' rabies or less commonly with a radiculomyelitic 'paralytic' form. These clinical presentations seem to be determined by whether the initial burden of disease occurs in the brain or the spinal cord. Both forms are usually fatal within days, although time to death in patients with the paralytic form is approximately twice that of encephalitic form [46].

Rabies virus enters the nervous system through the neuro-muscular junction and travels by retrograde tran-synaptic transmission via motor neurons to the CNS [47, 48]. The virus is also thought to spread to peripheral sensory ganglia and peripheral sensory nerves via centrifugal propagation and anterograde axonal transport [47, 49]. The predilection of rabies virus for neurons and its rapid spread through the nervous system may be related to the expression of specific neuronal membrane molecules which bind the virus, and the ability of virally-infected neurons to evade apoptosis [48, 50]. Electrophysiologic and pathophysiologic studies suggest significant peripheral nerve and nerve root dysfunction in paralytic rabies, compared to prominent anterior horn cell dysfunction in furious rabies [44, 51]. The pathogenetic reasons for these differences in clinical presentation are not completely understood, but may relate to host immunological factors [51].

Clinical presentation of paralytic rabies is with flaccid areflexic paralysis which can begin in one limb before evolving to quadriparesis, respiratory failure and dysautonomia. Neuropathic pain can occur and presentation can be mistaken for Guillain-Barre Syndrome. Radiculomyelitis also occurs in the encephalitic form of rabies, but is a later and less clinically important feature in this form as the patient is typically already comatose and severely ill [46].

MRI spinal cord typically shows T2 hyperintensity of the nerve roots and grey matter [46, 52, 53]. MRI brain shows similar non-enhancing increased T2 signal in the brainstem, thalamus, limbic system and white matter of the cerebral hemispheres [46]. Lymphocytic pleocytosis is seen in CSF. Rabies virus RNA can be isolated in CSF, saliva or skin biopsy and anti-rabies virus antibodies can be detected in serum [44]. Rabies virus antigen can also be isolated in skin biopsy taken from a region with hair follicles (viral antigen can be identified in adjacent small sensory nerves) [54].

There is no proven treatment for human rabies, although multiple strategies including rabies vaccination, immunoglobulin, ribavirin, sedatives and interferon-alpha have been attempted. Survival is extremely rare but has occurred with bat-variant rabies. Survival in these rare cases has not been consistently associated with given treatments, and may instead be determined by host immune response [46].

Flaviviruses

West Nile Virus

West Nile virus is an RNA virus transmitted to humans by the *Culex* mosquito [55]. The virus was first isolated from a female patient in the West Nile region of Uganda in 1937 and was named accordingly [56]. However, this nomenclature is misleading as outbreaks were quickly recognized in other regions such as the Mediterranean, Israel, North Africa, Russia and India [57]. Over the past 20 years, the epidemiology and clinical characteristics of West Nile virus have evolved [57]. Outbreaks of symptomatic disease have become more frequent in diverse locations, and CNS manifestations have become more widely recognized [57]. The first cases in the US were seen in 1999 in New York, and since then the virus has spread across the country [55]. In 2016, 2149 US cases from 46 states were reported to the Centers for Disease Control and Prevention, of which 1309 were reported to be neuro-invasive [58]. Highest incidence occurred in central states including North and South Dakota, Wyoming and Montana [58]. While North America currently has the highest global incidence of West Nile virus, presentations also remain frequent in areas of North Africa, Eastern Europe and France [59].

Symptomatic West Nile virus can be either neuroinvasive or non-neuroinvasive. As many infections are asymptomatic, neuroinvasive disease with direct infection of the nervous system only occurs in approximately 1% of overall infection [60]. Clinical presentation of neuroinvasive disease is with meningitis, encephalitis, myelitis, and radiculitis, either alone or in combination. Infectious symptoms (fever with or without maculopapular rash) usually occur 1–2 days prior to onset of West Nile myelitis, and neurological presentation is with acute flaccid paralysis due to involvement of the anterior horn cells of the spinal cord [60]. Rapid evolution of asymmetric weakness is seen, often with monoplegia, however severe presentations with quadriplegia and respiratory failure can occur [61]. Weakness usually reaches a nadir within 72 h of onset [61]. Cranial nerve manifestations such as facial weakness, extraocular muscle weakness, dysarthria and dysphagia are seen in the majority of patients [61]. Pain in affected limbs is frequent, but sensory loss or paresthesia are uncommon [60]. In rare cases, where polyradiculopathy is more prominent than myelitis, presentation with a Guillain-Barre-like syndrome of ascending weakness and sensory symptoms can occur, and a demyelinating sensorimotor neuropathy can be seen on nerve conduction studies in these patients [60, 61]. Encephalitis is frequently concurrent with other neurological involvement, which can make clinical assessment challenging.

CSF in neuroinvasive West Nile virus demonstrates a pleocytosis (typically a mixed population of lymphocytes and neutrophils with median white cell count of

100 or 200), while protein is usually elevated to the range of 100 mg/dL [61, 62]. The yield of serological and PCR tests varies depending on the stage of infection. West Nile virus replicates at the site of inoculation then spreads to lymph nodes to cause primary viremia, so in early infection viral RNA may be detectable in the serum [63, 64]. By the time symptoms of neuroinvasive infection occur, West Nile virus has typically been cleared from the serum and peripheral organs, and West Nile virus IgM antibody is typically detectable in both serum and CSF [62, 63]. In some cases, viral RNA may also be isolated in CSF with PCR, however sensitivity of this test is low [55]. MRI spinal cord in patients with myelitis shows T2 hyperintensity most prominent in the ventral horn grey matter, with or without enhancement of the conus medullaris and cauda equina) [65–67].

Prevention of outbreaks relies on protection from mosquito bites. There is no definitively proven effective treatment for West Nile virus, although case series suggest that IVIG may be beneficial [68]. IVIG is hypothesized to be therapeutic due to the presence of anti-West Nile virus antibodies, which can be detected at high titers in products pooled from endemic regions [69]. Moreover, a preparation of IVIG developed in Israel using only plasma from donors with anti-West Nile virus antibodies has shown promise in animal models [70].

Outcome is variable, though most patients with polio-like presentations will have persistent weakness [60, 61]. Respiratory failure and quadriparesis are associated with the poorest outcomes and possibility of death [60].

Other Flaviviruses

Zika is an emerging mosquito-borne virus. Rare cases of human zika infection were described prior to 2007, when the first significant outbreak occurred in the Federated States of Micronesia [71]. Over subsequent years the virus has spread across pacific regions, South America, Central America and the Caribbean [72]. Multiple neurological complications have been recognized including congenital microcephaly, Guillain-Barre syndrome, myelitis and encephalitis. A handful of cases of myelitis have been reported in association with zika infection [73, 74]. Zika infection can be diagnosed with serum and/or CSF rRT-PCR or with anti-zika IgM (if cross-reactivity with dengue virus IgM can be excluded) [74]. Further research is required to determine whether myelitis associated with zika infection is a result of direct infection, or an immune-mediated para-infectious process.

Dengue virus is another mosquito-borne virus with a significant global disease burden. Neurological manifestations are uncommon, but include encephalopathy, encephalitis, myelitis and post-infectious peripheral nervous system complications [75]. While myelitis is thought to be immune-mediated in most cases, occurrence of myelitis in the acute infectious phase with detectable dengue virus in the CSF suggests the possibility of direct infection in rare cases [75, 76].

Japanese encephalitis predominantly affects children and young adults in southern and eastern Asia, while tick-borne encephalitis is seen in Europe, Russia and East Asia [77, 78]. Both viruses typically present with encephalitis, but the spinal cord may be involved in a minority of cases. Myelitis manifests with acute flaccid paralysis and motor recovery is typically poor. Vaccination is available for both viruses.

Polio Virus

Poliomyelitis caused by the polio virus has essentially become a historical diagnosis, and for this reason we will not provide a detailed description of this disease. Due to concerted global efforts towards eradication, there were only 20 reported cases worldwide in 2017, occurring in Pakistan and Afghanistan [79]. It is hoped that poliomyelitis will become completely eradicated in the coming years. The virus is usually acquired via the fecal-oral route, and poliomyelitis almost exclusively occurs in children [80]. Clinical presentation is characterized by a flu-like illness followed by fever, meningismus, nausea and vomiting. The next symptoms are myalgia and muscle spasms, followed by asymmetric flaccid areflexic paralysis predominantly affecting the lower limbs which evolves over 48 hours [80]. Bulbar involvement, respiratory failure and autonomic involvement result in higher morbidity and mortality, and encephalitis may rarely occur [81].

CSF is typically inflammatory. The virus can frequently be isolated from nasopharyngeal or stool samples. Serological studies and PCR studies on CSF or blood may also be useful in establishing the diagnosis [81]. MRI spine shows hyperintensity of the anterior horn cells, the neuronal cell type most prominently affected [82]. Treatment is supportive and therapy should be undertaken to reduce contractures and deformity. Survivors usually experience significant residual weakness, loss of muscle bulk and skeletal deformity. Some patients will experience functional decline decades later, named post-polio syndrome, the etiology of which is uncertain [80].

Pediatric Acute Flaccid Myelitis

Since 2014, clusters of cases of 'polio-like' illness in children have been reported in North America, Australia, South America and Europe [83–86]. Cases have typically occurred in seasonal and/or regional clusters and affected children ranging in age from 3 months to 15 years [85, 86]. Clinical presentation is associated with prodromal symptoms of infection such as fever, upper respiratory tract symptoms or gastroenteritis. Neurological manifestations occur 1–14 days after prodromal illness [83, 86]. Pain in affected limbs often precedes acute weakness, which reaches a nadir between 4 and 72 h [86]. Asymmetric flaccid paralysis is the hallmark of this clinical syndrome, with depressed or absent reflexes in affected limbs. Cranial nerves or respiratory muscles may be involved, with some patients requiring mechanical ventilation [83, 86]. Sensory deficits, bowel/bladder dysfunction and altered mental status occur in a minority of cases [87].

CSF shows a lymphocytic-predominant mild-to-moderate pleocytosis and mildly elevated protein [87]. MRI demonstrates T2 hyperintensity in the gray matter of the spinal cord which is often patchy/poorly defined in the early stage but becomes confluent as the disease progress, extending over multiple vertebral levels and in some cases involving the whole length of the spinal cord and brainstem (Fig. 8.1) [87]. MRI abnormalities are typically non-enhancing at onset, although nerve-root

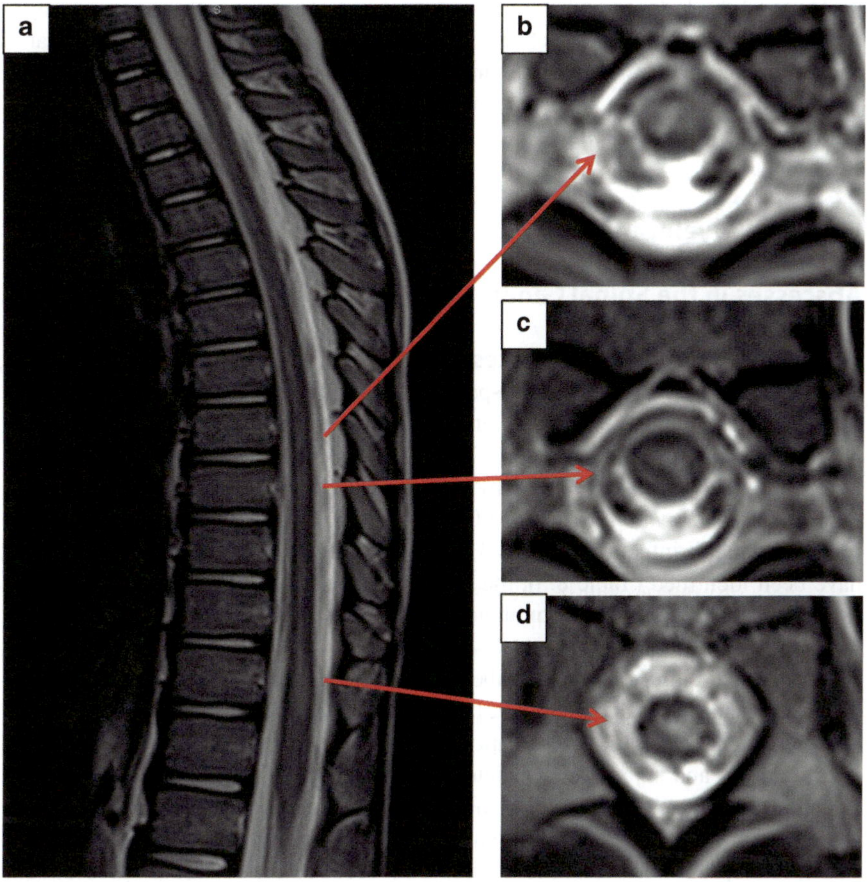

Fig. 8.1 Acute flaccid myelitis in a 3 year old male
Patchy asymmetric grey matter predominant hyperintensity can be seen throughout the spinal cord on sagittal (**a**) and (**b**–**d**) axial T2 sequences

enhancement may evolve later in the disease process [87]. Edema of the spinal cord may also be seen. Neurophysiology may demonstrate a motor neuropathy or neuronopathy in affected limbs, with electromyography changes persisting for a year or more [87].

The pathophysiology of AFM is not completely understood, but is thought to be primarily caused by non-polio enterovirus infection. Prodromal infectious symptoms are ubiquitous, and infectious organisms have been isolated in respiratory secretions or stool in many cases. The most frequently identified micro-organism in patients to date is enterovirus D68, with epidemiological evidence supporting an association between enterovirus D68 outbreaks and AFM clusters [87]. However, CSF PCR and next-generation sequencing studies have typically failed to identify viral organisms in the CNS of affected patients [87, 88].

There is no evidence-based treatment for AFM. Therapy with immunomodulatory or antiviral agents has been instituted in many cases, however it is unclear if any treatment affects the disease course [87]. Complete recovery following AFM is rare. Most patients have persistent motor deficits with muscle atrophy in affected limbs, and some patients may even remain ventilator dependent [87].

Bacterial Myelopathies

Abscesses in the Spinal Canal

Pyogenic Spinal Epidural Abscess

Abscess formation in the epidural space can result from hematogenous, lymphatic or contiguous sources of bacteria or from iatrogenic inoculation during medical procedures in the spinal region. The most common causative organism is *Staphylococcus aureus*, followed by gram-negative bacilli such as *Enterobacter, Klebsiella* and *Pseudomonas* [89, 90]. However, many other bacteria have been implicated in this infection (Table 8.3). Many risk factors for spinal epidural abscess have been identified (Table 8.3), the most important of which is diabetes mellitus [89, 91, 92]. However, in approximately 20% of cases there are no discernable risk factors [93].

The classic clinical triad described with spinal epidural abscess is back pain, fever and neurological deficits [92]. However, the full triad is only present in 10–15% of patients at first presentation [94]. Back pain is present in the vast majority of patients and is reported as acute, focal and severe. The pain may radiate in a radicular manner and the clinician may be able to elicit tenderness to palpation. A septic patient complaining of back pain should alert the physician to the possibility of a spinal epidural abscess. Meningism may occur as the disease progresses. The evolution of clinical symptoms ranges from days to weeks and neurological deficits usually follow other symptoms [94]. Findings on neurological examination will vary depending on the location of the abscess; from tetraparesis with cervical abscesses to cauda equina syndrome with lower lumbar abscesses.

Table 8.3 Pyogenic spinal epidural abscess: common organisms and risk factors

Causative bacteria	
Staphlyococcus aureus	*Escherichia coli*
Streptococcus	*Klebsiella*
Coagulase negative staphylococci	*Pseudomonas*
Brucella	*Mycobacterium tuberculosis*
Risk factors	
Diabetes mellitus	Recent surgery or procedure in spinal region
HIV	Intravenous drug use
Alcohol abuse	Trauma
Malignancy	Systemic infection (skin, soft tissue, UTI)
Other causes of immunosuppression	Indwelling catheters

Laboratory tests show raised inflammatory markers (C-reactive protein, erythrocyte sedimentation rate) and peripheral leukocytosis. MRI of the whole spine is the investigation of choice to diagnose spinal epidural abscess, as there may be multiple abscesses at different levels [90, 91]. Sensitivity of MRI is greater than 90%. Abscesses are most commonly seen in the thoracic and lumbar spine, specifically at the thoraco-lumbar junction [95]. The abscess is visualized as a T2 hyperintense, T1 hypointense mass in the epidural space, with associated thickening of overlying displaced dura. Post-contrast imaging is important as this demonstrates a rim-enhancing mass [90]. The spinal cord may show edema at the affected level, or there may be evidence of vascular compromise due to compressed or thrombosed vessels (arterial-pattern ischaemia or venous congestion can be seen). There may also be associated diskitis or facet joint infection, and fat-saturated images can be helpful in delineating areas of soft tissue and bone involvement [90, 94]. CSF is not particularly informative in spinal epidural abscess, and should be avoided in most scenarios due to the risk of creating further nidus of infection and the risk of downward spinal coning in cases with complete spinal subarachnoid block above the level of CSF sampling [96]. Instead, the causative organism should be isolated using other means. Positive blood cultures or sampling from another source of infection (e.g. cellulitis) may identify the culprit organism. However, blood cultures are negative in approximately 40% of cases, so direct sampling using CT-guided aspiration should not be delayed in cases where the organism cannot be quickly identified by other means [97]. In patients requiring urgent surgical decompression, microbiological samples can be obtained during the procedure. The decision on whether to withhold antibiotics until after a microbiological sample has been obtained depends on the patient's condition and the urgency of treatment.

In recent years, treatment of spinal epidural abscess has evolved, with approximately 40% of patients now treated by a primary medical approach rather than surgery [95]. Surgery (decompressive laminectomy and drainage) should be considered immediately in patients presenting with neurological deficits, and outcome is best with early intervention [98]. Medical therapy alone has a significant failure rate, with 10%–50% of these patients eventually requiring surgery [98]. Antibiotics are required in all cases, starting with broad-spectrum empiric treatment covering staphylococcus, streptococcus and gram-negative species, which can later be tailored according to culture and sensitivity findings.

Neurological deficits at presentation, older age (over 70 years) and co-morbid diabetes mellitus are predictors of poorer outcome in this patient group [98]. Recovery is particularly poor in patients with spinal cord injury secondary to vascular compromise [89].

Other Sites of Abscess Formation

Spinal intramedullary abscesses are extremely rare but can be a devastating neurological infection. They most frequently occur in association with an unrecognized congenital dermal sinus tract, often presenting in childhood [99, 100]. Intramedullary abscesses can also occur with penetrating trauma/procedure to the spinal canal [101], as a complication of bacterial or fungal meningitis [102, 103], or in association with infective endocarditis [104, 105]. Patients present with localized or radicular back pain and neurological deficits. MRI typically shows a rim-enhancing lesion with associated spinal cord edema [106].

Finally, bacterial infections in structures outside the spinal canal can also lead to compressive myelopathy e.g. diskitis and vertebral osteomyelitis.

Tuberculosis

Neurological complications of *mycobacterium tuberculosis* (TB) infection remain common in the developing world. In the developed world, TB cases predominantly occur in immigrants from regions of endemicity and in higher-risk subpopulations including prisoners, illicit drug users, homeless individuals, patients with HIV and patients treated with anti-TNF therapies [107, 108]. Almost 10,000 cases of TB are reported annually in the US [107].

Pott's Disease

Myelopathy in patients with TB most commonly results from skeletal vertebrae involvement, in the form of Pott's disease (tuberculous spondylitis). The spine is the most frequent location of skeletal TB, with Pott's disease occurring in 1–2% of TB cases [109]. Infection of the vertebrae arises after spread of mycobacteria from an active source (via blood, lymphatics or adjacent lung tissue), or occurs in situ as a result of latent reactivation [110]. Any region of the vertebrae may be involved, but the anterior or central portion of lower thoracic or upper lumbar vertebrae is characteristic [110, 111]. Myelopathy results from direct compression of the spinal cord or vascular compromise (inflammatory arterial thrombosis or venous obstruction). Clinical presentation is insidious, with patients often exhibiting advanced changes on imaging by the time of diagnosis. Back pain, fever and neurological deficits (gait disturbance, leg weakness or sensory changes) are the most frequent presenting symptoms [112–114]. Advanced cases may present with Gibbus deformity, an angulated thoracolumbar kyphosis due to wedge-shaped destruction of vertebral bodies. Involvement of cervical paravertebral regions may result in dysphagia or stridor. Systemic symptoms including fever, weight loss, night sweats and cough are present in approximately half of cases, and pulmonary TB is identified in less than half of patients presenting with Pott's disease [109, 112].

Plain x-ray films remain important for diagnosis in the developing world and may demonstrate loss of vertebral body height, bony erosion, wedge-shaped destruction, kyphosis or associated soft-tissue changes [110]. Computed tomography can identify bony changes with more accuracy and may also identify pulmonary involvement. However, MRI of the entire spine should be the imaging modality of choice in patients with Pott's disease. This allows evaluation of the extent of bone and soft tissue involvement, and assessment of the spinal canal and spinal cord. Multiple non-contiguous vertebrae may be involved or a well-defined paravertebral abscess may be identified. Involvement of the intervertebral disc occurs late in Pott's disease, and sparing of the disc may be helpful in differentiating TB from other pyogenic infections which typically arise from the disc [110]. Increased signal in the spinal cord can be a result of direct compression, or the pattern may suggest arterial compromise (prominent gray matter changes) or venous congestion (edematous lower spinal cord) [110]. Differential diagnosis includes other pyogenic infections, fungal infection, histiocytosis, lymphoma and bony metastases. Ancillary investigations for TB such as Mantoux test, serum interferon-gamma release assays, Ziehl-Neelsen staining or Lowenstein-Jensen culture of respiratory samples should be considered. However, diagnosis may be challenging and bone biopsy is frequently performed to identify caseating granulomas [109]. In addition to systemic anti-TB therapy, surgical decompression is usually required in individuals exhibiting neurological deficits.

Spinal Tuberculous Arachnoiditis

Tuberculous radiculomyelopathy results from inflammation of the arachnoid membrane and exiting nerve roots (spinal arachnoiditis). Spinal arachnoiditis can occur in association with TB meningitis, tuberculous spondylitis, or as the primary CNS TB manifestation [115]. Clinical presentation is characterized by subacute areflexic paralysis, often associated with radicular pain and sphincter disturbance [116]. Most patients present with a syndrome of polyradiculopathy, with less than 15% manifesting with myelitis [116]. Clinical findings may suggest cauda equina syndrome or conus medullaris syndrome. MRI spine demonstrates varying degrees of enhancing arachnoiditis, with possible loculated CSF spaces, cystic changes, clumping of nerve roots or spinal cord inflammation and edema [117, 118]. MRI brain should also be performed to assess for pachymeningitis, hydrocephalus or intracranial tuberculomas. Grossly elevated CSF protein (up to 8 g/L) is characteristic of TB meningitis and arachnoiditis [117]. CSF also demonstrates lymphocytic pleocytosis and low CSF glucose [117].

Other Causes of Myelopathy in TB

Cases of acute transverse myelitis (including longitudinally extensive transverse myelitis) have been reported with TB [119]. Intradural-extramedullary or intramedullary tuberculoma can also cause myelopathy and occur most frequently in the thoracic region; presentation is chronic and patients are usually not systemically unwell [116]. Epidural tuberculous abscess can result in compressive spinal cord injury [120]. Syringomyelia can occur as an early or late complication of TB meningitis or spinal arachnoiditis [121, 122]. TB can also trigger CNS vasculitis which can result in spinal cord infarction [116]. MRI and CSF studies are the cornerstone of diagnosis of CNS complications of TB. It is important to remember that patients with HIV are more likely to have disseminated TB with CNS involvement. Patients with CNS manifestations of TB may require longer courses of anti-TB therapy than patients with other manifestations. The addition of corticosteroids has been demonstrated to improve mortality in patients with TB meningitis [123].

Lyme Disease

Borrelia burgdorferi is transmitted by the Ixodes tick species and infection with the spirochete causes Lyme disease. Lyme disease is endemic in North America (particularly north-east and mid-Atlantic states), Europe (highest incidence in Central and North-Eastern Europe) and Asia (Russia, China, Mongolia and Japan) [124]. An estimated 30,000 people are diagnosed with Lyme disease annually in the US [125], with acute cases occurring in a seasonal manner (highest incidence in spring and summer) [126]. While a tick bite is necessary to acquire the infection, many patients do not report or recall this occurring.

Erythema Migrans is the initial presentation of Lyme infection, and is reported in the majority of patients [127]. EM usually occurs 1–2 weeks after the tick bite and is clinically characterized by single or multiple flat erythematous skin lesions which may be painful, itchy or associated with mild systemic symptoms such as malaise, fever and lymphadenopathy [126]. The rash may have a 'bull's eye' appearance or a clear central punctum, but these features are not always present. If early infection is untreated, Lyme disease may disseminate and result in cardiac, rheumatologic or neurologic involvement.

Neuroborreliosis occurs in around 10% of patients with Lyme disease, and can be divided into early and late manifestations [128]. Spinal cord involvement is uncommon in both phases. The most common early complications are cranial neuritis, lymphocytic meningitis and painful polyradiculitis [126, 129]. Very rarely, involvement of the spinal cord can occur during this phase in the form of acute transverse myelitis, which can be longitudinally extensive or can occur as a focal lesion in association with radiculitis [126, 130, 131]. This extension of radicular inflammation into the spinal cord to cause segmental myelitis has been reported with European subspecies of *Borrelia*. Late complications of Lyme disease (disease duration greater than 6 months) are an area of ongoing debate and some uncertainty, particularly in the case of neurological complications [132–134]. Rare cases of chronic progressive Lyme encephalomyelitis have been suggested with longstanding untreated infection, however there is a relative paucity of recent studies in this field [135–137]. Patients with late CNS complications arising from longstanding untreated Lyme disease demonstrate inflammatory CSF abnormalities and intrathecal production of *Borrelia* specific antibodies [128].

Diagnosis of Lyme disease (with or without neuroborreliosis) is also an area of some contention. Two-tier serologic testing is recommended (screening with enzyme immunoassay or indirect immunofluorescence assay followed by confirmation with reflexive immunoblotting for *Borrelia* IgM and IgG to increase specificity), however these tests may be negative in the earliest stages of infection [138]. Consideration of clinical context is crucial, as even *Borrelia* IgM may persist for years after infection [138]. CSF culture and PCR for *Borrelia* are both low yield, and therefore indirect serological studies remain the mainstay of diagnosis for neurological complications [129]. In Europe, the European Academy of Neurology requires fulfillment of 3 of the following criteria for definite neuroborreliosis, and 2 of 3 for possible neuroborreliosis; [1] neurological symptoms suggestive of neuroborreliosis, [2] CSF pleocytosis, and [3] intrathecal production of *borrelia burgdorferi*-specific antibodies [139]. In the US, which has less heterogeneity of *Borrelia* subspecies, some groups suggest that positive two-tier serology in the context of a characteristic neurological syndrome may be sufficient for diagnosis [138]. Regardless, CSF study should be performed. The vast majority of patients with neuroborreliosis demonstrate lymphocytic pleocytosis, while elevated CSF protein, and positive oligoclonal bands are also common. Intrathecal *Borrelia*-specific antibody production is the most specific test for neuroborreliosis. CSF levels should be compared to serum antibody levels, with ratio >1.0 supportive of intrathecal synthesis rather than passive transfer from serum [138]. MRI may demonstrate a segmental or longitudinally extensive enhancing lesion in cases of acute transverse myelitis (Fig. 8.2).

Treatment of neuroborreliosis should be in accordance with regional guidelines; intravenous ceftriaxone for 2 weeks is a typical recommended treatment, while other options include intravenous penicillin or oral doxycycline [138].

Syphilis

Syphilitic infection is caused by the bacterium *Treponema pallidum*. Almost 30,000 cases of syphilis were reported in the US in 2016 and disease rates have been increasing over the past 15 years, particularly amongst men who have sex with men [140].

T. pallidum is thought to invade the CNS at an early stage of infection, with asymptomatic CSF abnormalities detectable in up to 48% of early syphilis cases [141]. Early or late neurosyphilis can occur in patients who do not clear the organism from the CNS in this early phase (either by immune response or antibiotic treatment) [142]. Neurosyphilis occurs more frequently in patients with syphilis who are HIV-positive than in those who are HIV-negative [141]. Myelopathy as a result of syphilis infection has become rare in the antibiotic era, however it can still occur at any stage in the illness due to a variety of underlying pathologies.

Symptomatic syphilitic meningitis is the most common early CNS manifestation and typically occurs within a year of infection [142]. Spinal cord involvement can occur at this stage in the form of syphilitic meningomyelitis [143–145]. Clinical presentation is with an acute or subacute myelopathic syndrome, with or without concurrent symptoms of meningitis. MRI spine shows a T2 hyperintense lesion in the cord which is often central and longitudinally extensive, associated with cord expansion, and demonstrates areas of focal enhancement [144].

Tabes dorsalis is a late complication of untreated syphilis infection which has become very rare. It usually manifests insidiously 15 to 30 years following initial infection [141]. The first symptom is usually severe 'lightning-like' pains in the limbs or trunk with associated allodynia. Associated Argyll-Robertson pupils demonstrating light-near dissociation are characteristic. Proprioceptive deficits follow and cause sensory ataxia which can result in Charcot joints [141]. Interestingly, Romberg's sign was first described based on findings in patients with tabes dorsalis

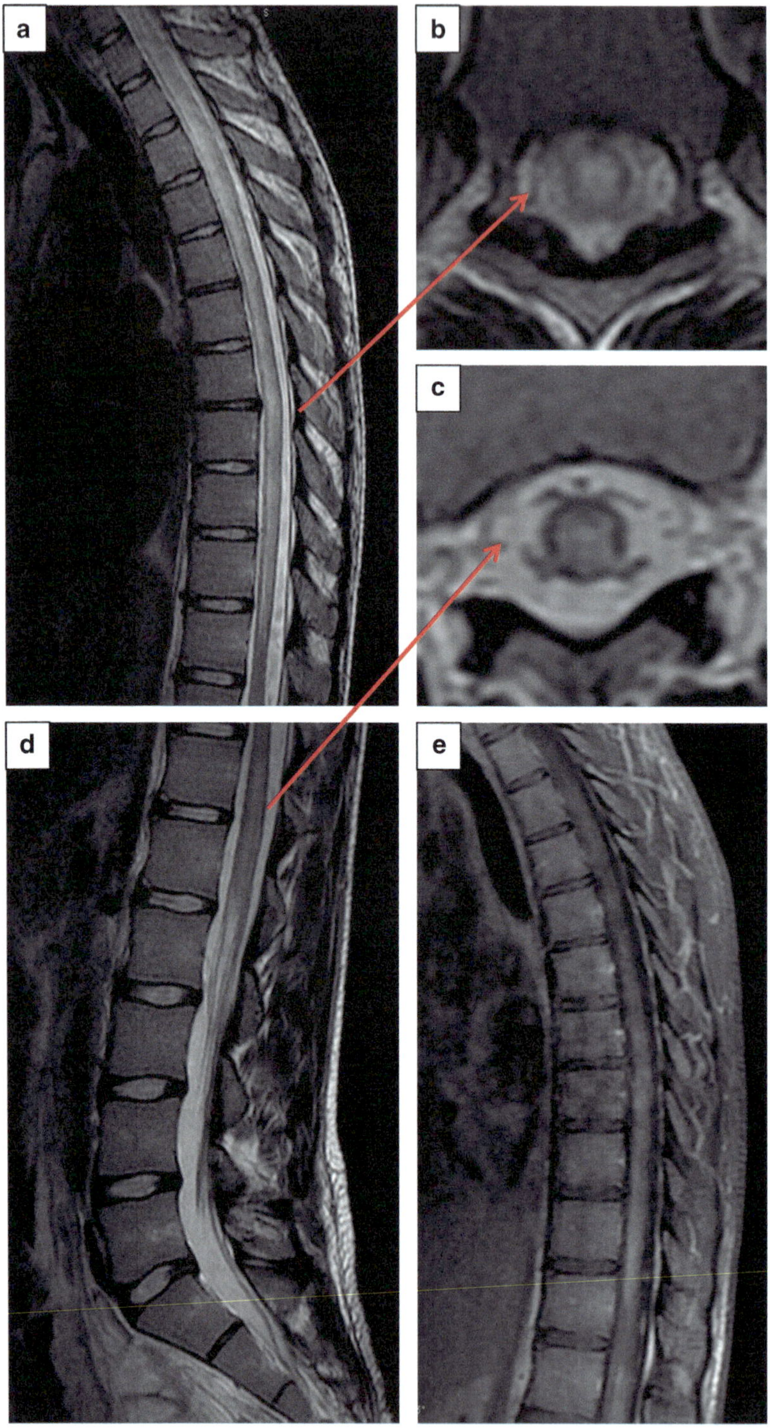
a
b
c
d
e

[146]. Loss of deep pain sensation can be demonstrated with a number of eponymous signs such as Abadie sign (absence of pain on squeezing the Achilles tendon) [141]. Loss of muscle stretch reflexes results in absent lower extremity reflexes. Autonomic impairment manifests with erectile dysfunction, bladder and bowel symptoms [141]. End-stage tabes dorsalis is characterized by painful spastic paraplegia with incontinence. MRI spine in untreated tabes dorsalis may show spinal cord atrophy and high signal in the posterior cord [147].

Myelopathy can also occur due to syphilitic gumma in the spinal canal (intramedullary or extramedullary) [148, 149]. Meningovascular syphilis can cause cerebral stroke, and rarely may cause spinal cord infarction [150].

Diagnosis of neurosyphilis is supported by serological tests and CSF findings in the appropriate clinical context, and there are no broadly accepted diagnostic criteria. Non-treponemal serology tests such as the rapid plasma reagin (RPR) test or the venereal disease research laboratory (VDRL) test detect IgM and IgG antibodies to a cardiolipin-lecithin-cholesterol antigen [142]. However, levels may be undetectable in late neurosyphilis, and by contrast, false positives can occur due to a range of other conditions including pregnancy, autoimmune disease and other infections such as malaria [142, 151]. Treponemal tests such as the *T. pallidum* particle agglutination assay (TPPA) measure IgM and IgG antibodies to the treponemal bacteria [142]. Treponemal test reactivity usually persists after treatment, while non-treponemal titers fall with treatment. Non-treponemal tests are usually used as a screening tool followed by treponemal tests if positive.

CSF findings can be very helpful in diagnosing neurosyphilis. Lymphocytic pleocytosis is seen in most cases, but white cell counts drop as the disease progresses and may even normalize in late disease [142]. There may also be elevated CSF protein, elevated IgG index or positive oligoclonal bands [141]. A positive CSF-VDRL test is very specific for diagnosing neurosyphilis, but less than 70% sensitive [142]. Treponemal tests can be performed on CSF but may be positive in patients with latent or asymptomatic syphilis, and therefore lack specificity in diagnosing neurosyphilis [141]. Overall, physicians should remember that there are multiple treponemal and non-treponemal tests that can be performed on serum and CSF, with varying sensitivity and specificity, so results should be considered in the context of the type of laboratory test used and the clinical scenario.

T. pallidum is highly sensitive to penicillin, and treatment should be instituted upon diagnosis. Guidelines for treatment of neurosyphilis typically suggest intravenous or intramuscular penicillin preparations for 10–21 days [141]. Early neurosyphilis (e.g. syphilitic meningomyelitis) may respond well to treatment, but late complications such as tabes dorsalis may not improve. Non-treponemal serum and

Fig. 8.2 Lyme myelitis in an 18 year old male
Longitudinally extensive central cord hyperintensity is demonstrated on sagittal (**a**, **d**) and axial (**b**, **c**) T2 sequences. Extensive contrast enhancement can be seen in the thoracic spinal cord on sagittal T1 post-gadolinium sequence (**e**)

CSF (e.g. VDRL) titers can be monitored and should fall after treatment, but it can take from 3 months to 5 years to convert to 'seronegativity' [141, 142].

Fungal Myelopathies

Fungal infections of the CNS are uncommon, and most frequently occur in immunocompromised patients.

Cryptococcus neoformans myelitis or myeloradiculitis has been reported in patients with HIV/AIDS, particularly in areas of endemicity, and rarely in immunocompetent hosts [152–154]. Formation of intramedullary or extramedullary cryptococcal granulomas is also possible [155–158], and may occur in association with cryptococcal meningitis or osteomyelitis. CSF should be stained with India ink and can be cultured with Sabouraud dextrose agar to isolate *C. neoformans*. Rapid screening for cryptococcal antigen in the CSF can also be performed, with sensitivity of over 90% in cases of cryptococcal meningitis [159].

CNS aspergillosis (most commonly due to *aspergillus fumigatus*) occurs almost exclusively in patients who are markedly immunocompromised e.g. patients with hematological malignancy, bone marrow or solid organ transplant recipients. CNS infection tends to occur in association with systemic sites of infection such as the lung. Rarely, the spinal cord may be involved in CNS aspergillosis, in the form of necrotizing transverse myelitis with or without associated spinal cord infarction [160]. CSF galactomannan testing has high sensitivity and specificity for CNS aspergillosis [161]. PCR can also be performed for *aspergillus* species in the CSF. CSF fungal cultures are frequently negative [162], and some patients with CNS aspergillosis undergo biopsy for histopathological examination [159].

Fungal infection may also result in spinal cord compromise due to the formation of epidural abscess, vertebral osteomyelitis and spondylodiskitis. These complications have been reported with *aspergillus, cryptococcus, candida, blastomycoses* and *histoplasma* species, among others [163–171], though it should be emphasized that these manifestations are exceedingly rare.

Parasitic Myelopathies

Schistosomiasis

Schistosomiasis is a parasitic infection acquired through contact with fresh water containing larval forms of *Schistosoma* parasites (cerceriae) which penetrate human skin. The disease occurs in Sub-Saharan Africa, Asia (China, Japan and South-East Asia) and South America (particularly Brazil and Venezuela), and different subspecies of the parasite have regional preponderances [172]. However, outbreaks in Europe have also been recognized in recent years and traced to Southern European fresh-water locations such as Corsica [173]. It is estimated that over 200 million people are infected worldwide [174].

Clinical manifestations of acute *schistosoma* infection are most frequently seen in individuals visiting endemic areas with no prior exposure to *schistosoma* species i.e. travelers [175]. A pruritic maculopapular rash at the site of larval penetration, 'cercarial dermatitis', may occur within 24 h of exposure. Acute schistosomiasis occurs several weeks later and manifests with cough, fever, cough, gastrointestinal symptoms and urticarial or angioedema [175]. This phase of disease is thought to be an allergic/toxic reaction to circulating parasites. However, many patients also proceed to chronic infection without any acute symptoms [175]. Chronic infection typically causes inflammation and fibrosis of gastrointestinal, hepatic or urinary tract structures.

Neurological manifestations are rare, but can occur at any stage of schistosomiasis and usually occur without other systemic symptoms. Cerebral involvement is seen with *S. japonicum*, while spinal cord involvement is seen most commonly with *S. mansoni* and less frequently with *S. haematobium* [172]. Myeloradiculopathy is the most frequent presentation, with a minority of patients presenting with either isolated myelitis or cauda equina involvement [172]. Neurological symptoms evolve over less than 2 weeks [176]. Back pain or radicular pain is the most frequent initial symptom, followed by sphincter dysfunction, leg weakness and sensory symptoms. Weakness is usually severe, with most patients unable to walk at clinical nadir. The full complement of motor, sensory and autonomic involvement are seen in the vast majority of patients [176].

CSF examination shows elevated protein and lymphocytic pleocytosis, however eosinophils are also seen in up to 50% of cases and may be a clue to the diagnosis [172, 176]. Oligoclonal bands may be present [177]. MRI typically shows a T2 hyperintense lesion with spinal cord enlargement and nerve root thickening, with associated contrast enhancement in affected regions [172]. Nearly all lesions occur in the lower thoracic or lumbar region, which may be related to venous anastomoses linking the portal venous system (a reservoir for schistosomal parasites) in this spinal region [172].

Establishing a definitive diagnosis can be challenging. *S. mansoni* ova can be identified with stool examination in less than half of cases, or with rectal biopsy which has higher sensitivity [172]. Serological studies are only useful in patients from non-endemic regions i.e. travellers. CSF ELISA for antibodies to *S. mansoni* and CSF PCR for *S. Mansoni* DNA have both been suggested as tests with high specificity [177, 178].

Treatment is with anti-schistosomal therapy such as Praziquantel, and the addition of steroids is probably beneficial (high-dose initially, followed by a taper over at least 2 months) [179]. Most patients have a good functional recovery after treatment. Outcome is worst with delayed diagnosis and with isolated myelitis [172, 180].

Neurocysticercosis

Neurocysticercosis is caused by the larval form of the tapeworm *Taenia solium*, and is the most common parasitic CNS infection [181]. The tapeworm develops in humans after ingestion of viable larval cysts in contaminated pork, resulting in taeniasis [181]. When the tapeworm matures to adulthood, eggs are released in the host's feces. Cysticercosis develops after humans become infected with *T. solium* eggs via the fecal-oral route (typically due to contaminated food or water due to poor hygiene). Eggs penetrate the intestinal wall and travel hematogenously to distant sites – typically the brain, eye, subcutaneous tissues and muscle [181]. This infection is endemic in countries lacking sanitation and clean water supplies, such as South and Central America, Sub-Saharan Africa, China, India and Southeast Asia [181, 182]. Cases in North America and Europe occur predominantly in people who have previously lived in endemic regions [181], although outbreaks have also been reported in those who have never travelled and have been traced to tapeworm carriage in infected food handlers or domestic workers [183].

Neurocysticercosis is an important cause of seizures in endemic countries [184], but other intracranial manifestations include hydrocephalus, meningitis, arachnoiditis, psychiatric disturbance, cranial neuropathies and vasculitis [181]. Spinal cord involvement is rare (occurring in less than 3% of cases of neurocysticercosis) [185] and accompanies basal subarachnoid intracranial disease more frequently than intraparenchymal cerebral disease [186]. Spinal cord involvement without intracranial disease is exceptionally rare [187]. Spinal involvement is most frequently intradural-extramedullary [186, 188], but can also be intramedullary [187, 189].

Clinical presentation is typically with a subacute or chronic myelopathic syndrome or cauda equina syndrome, depending on lesion location [187, 189, 190]. Symptoms may include radicular pain in addition to motor, sensory or sphincter dysfunction [181]. Spinal involvement may also be asymptomatic but detectable on MRI imaging of patients presenting with intracranial manifestations [186].

Diagnosis is difficult, with diagnostic criteria including findings from histology, neuroimaging and clinical/exposure history [191]. Characteristic CNS lesions may be seen on MRI such as demonstration of a high-density scolex (the tapeworm's head) within a cystic lesion, or a 'starry sky' pattern caused by multiple intraparenchymal cysts [181]. CT may demonstrate calcifications in up to half of patients [181]. Spinal MRI findings are usually less specific. Multiple spinal segments are often involved [186], and extramedullary cystic lesions may mimic an arachnoid cyst [190] or Tarlov cyst [192]. Intramedullary involvement is characterized by well-demarcated enhancing cystic lesions with surrounding edema [187]. Subretinal cysticerci can be visualized on ophthalmologic examination in some cases, confirming CNS involvement [191]. Biopsy can be considered for brain lesions, but is not usually undertaken with spinal cord lesions.

CSF shows elevated protein and pleocytosis, with eosinophils frequently present [193]. Antibodies to *T. solium* antigens can be detected in serum or CSF using enzyme-linked immunoelectrotransfer blot (EITB), however seroprevalence may be up to 20% in endemic regions, and EITB testing may give false-negative results in patients with a single CNS lesion or calcified lesions [191]. ELISA testing for cysticercal antigen in serum or CSF is a recently described method which may also be useful [191]. The diagnosis may also be supported by identification of extra-CNS cysticercosis, for example in subcutaneous nodules [191].

Treatment is with cysticidal drugs such as albendazole and praziquantel. However, rapid death of tapeworms can trigger extensive inflammatory response in the CNS, potentially precipitating neurological deterioration, or hydrocephalus in patients with arachnoiditis or intraparenchymal lesions [181]. Furthermore, anti-cysticercal therapy does not affect calcified cysts containing dead parasites. Therefore, the full burden of CNS disease should be assessed carefully prior to consideration of treatment, and steroids should be initiated prior to anti-cysticercal therapy (and continued throughout treatment) [181]. Lastly, parenchymal neurocysticercosis lesions may self-resolve with time, and so there is some debate about whether all patients actually require treatment [194]. Surgery may be required on some spinal cases, to reduce compression of the spinal cord [190, 192].

Case reports of spinal disease suggest good clinical outcomes with both medical and surgical treatment [187, 189, 190, 192].

Other Parasites

Other parasitic causes of myelopathy are extremely rare. Intramedullary *Toxoplasma gondi* lesions have been reported in patients with HIV/AIDS [195–197]. Hydatid cysts resulting from *Echinococcus granulosus* infection can occur in vertebral bodies, paraspinal, extradural or intradural-extramedullary locations resulting in progressive compressive myelopathy or cauda equina syndrome [198–202]. Myelitis or myeloradiculitis can occur with visceral larva migrans due to *ascaris suum* or *toxocara canis* infection [203–205].

Para-infectious Myelitis

Para-infectious myelitis, one of the causes of the syndrome 'acute transverse myelitis', may be provoked by systemic infection with a range of micro-organisms, most of which are not known to cause direct infection of the spinal cord. Para-infectious myelitis is felt to be an immune-mediated process, with hypotheses such as molecular mimicry or superantigen effect proposed as pathophysiologic mechanisms [206]. Numerous micro-organisms have been implicated in triggering this process, including (but not limited to) *mycoplasma pneumonia*, *enteroviruses*, influenza, *adenoviruses*, measles virus, mumps virus, *haemophilus influenza*, *streptococcus pneumonia*, hepatitis A, rubeola, rubella, *legionella* and *bartonella* [206–209]. In many cases the organism is never identified, despite the presence of infectious symptoms prior to myelitis [210].

Patients present with an acute or subacute myelopathy with first neurological symptoms occurring 3–21 days after onset of infectious symptoms such as fever, upper respiratory symptoms, gastroenteritis or flu-like illness [211]. Sensory symptoms are most frequent, followed by motor symptoms and autonomic symptoms. A sensory level is often elicited on examination [210]. Around half of patients experience severe paraplegia at clinical nadir [212]. Reflexes are often depressed in the initial days of neurological illness, but become brisk as the disease process is established.

Non-specific inflammatory markers such as serum C-reactive protein (CRP) or white blood cell counts may be elevated, supporting recent or ongoing systemic infection. MRI typically shows a T2 hyperintense lesion which may be longitudinally extensive and enhances post-contrast. In some cases there may be multiple lesions [210]. CSF typically shows evidence of inflammation with pleocytosis, elevated protein, positive oligoclonal bands or elevated CSF IgG index [210, 211], though these studies may be normal particularly if obtained early on. Cultures, PCR or antibody studies of blood, stool, or nasopharyngeal swabs should be considered in an attempt to identify the infectious agent.

It is important to consider direct causes of infection such as those discussed in this chapter, prior to proceeding with diagnosis and treatment of immune-mediated para-infectious myelitis. Other disorders that cause myelitis (such as neuromyelitis optica, multiple sclerosis or neurosarcoidosis) should be excluded as far as practicable.

Patients are treated with short course high-dose intravenous steroids (e.g. intravenous methylprednisolone 1 g daily for 3–5 days) and/or intravenous immunoglobulin. Plasma exchange can be considered for severe cases or if there is a poor response to initial steroid treatment [212].

Prognosis is varied and difficult to describe, as case series of transverse myelitis often include a wide variety of underlying etiologies [212]. By natural history, para-infectious myelitis should be a monophasic illness. Recurrent or relapsing myelitis should prompt consideration of other etiologies.

Conclusions

A wide range of infections can cause myelopathy through a number of pathological processes including direct infection, spinal cord compression, or para-infectious etiology. Some infections are endemic in certain regions or are seen more frequently in certain populations e.g. the immunocompromised. These factors should be considered when evaluating a patient with a potential infectious cause of myelopathy. Physicians should also pay careful attention to elements of the clinical presentation such as the temporal profile, prodromal symptoms, and type of neurological deficits. MRI and CSF study are the cornerstone of investigation in most cases, while further laboratory tests such as serological or PCR studies should be tailored to the specific micro-organism(s) suspected. In many cases, clinical outcome may improve with prompt diagnosis and treatment, often with specific anti-microbials.

References

1. Petito CK, Navia BA, Cho ES, Jordan BD, George DC, Price RW. Vacuolar myelopathy pathologically resembling subacute combined degeneration in patients with the acquired immunodeficiency syndrome. N Engl J Med. 1985 Apr 04;312(14):874–9.
2. Eyer-Silva WA, Auto I, Pinto JF, Morais-de-Sá CA. Myelopathy in a previously asymptomatic HIV-1-infected patient. Infection. 2001 Mar-Apr;29(2):99–102.
3. Berger J, Sabet A. Infectious myelopathies. Semin Neurol. 2002;22(2):133–42.
4. Berger JR. Infectious myelopathies. Continuum (Minneap Minn). 2011 Aug;17(4):761–75.
5. Oshinaike O, Akinbami A, Ojo O, Ogbera A, Okubadejo N, Ojini F, et al. Influence of age and neurotoxic HAART use on frequency of HIV sensory neuropathy. AIDS Research and Treatment. 2012;2012:1–5.
6. Sartoretti-Schefer S, Blättler T, Wichmann W. Spinal MRI in vacuolar myelopathy, and correlation with histopathological findings. Neuroradiology. 1997 Dec;39(12):865–9.
7. Dhasmana D, Taylor GP. Human T-lymphotropic virus/HIV co-infection: a clinical review. Curr Opin Infect Dis. 2014 Feb;27(1):16–28.
8. Cho TA, Vaitkevicius H. Infectious myelopathies. Continuum (Minneap Minn). 2012 Dec;18(6 Infectious Disease):1351–73.
9. Di Rocco A, Bottiglieri T, Werner P, Geraci A, Simpson D, Godbold J, et al. Abnormal cobalamin-dependent transmethylation in AIDS-associated myelopathy. Neurology. 2002 Mar 12;58(5):730–5.
10. Hamada Y, Watanabe K, Aoki T, Arai N, Honda M, Kikuchi Y, et al. Primary HIV infection with acute transverse myelitis. Intern Med. 2011;50(15):1615–7.
11. Bangham CRM, Araujo A, Yamano Y, Taylor GP. HTLV-1-associated myelopathy/tropical spastic paraparesis. Nat Rev Dis Primers. 2015 June 18;1:15012.
12. Lyons JL. Myelopathy associated with microorganisms. Continuum (Minneap Minn). 2015 Feb;21(1 Spinal Cord Disorders):100–20.
13. Khabbaz RF, Darrow WW, Hartley TM, Witte J, Cohen JB, French J, et al. Seroprevalence and risk factors for HTLV-I/II infection among female prostitutes in the United States. JAMA, 1990 Jan 05. 263(1):60–4.
14. Lehky TJ, Flerlage N, Katz D, Houff S, Hall WH, Ishii K, et al. Human T-cell lymphotropic virus type II-associated myelopathy: clinical and immunologic profiles. Ann Neurol. 1996 Nov;40(5):714–23.
15. Orland JR, Engstrom J, Fridey J, Sacher RA, Smith JW, Nass C, et al. Prevalence and clinical features of HTLV neurologic disease in the HTLV outcomes study. Neurology. 2003 Dec 09;61(11):1588–94.
16. Maloney EM, Cleghorn FR, Morgan OS, Rodgers-Johnson P, Cranston B, Jack N, et al. Incidence of HTLV-I-associated myelopathy/tropical spastic paraparesis (HAM/TSP) in Jamaica and Trinidad. J Acquir Immune Defic Syndr Hum Retrovirol. 1998 Feb 01;17(2):167–70.
17. Akizuki S, Nakazato O, Higuchi Y, Tanabe K, Setoguchi M, Yoshida S, et al. Necropsy findings in HTLV-I associated myelopathy. Lancet. 1987 Jan 17;1(8525):156–7.
18. San-Martin DL, Santos DND, Baptista AF. Pain prevalence, characteristics and associated factors in human T-cell lymphotropic virus type 1 infected patients: a systematic review of the literature. Braz J Infect Dis. 2016 Nov – Dec;20(6):592–8.
19. Malm K, Kjerstadius T, Andersson S. Evaluation of a new screening assay for HTLV-1 and -2 antibodies for large-scale use. J Med Virol. 2010 Sep;82(9):1606–11.
20. Takatani M, Crispim ME, Fraiji N, Stefani MMA, Kiesslich D. Clinical and laboratory features of HTLV-I asymptomatic carriers and patients with HTLV-I-associated myelopathy/tropical spastic paraparesis from the Brazilian Amazon. Rev Inst Med Trop Sao Paulo. 2017 Apr 03;59:e5.

21. Bagnato F, Butman JA, Mora CA, Gupta S, Yamano Y, Tasciyan TA, et al. Conventional magnetic resonance imaging features in patients with tropical spastic paraparesis. J Neurovirol. 2005 Dec;11(6):525–34.
22. Liu W, Nair G, Vuolo L, Bakshi A, Massoud R, Reich DS, et al. In vivo imaging of spinal cord atrophy in neuroinflammatory diseases. Ann Neurol. 2014 Sep;76(3):370–8.
23. Nakagawa M, Nakahara K, Maruyama Y, Kawabata M, Higuchi I, Kubota H, et al. Therapeutic trials in 200 patients with HTLV-I-associated myelopathy/ tropical spastic paraparesis. J Neurovirol. 1996 Oct;2(5):345–55.
24. Berger JR, Houff S. Neurological complications of herpes simplex virus type 2 infection. Arch Neurol. 2008 May 1;65(5):596–600.
25. Nakajima H, Furutama D, Kimura F, Shinoda K, Ohsawa N, Nakagawa T, et al. Herpes simplex virus myelitis: clinical manifestations and diagnosis by the polymerase chain reaction method. Eur Neurol. 1998;39(3):163–7.
26. Wiley CA, VanPatten PD, Carpenter PM, Powell HC, Thal LJ. Acute ascending necrotizing myelopathy caused by herpes simplex virus type 2. Neurology. 1987 Jan 11;37(11):1791.
27. Nardone R, Versace V, Brigo F, Tezzon F, Zuccoli G, Pikija S, et al. Herpes simplex virus type 2 myelitis: case report and review of the literature. Front Neurol. 2017;8:199.
28. Savoldi F, Kaufmann T, Flanagan E, Toledano M, Weinshenker B. Elsberg syndrome: a rarely recognized cause of cauda equina syndrome and lower thoracic myelitis. Neurology: Neuroimmunology & Neuroinflammation. 2017 Jul:4(4).
29. Figueroa D, Isache C, Sands M, Guzman N. An unusual case of acute transverse myelitis caused by HSV-1 infection. IDCases. 2016;5:29–31.
30. Nagel MA, Gilden D. Neurological complications of VZV reactivation. Curr Opin Neurol. 2014 June;27(3):356–60.
31. Steiner I, Kennedy PG, Pachner AR. The neurotropic herpes viruses: herpes simplex and varicella-zoster. Lancet Neurol. 2007 November 1;6(11):1015–28.
32. Manian FA, Kindred M, Fulling KH. Chronic varicella-zoster virus myelitis without cutaneous eruption in a patient with AIDS: report of a fatal case. Clin Infect Dis. 1995;21(4):986–8.
33. Nagel MA, Forghani B, Mahalingam R, Wellish MC, Cohrs RJ, Russman AN, et al. The value of detecting anti-VZV IgG antibody in CSF to diagnose VZV vasculopathy. Neurology. 2007 Mar 27;68(13):1069–73.
34. Takahashi T, Tamura M, Miki K, Yamaguchi M, Kanno A, Nunomura S, et al. Varicella zoster virus myelitis in two elderly patients: diagnostic value of nested polymerase chain reaction assay and antibody index for cerebrospinal fluid specimens. Case Rep Neurol. 2013 Jan;5(1):81–90.
35. Staras SAS, Dollard SC, Radford KW, Flanders WD, Pass RF, Cannon MJ. Seroprevalence of Cytomegalovirus Infection in the United States, 1988–1994. Clin Infect Dis. 2006 Jan 11;43(9):1143–51.
36. Seale H, Raina MacIntyre C, Gidding HF, Backhouse JL, Dwyer DE, Gilbert L. National serosurvey of cytomegalovirus in Australia. Clin Vacc Immunol. 2006 Nov 1;13(11):1181–4.
37. Saraswathy TS, Az-Ulhusna A, Asshikin RN, Suriani S, Zainah S. Seroprevalence of cytomegalovirus infection in pregnant women and associated role in obstetric complications: a preliminary study. Southeast Asian J Trop Med Public Health. 2011 Mar;42(2):320–2.
38. Krech U, Tobin J. A collaborative study of cytomegalovirus antibodies in mothers and young children in 19 countries. Bull World Health Organ. 1981;59(4):605.
39. Cohen BA, McArthur JC, Grohman S, Patterson B, Glass JD. Neurologic prognosis of cytomegalovirus polyradiculomyelopathy in AIDS. Neurology. 1993 Mar;43(3 Pt 1):493–9.
40. Maschke M, Kastrup O, Diener H. CNS manifestations of cytomegalovirus infections: diagnosis and treatment. CNS Drugs. 2002;16(5):303–15.
41. Fux CA, Pfister S, Nohl F, Zimmerli S. Cytomegalovirus-associated acute transverse myelitis in immunocompetent adults. Clin Microbiol Infect. 2003 Dec;9(12):1187–90.
42. Karunarathne S, Govindapala D, Udayakumara Y, Fernando H. Cytomegalovirus associated transverse myelitis in an immunocompetent host with DNA detection in cerebrospinal fluid; a case report. BMC Research Notes. 2012 Jan 1;5(1):364.

43. Scheld WM, Whitley RJ, Marra CM. Infections of the central nervous system. Lippincott Williams & Wilkins; 2014.
44. Jackson A. Human rabies: a 2016 update. Curr Infect Dis Rep. 2016 Nov;18(11):1–6.
45. Hampson K, Coudeville L, Lembo T, Sambo M, Kieffer A, Attlan M, et al. Estimating the global burden of endemic canine rabies. PLoS Negl Trop Dis. 2015 Apr;9(4):e0003709.
46. Hemachudha T, Ugolini G, Wacharapluesadee S, Sungkarat W, Shuangshoti S, Laothamatas J. Human rabies: neuropathogenesis, diagnosis, and management. Lancet Neurol. 2013 May 1;12(5):498–513.
47. Ugolini G. Chapter 10: Rabies virus as a transneuronal tracer of neuronal connections. In: Jackson AC, editor. Advances in virus research. Academic Press; 2011. p. 165–202.
48. Lafon M. Rabies virus receptors. J Neurovirol. 2005 Feb;11(1):82–7.
49. Bauer A, Nolden T, Schröter J, Römer-Oberdörfer A, Gluska S, Perlson E, et al. Anterograde glycoprotein-dependent transport of newly generated rabies virus in dorsal root ganglion neurons. J Virol. 2014 Dec 15;88(24):14172–83.
50. Reiss CS. Neurotropic viral infections. Cambridge University Press; 2008.
51. Mitrabhakdi E, Shuangshoti S, Wannakrairot P, Lewis RA, Susuki K, Laothamatas J, et al. Difference in neuropathogenetic mechanisms in human furious and paralytic rabies. J Neurol Sci. 2005 Nov 15;238, 3(1–2):–10.
52. Desai RV, Jain V, Singh P, Singhi S, Radotra BD. Radiculomyelitic rabies: can MR imaging help? AJNR Am J Neuroradiol. 2002 Apr;23(4):632–4.
53. Kalita J, Bhoi SK, Bastia JK, Lashkar S, Mahadevan A, Misra UK. Paralytic rabies: MRI findings and review of literature. Neurol India. 2014 Nov–Dec;62(6):662–4.
54. Bryceson ADM, Greenwood BM, Warrell DA, Davidson NM, Pope HM, Lawrie JH, et al. Demonstration during life of rabies antigen in humans. J Infect Dis. 1975 Jan 01;131(1):71–4.
55. Lyons J, McArthur J. Emerging infections of the central nervous system. Curr Infect Dis Rep. 2013 Dec;15(6):576–82.
56. Smithburn KC, Hughes TP, Burke AW, Paul JH. A neurotropic virus isolated from the blood of a native of Uganda. American Journal of Tropical Medicine. 1940;20:471–2.
57. Sejvar JJ. West Nile virus: an historical overview. Ochsner J. 2003;5(3):6–10.
58. Centers for Disease Control and Prevention. West Nile virus, cumulative data 1999–2016; 2017. Available at https://www.cdc.gov/westnile/statsmaps/cumMapsData.html. Accessed 24 Oct 2017
59. WHO GIDEON (Global Infectious Diseases and Epidemiology Online). West Nile fever; 2017. Available at https://www.gideononline.com/cases/westnilefever/. Accessed 24 Oct 2017
60. Sejvar JJ. Clinical manifestations and outcomes of West Nile virus infection. Viruses. 2014 Feb;6(2):606–23.
61. Sejvar JJ, Bode AV, Marfin AA, Campbell GL, Ewing D, Mazowiecki M, et al. West Nile virus-associated flaccid paralysis. Emerging Infect Dis. 2005 Jul;11(7):1021–7.
62. Tyler KL, Pape J, Goody RJ, Corkill M, Kleinschmidt-DeMasters BK. CSF findings in 250 patients with serologically confirmed West Nile virus meningitis and encephalitis. Neurology. 2006 Feb 14;66(3):361–5.
63. Sambri V, Capobianchi MR, Cavrini F, Charrel R, Donoso-Mantke O, Escadafal C, et al. Diagnosis of West Nile virus human infections: overview and proposal of diagnostic protocols considering the results of external quality assessment studies. Viruses. 2013 Sept 25;5(10):2329–48.
64. Samuel MA, Diamond MS. Pathogenesis of West Nile virus infection: a balance between virulence, innate and adaptive immunity, and viral evasion. J Virol. 2006 Oct;80(19):9349–60.
65. Petropoulou KA, Gordon SM, Prayson RA, Ruggierri PM. West Nile virus meningoencephalitis: MR imaging findings. AJNR Am J Neuroradiol. 2005 Sep;26(8):1986–95.
66. Maramattom BV, Philips G, Sudheesh N, Arunkumar G. Acute flaccid paralysis due to West nile virus infection in adults: a paradigm shift entity. Ann Indian Acad Neurol. 2014 Jan;17(1):85–8.

67. Ali M, Safriel Y, Sohi J, Llave A, Weathers S. West Nile virus infection: MR imaging findings in the nervous system. AJNR Am J Neuroradiol. 2005 Feb;26(2):289–97.
68. Shimoni Z, Bin H, Bulvik S, Niven M, Hazzan R, Mendelson E, et al. The clinical response of West Nile virus neuroinvasive disease to intravenous immunoglobulin therapy. Clin Pract. 2012 Jan 27;2(1)
69. Haley M, Retter AS, Fowler D, Gea-Banacloche J, O'Grady NP. The role for intravenous immunoglobulin in the treatment of West Nile virus encephalitis. Clin Infect Dis. 2003 Sep 15;37(6):88.
70. Ben-Nathan D, Gershoni-Yahalom O, Samina I, Khinich Y, Nur I, Laub O, et al. Using high titer West Nile intravenous immunoglobulin from selected Israeli donors for treatment of West Nile virus infection. BMC Infect Dis. 2009 Feb 17;9:18.
71. Duffy MR, Chen T, Hancock WT, Powers AM, Kool JL, Lanciotti RS, et al. Zika Virus outbreak on Yap Island, Federated States of Micronesia. New England Journal of Medicine. 2009 June 11;360(24):2536–43.
72. Muñoz L, Barreras P, Pardo C. Zika Virus – associated neurological disease in the adult: Guillain–Barré syndrome, encephalitis, and myelitis. Semin Reprod Med. 2016 Sep 9;34(5):273–9.
73. Mécharles S, Herrmann C, Poullain P, Tran T, Deschamps N, Mathon G, et al. Acute myelitis due to Zika virus infection. The Lancet. 2016 April 02;387(10026):1481.
74. da Silva IRF, Frontera JA, de Filippis AMB, do Nascimento OJM. Neurologic complications associated with the Zika Virus in Brazilian adults. JAMA Neurol. 2017 Oct 01;74(10):1190–8.
75. Carod-Artal FJ, Wichmann O, Farrar J, Gascón J. Neurological complications of dengue virus infection. Lancet Neurol. 2013 Sept 01;12(9):906–19.
76. Kunishige M, Mitsui T, Tan BH, Leong HN, Takasaki T, Kurane I, et al. Preferential gray matter involvement in dengue myelitis. Neurology. 2004 Nov 23;63(10):1980–1.
77. Solomon T, Dung NM, Kneen R, Gainsborough M, Vaughn DW, Khanh VT. Japanese encephalitis. J Neurol Neurosurg Psych. 2000 April 01;68(4):405–15.
78. Taba P, Schmutzhard E, Forsberg P, Lutsar I, Ljøstad U, Mygland Å, et al. EAN consensus review on prevention, diagnosis and management of tick-borne encephalitis. Eur J Neurol. 2017 Oct;24(10):e61.
79. Polio Global Eradication Initiative. Polio now; 2017. Available at: http://polioeradication.org/polio-today/polio-now/this-week/. Accessed 5 Jan 2018
80. Howard RS. Poliomyelitis and the postpolio syndrome. BMJ. 2005 Jun 04;330(7503):1314–8.
81. Howard RS. Poliomyelitis. In: Hilton-Jones D, Turner MR, editors. Oxford textbook of neuromuscular disorders. Oxford University Press; 2014. p. 51–7.
82. Haq A, Wasay M. Magnetic resonance imaging in poliomyelitis. Arch Neurol. 2006 May 01;63(5):778.
83. Ruggieri V, Paz MI, Peretti MG, Rugilo C, Bologna R, Freire C, et al. Enterovirus D68 infection in a cluster of children with acute flaccid myelitis, Buenos Aires, Argentina, 2016. Eur J Paediatr Neurol. 2017 Nov;21(6):884–90.
84. Andersen EW, Kornberg AJ, Freeman JL, Leventer RJ, Ryan MM. Acute flaccid myelitis in childhood: a retrospective cohort study. Eur J Neurol. 2017 August 1;24(8):1077–83.
85. Hübner J, Kruse B, Christen HJ, Weidenmann J, Weiner V, Schöne-Bake JC, et al. Acute flaccid myelitis in German children in 2016-the return of polio? Dtsch Arztebl Int. 2017 August;114(33–34):557.
86. Messacar K, Schreiner TL, Maloney JA, Wallace A, Ludke J, Oberste MS, et al. A cluster of acute flaccid paralysis and cranial nerve dysfunction temporally associated with an outbreak of enterovirus D68 in children in Colorado, USA. Lancet. 2015 Apr 25;385(9978):1662–71.
87. Messacar K, Schreiner TL, Van Haren K, Yang M, Glaser CA, Tyler KL, et al. Acute flaccid myelitis: a clinical review of US cases 2012–2015. Ann Neurol. 2016 Sep;80(3):326–38.
88. Sejvar JJ, Lopez AS, Cortese MM, Leshem E, Pastula DM, Miller L, et al. Acute flaccid myelitis in the United States, August–December 2014: results of nationwide surveillance. Clin Infect Dis. 2016 Sept 15;63(6):737–45.

89. Roos KL. Bacterial infections of the central nervous system. Continuum: Lifelong Learning in Neurology. 2015 Dec 01;21(6, Neuroinfectious Disease):1679–91.
90. Tali ET, Oner AY, Koc AM. Pyogenic spinal infections. Neuroimaging Clinics of North America. 2015 May 1;25(2):193–208.
91. Bond A, Manian FA. Spinal epidural abscess: a review with special emphasis on earlier diagnosis. BioMed Research International. 2016 Jan 1;2016:1–6.
92. Alerhand S, Wood S, Long B, Koyfman A. The time-sensitive challenge of diagnosing spinal epidural abscess in the emergency department. Intern Emerg Med. 2017 Dec;12(8):1179–83.
93. Patel AR, Alton TB, Bransford RJ, Lee MJ, Bellabarba CB, Chapman JR. Spinal epidural abscesses: risk factors, medical versus surgical management, a retrospective review of 128 cases. The Spine Journal. 2014 February 1;14(2):326–30.
94. Sendi P, Bregenzer T, Zimmerli W. Spinal epidural abscess in clinical practice. QJM. 2008 Jan 01;101(1):1–12.
95. Arko L, Quach E, Nguyen V, Chang D, Sukul V, Kim B. Medical and surgical management of spinal epidural abscess: a systematic review. Neurosurg Focus. 2014 Aug;37(2):E4.
96. Hollis PH, Malis LI, Zappulla RA. Neurological deterioration after lumbar puncture below complete spinal subarachnoid block. J Neurosurg. 1986 Feb;64(2):253–6.
97. Curry WT, Hoh BL, Amin-Hanjani S, Eskandar EN. Spinal epidural abscess: clinical presentation, management, and outcome. Surg Neurol. 2005;63(4):371. discussion 371
98. Suppiah S, Meng Y, Fehlings MG, Massicotte EM, Yee A, Shamji MF. How best to manage the spinal epidural abscess? A current systematic review. World Neurosurg. 2016 Sep;93:20–8.
99. Kanaheswari Y, Lai C, Raja Lope RJ, Azizi AB, Zulfiqar MA. Intramedullary spinal cord abscess: the result of a missed congenital dermal sinus. J Paediatr Child Health. 2015 Feb;51(2):223–5.
100. Papaevangelou G, Tsitsopoulos PP, Flaris N, Iliadis C, Tsonidis C. Dermal sinus tract of the thoracic spine presenting with intramedullary abscess and cranial nerve deficits. Pediatr Neurosurg. 2015;50(6):339–43.
101. da Silva PSL, de Souza Loduca RD. Intramedullary spinal cord abscess as complication of lumbar puncture: a case-based update. Childs Nerv Syst. 2013 July;29(7):1061–8.
102. Vo DT, Cravens GF, Germann RE. Streptococcus pneumoniae meningitis complicated by an intramedullary abscess: a case report and review of the literature. J Med Case Rep. 2016 Dec;10(1)
103. Bajema KL, Dalesandro MF, Fredricks DN, Ramchandani M. Disseminated coccidioidomycosis presenting with intramedullary spinal cord abscesses: management challenges. Med Mycol Case Rep. 2017 Mar;15:1–4.
104. Fernández-Ruiz M, López-Medrano F, García-Montero M, Hornedo-Muguiro J, Aguado J. Intramedullary cervical spinal cord abscess by viridans group streptococcus secondary to infective endocarditis and facilitated by previous local radiotherapy. Intern Med. 2009;48(1):61–4.
105. Arnáiz-García ME, González-Santos JM, López-Rodriguez J, Dalmau-Sorli MJ, Bueno-Codoñer M, Arévalo-Abascal A. Intramedullary cervical abscess in the setting of aortic valve endocarditis. Asian Cardiovasc Thorac Ann. 2015 Jan;23(1):64–6.
106. Dörflinger-Hejlek E, Kirsch EC, Reiter H, Opravil M, Kaim AH. Diffusion-weighted MR imaging of intramedullary spinal cord abscess. AJNR Am J Neuroradiol. 2010 Oct;31(9):1651–2.
107. Centers for Disease Control and Prevention Trends in tuberculosis – United States; 2017. Available at https://www.cdc.gov/tb/publications/factsheets/statistics/tbtrends.htm. Accessed 20 Nov 2017
108. Xie X, Li F, Chen J, Wang J. Risk of tuberculosis infection in anti-TNF-α biological therapy: from bench to bedside. Journal of Microbiology, Immunology and Infection. 2014 August 1;47(4):268–74.
109. Schlesinger N, Lardizabal A, Rao J, Rao J, McDonald R. Tuberculosis of the spine: experience in an inner city hospital. J Clin Rheumatol. 2005 Feb;11(1):17–20.

110. Kilborn T, van Rensburg PJ, Candy S. Pediatric and adult spinal tuberculosis: imaging and pathophysiology. Neuroimaging Clinics of North America. 2015 May 1;25(2):209–31.
111. Hogan JI, Hurtado RM, Nelson SB. Mycobacterial musculoskeletal infections. Infectious Disease Clinics of North America. 2017 June 1;31(2):369–82.
112. Johansen IS, Nielsen SL, Hove M, Kehrer M, Shakar S, Wøyen AVT, et al. Characteristics and clinical outcome of bone and joint tuberculosis from 1994 to 2011: a retrospective register-based study in Denmark. Clin Infect Dis. 2015 Aug 15;61(4):554–62.
113. Turgut M. Spinal tuberculosis (Pott's disease): its clinical presentation, surgical management, and outcome. A survey study on 694 patients. Neurosurg Rev. 2001 Apr;24(1):8–13.
114. Moghtaderi A, Alavi-Naini R, Rahimi-Movaghar V. Tuberculous myelopathy: current aspects of neurologic sequels in the southeast of Iran. Acta Neurol Scand. 2006 Apr;113(4):267–72.
115. Hernández-Albújar S, Arribas JR, Royo A, González-García JJ, Peña JM, Vázquez JJ. Tuberculous radiculomyelitis complicating tuberculous meningitis: case report and review. Clin Infect Dis. 2000 June 01;30(6):915–21.
116. Garg RK, Malhotra HS, Gupta R. Spinal cord involvement in tuberculous meningitis. Spinal Cord, 2015 Sep 1. 53(9):649.
117. Abdelmalek R, Kanoun F, Kilani B, Tiouiri H, Zouiten F, Ghoubantini A, et al. Tuberculous meningitis in adults: MRI contribution to the diagnosis in 29 patients. International Journal of Infectious Diseases. 2006 September 1;10(5):372–7.
118. Srivastava T, Kochar D. Asymptomatic spinal arachnoiditis in patients with tuberculous meningitis. Neuroradiology. 2003 Oct;45(10):727–9.
119. Sahu SK, Giri S, Gupta N. Longitudinal extensive transverse myelitis due to tuberculosis: a report of four cases. J Postgrad Med. 2014 Oct–Dec;60(4):409–12.
120. Metta H, Corti M, Redini L, Yampolsky C, Schtirbu R. Spinal epidural abscess due to Mycobacterium tuberculosis in a patient with AIDS: case report and review of the literature. Brazilian Journal of Infectious Diseases. 2006 Apr 1;10(2):146–8.
121. Kaynar MY, Koçer N, Gençosmanoğlu BE, Hancı M. Syringomyelia – as a late complication of tuberculous meningitis. Acta Neurochir. 2000 Aug;142(8):935–9.
122. Daif AK, al Rajeh S, Ogunniyi A, al Boukai A, al Tahan A. Syringomyelia developing as an acute complication of tuberculous meningitis. Can J Neurol Sci. 1997 Feb;24(1):73–6.
123. Prasad K, Singh MB, Ryan H. Corticosteroids for managing tuberculous meningitis. Cochrane Database Syst Rev. 2016;4:CD002244.
124. Mead PS. Epidemiology of Lyme disease. Infectious Disease Clinics of North America. 2015 June 1;29(2):187–210.
125. Nelson C, Saha S, Kugeler K, Delorey M, Shankar M, Hinckley A, et al. Incidence of clinician-diagnosed Lyme disease, United States, 2005–2010. Emerg Infect Dis. 2015;21(9):1625–31. https://doi.org/10.3201/eid2109.150417.
126. Marques AR. Lyme neuroborreliosis. Continuum: Lifelong Learning in Neurology. 2015 Dec 01;21(6, Neuroinfectious Disease):1729–44.
127. Allen HB, Vin H. Lyme disease: beyond erythema migrans. Journal of Clinical & Experimental Dermatology Research. 2016;7(2)
128. Koedel U, Pfister H. Lyme neuroborreliosis. Curr Opin Infect Dis. 2017 Feb;30(1):101–7.
129. Koedel U, Fingerle V, Pfister H. Lyme neuroborreliosis-epidemiology, diagnosis and management. Nat Rev Neurol. 2015 Aug;11(8):446.
130. Bigi S, Aebi C, Nauer C, Bigler S, Steinlin M. Acute transverse myelitis in Lyme neuroborreliosis. Infection. 2010 Oct 1;38(5):413–6.
131. Rousseau JJ, Lust C, Zangerle PF, Bigaignon G. Acute transverse myelitis as presenting neurological feature of Lyme disease. Lancet. 1986 Nov 22;2(8517):1222–3.
132. Halperin JJ. Chronic Lyme disease: misconceptions and challenges for patient management. Infection and Drug Resistance. 2015;8:119–28.
133. Ballantyne C. The chronic debate over Lyme disease. Nature Medicine. 2008 Nov 01;14(11):1135.
134. Rowe PM. Chronic Lyme disease: the debate goes on. The Lancet. 2000 April 22;355(9213):1436.

135. Halperin JJ. Nervous system Lyme disease. Curr Infect Dis Rep. 2015 Jan;17(1):445.
136. Oschmann P, Dorndorf W, Hornig C, Schäfer C, Wellensiek HJ, Pflughaupt KW. Stages and syndromes of neuroborreliosis. J Neurol. 1998 May;245(5):262–72.
137. Logigian EL, Kaplan RF, Steere AC. Chronic neurologic manifestations of Lyme disease. N Engl J Med. 1990;323(21):1438–44.
138. Moore A, Nelson C, Molins C, Mead P, Schriefer M. Current guidelines, common clinical pitfalls, and future directions for laboratory diagnosis of Lyme disease. United States Emerging Infect Dis. 2016;07:22(7).
139. Mygland A, Ljøstad U, Fingerle V, Rupprecht T, Schmutzhard E, Steiner I. EFNS guidelines on the diagnosis and management of European Lyme neuroborreliosis. Eur J Neurol. 2010 Jan;17(1):4.
140. Centers for Disease Control and Prevention Syphilis – 2016 STD surveillance report. 10-17T05:35:17Z; 2017
141. Berger JR, Dean D. Neurosyphilis. In: Biller J, Ferro JM, editors. Handbook of clinical neurology. Elsevier; 2014. p. 1461–72.
142. Marra CM. Neurosyphilis. Continuum: Lifelong Learning in Neurology. 2015 Dec 01;21(6, Neuroinfectious Disease):1714–28.
143. Tohge R, Shinoto Y, Takahashi M. Longitudinally extensive transverse myelitis and optic neuropathy associated with syphilitic meningomyelitis and human immunodeficiency virus infection: a case report and review of the literature. Intern Med. 2017;56(15):2067–72.
144. Chilver-Stainer L, Fischer U, Hauf M, Fux CA, Sturzenegger M. Syphilitic myelitis: rare, nonspecific, but treatable. Neurology. 2009 Feb 17;72(7):673–5.
145. Siu G. Syphilitic meningomyelitis. J Am Osteopath Assoc. 2017 Dec 01;117(10):671.
146. Pearce JMS. Romberg and his sign. Eur Neurol. 2005;53(4):210–3.
147. Pandey S. Magnetic resonance imaging of the spinal cord in a man with tabes dorsalis. J Spinal Cord Med. 2011 Nov;34(6):609–11.
148. Yang C, Li G, Fang J, Liu H, Yang B, Xu Y. Spinal intramedullary syphilitic gumma: an unusual presentation of neurosyphilis. World Neurosurgery. 2016 November 1;95(Supplement C):622.e23.
149. Zhou H, Zhan R, Chen M, Cao F, Zheng X. Solitary spinal dural syphilis granuloma mimicking a spinal meningioma. Turk Neurosurg. 2014;24(2):288–91.
150. Terry PM, Glancy GR, Graham A. Meningovascular syphilis of the spinal cord presenting with incomplete Brown-Séquard syndrome: case report. Genitourin Med. 1989 Jun;65(3):189–91.
151. Maves RC, Dean K, Gadea N, Halsey ES, Graf PCF, Lescano AG. False-positive rapid plasma reagin testing in patients with acute Plasmodium vivax malaria: a case control study. Travel Med Infect Dis. 2014 May–Jun;12(3):268–73.
152. Gumbo T, Hakim JG, Mielke J, Siwji S, Just-Nübling G, Ismail A. Cryptococcus myelitis: atypical presentation of a common infection. Clin Infect Dis. 2001 Apr 15;32(8):1235–6.
153. Dromer F, Moulignier A, Dupont B, Guého E, Baudrimont M, Improvisi L, et al. Myeloradiculitis due to cryptococcus curvatus in AIDS. AIDS. 1995 Apr;9(4):395–6.
154. Rai AK, Synmon B, Basumatary LJ, Das M, Goswami M, Kayal AK. Cryptococcal myelitis: a rare manifestation in immunocompetent patients. Neurol India. 2014 May–Jun;62(3):321–2.
155. Su MC, Ho WL, Chen JH. Intramedullary cryptococcal granuloma of spinal cord: a case report. Zhonghua Yi Xue Za Zhi (Taipei). 1994 Jan;53(1):58–61.
156. Ramamurthi B, Anguli VC. Intramedullary cryptococcic granuloma of the spinal cord. Journal of Neurosurgery. 1954 November 1;11(6):622–4.
157. Asanuma Y, Fujimoto H, Nakabayashi H, Akeda K, Asanuma K, Tanaka M, et al. Extradural cryptococcoma at the sacral spine without bone involvement in an immunocompetent patient. J Orthop Sci. 2014;19(6):1040.
158. Rao SB, Rao KS, Dinakar I. Spinal extradural cryptococcal granuloma. A case report. Neurol India. 1970 Sep;18(3):192–3.
159. Murthy JMK, Sundaram C. Fungal infections of the central nervous system. In: Biller J, Ferro JM, editors. Handbook of clinical neurology. Elsevier; 2014. p. 1383–401.

160. Kleinschmidt-DeMasters BK. Central nervous system aspergillosis: a 20-year retrospective series. Hum Pathol. 2002 Jan;33(1):116–24.
161. Chong GM, Maertens JA, Lagrou K, Driessen GJ, Cornelissen JJ, Rijnders BJA. Diagnostic performance of galactomannan antigen testing in cerebrospinal fluid. J Clin Microbiol. 2016 Feb;54(2):428–31.
162. Sonneville R, Magalhaes E, Meyfroidt G. Central nervous system infections in immunocompromised patients. Current Opinion in Critical Care. 2017 Apr 01;23(2):128–33.
163. N'dri Oka D, Varlet G, Kakou M, Zunon-Kipre Y, Broalet E, Ba ZV. Spondylodiscitis due to Histoplasma duboisii. Report of two cases and review of the literature. Neurochirurgie. 2001 Sep;47(4):431–4.
164. Ozdemir N, Celik L, Oğuzoğlu S, Yildirim L, Bezircioğlu H. Cervical vertebral osteomyelitis and epidural abscess caused by Candida albicans in a patient with chronic renal failure. Turk Neurosurg. 2008 Apr;18(2):207–10.
165. Chia SL, Tan BH, Tan CT, Tan SB. Candida spondylodiscitis and epidural abscess: management with shorter courses of anti-fungal therapy in combination with surgical debridement. J Infect. 2005 Jul;51(1):17–23.
166. Garbino J, Schnyder I, Lew D, Bouchuiguir-Wafa K, Rohner P. An unusual cause of vertebral osteomyelitis: Candida species. Scand J Infect Dis. 2003;35(4):288–91.
167. Dimar JR, Puno RM, Nowacki MR, Carreon LY. Surgery for blastomycosis of the spine. Am J Orthop. 2014 Nov;43(11):266.
168. Makary CA, Roberts TD, Wetmore SJ. Disseminated blastomycosis presenting as mastoiditis and epidural abscess. W V Med J. 2014 Jan-Feb;110(1):46–7.
169. Gupta SK, Chhabra R, Sharma BS, Das A, Khosla VK. Vertebral cryptococcosis simulating tuberculosis. Br J Neurosurg. 2003 Dec;17(6):556–9.
170. Raj KA, Srinivasamurthy BC, Nagarajan K, Sinduja MGI. A rare case of spontaneous aspergillus spondylodiscitis with epidural abscess in a 45-year-old immunocompetent female. J Craniovertebr Junction Spine. 2013 Jul;4(2):82–4.
171. Jiang Z, Wang Y, Jiang Y, Xu Y, Meng B. Vertebral osteomyelitis and epidural abscess due to Aspergillus nidulans resulting in spinal cord compression: case report and literature review. J Int Med Res. 2013 Apr;41(2):502–10.
172. Coyle CM. Chapter 22 - schistosomiasis of the nervous system. In: Garcia HH, Tanowitz HB, Del Brutto OH, editors. Handbook of clinical neurology. Elsevier; 2013. p. 271–81.
173. Boissier J, Moné H, Mitta G, Bargues MD, Molyneux D, Mas-Coma S. Schistosomiasis reaches Europe. The Lancet Infectious Diseases. 2015 July 1;15(7):757–8.
174. Centers for Disease Control and Prevention. Neglected tropical diseases: the burden of schistosomiasis; 2011. Available at https://www.cdc.gov/globalhealth/ntd/diseases/schisto_burden.html. Accessed 18 Dec 2017
175. Jauréguiberry S, Paris L, Caumes E. Acute schistosomiasis, a diagnostic and therapeutic challenge. Clinical Microbiology and Infection. 2010 March 1;16(3):225–31.
176. Ferrari TCA, Moreira PRR, Cunha AS. Spinal cord schistosomiasis: a prospective study of 63 cases emphasizing clinical and therapeutic aspects. Journal of Clinical Neuroscience. 2004 April 1;11(3):246–53.
177. Pammenter MD, Haribhai HC, Epstein SR, Rossouw EJ, Bhigjee AI, Bill PLA. The value of immunological approaches to the diagnosis of schistosomal myelopathy. The American Journal of Tropical Medicine and Hygiene. 1991 March 01;44(3):329–35.
178. Bruscky IS, de Melo FL, de Medeiros ZM, Albuquerque FF, Wanderley LB, da Cunha-Correia C. Nested polymerase chain reaction in cerebrospinal fluid for diagnosing spinal cord schistosomiasis: a promising method. J Neurol Sci. 2016 Jul 15;366:87–90.
179. Silva LCS, Maciel PE, Ribas JGR, Souza-Pereira SR, Antunes CM, Lambertucci JR. Treatment of schistosomal myeloradiculopathy with praziquantel and corticosteroids and evaluation by magnetic resonance imaging: a longitudinal study. Clin Infect Dis. 2004 Dec 01;39(11):1618–24.
180. Alsomaili M, Abulaban AA. Spinal cord schistosomiasis: two different outcomes. Case Reports in Neurology. 2016 Jan;8(1):47–52.

181. Gripper LB, Welburn SC. Neurocysticercosis infection and disease – a review. Acta Trop. 2017 Feb;166:218–24.
182. Webb CM, White AC. Update on the diagnosis and management of neurocysticercosis. Curr Infect Dis Rep. 2016 Dec;18(12):44.
183. Schantz PM, Moore AC, Muñoz JL, Hartman BJ, Schaefer JA, Aron AM, et al. Neurocysticercosis in an orthodox Jewish community in New York City. N Engl J Med. 1992 Sep 03;327(10):692–5.
184. Ndimubanzi PC, Carabin H, Budke CM, Nguyen H, Qian Y, Rainwater E, et al. A systematic review of the frequency of neurocyticercosis with a focus on people with epilepsy. PLoS Negl Trop Dis. 2010 Nov 02;4(11):e870.
185. Canelas HM, Ricciardi-Cruz O, Escalante AD. Cysticercosis of the nervous system: less frequent clinical forms III, spinal cord forms. Arq Neuropsiquiatr. 1963 Jun;21:77–86.
186. Callacondo D, Garcia HH, Gonzales I, Escalante D, Nash TE. High frequency of spinal involvement in patients with basal subarachnoid neurocysticercosis. Neurology. 2012 May 01;78(18):1394–400.
187. Datta SGS, Mehta R, Macha S, Tripathi S. Primary spinal intramedullary neurocysticercosis: a report of 3 cases. World Neurosurg. 2017 Sep;105:1037.e7.
188. Jongwutiwes U, Yanagida T, Ito A, Kline SE. Isolated intradural-extramedullary spinal cysticercosis: a case report. J Travel Med. 2011 July 01;18(4):284–7.
189. Salazar Noguera EM, Pineda Sic R, Escoto SF. Intramedullary spinal cord neurocysticercosis presenting as Brown-Séquard syndrome. BMC Neurol. 2015 Jan 16;15:1.
190. Pal A, Biswas C, Ghosh TR, Deb P. A rare case of recurrence of primary spinal neurocysticercosis mimicking an arachnoid cyst. Asian J Neurosurg. 2017 Apr–Jun;12(2):250–2.
191. Del Brutto OH, Nash TE, White AC, Rajshekhar V, Wilkins PP, Singh G, et al. Revised diagnostic criteria for neurocysticercosis. J Neurol Sci. 2017 Jan 15, 372:202–10.
192. Bansal S, Suri A, Sharma MC, Kakkar A. Isolated lumbar intradural extra medullary spinal cysticercosis simulating tarlov cyst. Asian J Neurosurg. 2017 Apr–Jun;12(2):279–82.
193. dos Reis JB, Bei A, Reis-Filho JB, Nasser J. Cerebrospinal fluid in cysticercosis of the brain. Arq Neuropsiquiatr. 1979 Jun;37(2):113–26.
194. García HH, Evans CAW, Nash TE, Takayanagui OM, White AC, Botero D, et al. Current Consensus Guidelines for Treatment of Neurocysticercosis. Clin Microbiol Rev. 2002 Oct 01;15(4):747–56.
195. Agrawal SR, Singh V, Ingale S, Jain AP. Toxoplasmosis of spinal cord in acquired immunodeficiency syndrome patient presenting as paraparesis: a rare entity. J Glob Infect Dis. 2014 Oct;6(4):178–81.
196. García-García C, Castillo-Álvarez F, Azcona-Gutiérrez JM, Herraiz MJ, Ibarra V, Oteo JA. Spinal cord toxoplasmosis in human immunodeficiency virus infection/acquired immunodeficiency syndrome. Infect Dis (Lond). 2015 May;47(5):277–82.
197. Pérez-Lazo G, Castillo-Córdova R, Maquera-Afaray J. Intramedullary toxoplasmosis in HIV-tuberculosis co-infected patient. Rev Chil Infectol. 2017 Feb;34(1):77–80.
198. Sridharan S, Jagan Narayana GS, Chidambaram K, Jayachandiran AP. Primary Paraspinal Hydatidosis causing acute paraplegia. J Neurosci Rural Pract. 2017 Jul–Sep;8(3):472–4.
199. Gennari A, Almairac F, Litrico S, Albert C, Marty P, Paquis P. Spinal cord compression due to a primary vertebral hydatid disease: a rare case report in metropolitan France and a literature review. Neurochirurgie. 2016 Aug;62(4):226–8.
200. Celik C, Sasmaz MF, Oktay F, Ucan H, Kaptanoglu E. Paraplegia associated with spinal hydatid cyst: a case report. Spine. 2010 Apr 20;35(9):356.
201. Kalkan E, Cengiz SL, Ciçek O, Erdi F, Baysefer A. Primary spinal intradural extramedullary hydatid cyst in a child. J Spinal Cord Med. 2007;30(3):297–300.
202. Prabhakar MM, Acharya AJ, Modi DR, Jadav B. Spinal hydatid disease: a case series. J Spinal Cord Med. 2005;28(5):426–31.
203. Osoegawa M, Matsumoto S, Ochi H, Yamasaki K, Horiuchi I, Kira YO, et al. Localised myelitis caused by visceral larva migrans due to Ascaris suum masquerading as an isolated spinal cord tumour. J Neurol Neurosurg Psychiatry. 2001 Feb;70(2):265–6.

204. Yoshida S, Matsui M, Wang H, Oeda T, Sasaki T, Komure O, et al. A case of myeloradiculitis as a complication of visceral larva migrans due to Ascaris suum. Rinsho Shinkeigaku. 2004 Mar;44(3):198–202.
205. Umehara F, Ookatsu H, Hayashi D, Uchida A, Douchi Y, Kawabata H, et al. MRI studies of spinal visceral larva migrans syndrome. J Neurol Sci. 2006 Nov 01;249(1):7–12.
206. Awad A, Stuve O. Idiopathic transverse myelitis and neuromyelitis optica: clinical profiles. Pathophysiology and Therapeutic Choices Current Neuropharmacology. 2011 Sep;9(3):417–28.
207. Yeshokumar AK, Waubant E. Pediatric demyelinating diseases of the central nervous system and their mimics. 1st ed. Springer; 2017.
208. Williams T, Thorpe J. Post-infective transverse myelitis following Streptococcus pneumoniae meningitis with radiological features of acute disseminated encephalomyelitis: a case report. J Med Case Rep. 2012 Sep 19;6:313.
209. Candler PM, Dale RC. Three cases of central nervous system complications associated with mycoplasma pneumoniae. Pediatr Neurol. 2004 Aug;31(2):133–8.
210. Harzheim M, Schlegel U, Urbach H, Klockgether T, Schmidt S. Discriminatory features of acute transverse myelitis: a retrospective analysis of 45 patients. J Neurol Sci. 2004 Feb 15;217(2):217–23.
211. Jeffery DR, Mandler RN, Davis LE. Transverse myelitis. Retrospective analysis of 33 cases, with differentiation of cases associated with multiple sclerosis and parainfectious events. Arch Neurol. 1993 May;50(5):532–5.
212. Krishnan C, Kaplin AI, Deshpande DM, Pardo CA, Kerr DA. Transverse Myelitis: pathogenesis, diagnosis and treatment. Front Biosci. 2004 May 01;9:1483–99.

Malignancies of the Spinal Cord

9

Sohail Syed, Jared S. Fridley, Matthew N. Andersen,
Thomas Kosztowski, Adetokunbo A. Oyelese,
and Ziya L. Gokaslan

Contents

Introduction

Epidemiology

While tumors of the spine are a rare cause of myelopathy, a missed or delayed diagnosis can be devastating. Spinal column tumors can be categorized based on their anatomic location within the spine: extradural, intradural extramedullary, and intramedullary and on whether they are primary tumors or metastases. Extradural and intradural masses occur in roughly the same incidence with a slight predilection for extradural masses (60% vs 40% respectively) [1]. Intramedullary or spinal cord tumors however, are very uncommon, constituting only about 5% of the tumors encountered clinically in adults, and up to as many as 30% of tumors in children [2]. The focus of this chapter will be tumors arising or involving the spinal cord itself and unless otherwise specified spinal cord tumors will refer only to intramedullary lesions.

S. Syed · J. S. Fridley · M. N. Andersen · T. Kosztowski · A. A. Oyelese · Z. L. Gokaslan (✉)
Department of Neurosurgery, Warren Alpert School of Medicine, Brown University, Rhode Island Hospital, Providence, RI, USA
e-mail: ziya_gokaslan@brown.edu

B. Greenberg (ed.), *Myelopathy*, https://doi.org/10.1007/978-3-030-99906-3_9

Spinal cord tumors can be divided into primary spinal cord tumors and metastatic lesions to the spinal cord. It is important to note that in general while metastatic lesions are very common, metastases to the spinal cord are rare and account for <5% of spinal cord tumors [2]. Of the primary spinal cord tumors the majority are either ependymomas, astrocytomas (with an approximately 2:1 preference for ependymomas), or hemangioblastomas [2].

Presentation

Symptomatic presentation from a spinal cord malignancy can vary based on location, number of lesions, and the rate of tumor progression. Patients with metastatic spinal cord tumors patient may exhibit additional systemic signs of illness such as fever, chills, and/or weight loss, or symptoms of disease from additional organ system involvement. In general, spinal pain is the most common symptom of malignancy within the spinal cord. The relative non-specific nature of pain, especially in older populations where spondylotic degeneration is a common cause of back may lead to delay in diagnosis. Pain may occur from both neural and non-neural involvement. Nerve root involvement, specifically pain from the dorsal rootlets, may lead to radiculopathic pain. Tumor expansion can stretch and irritate the spinal dura or associated vasculature, and tumor secreted inflammatory factors all can lead to local inflammation and subsequent pain.

Sensorimotor and other white matter tract signs may arise from direct tumor invasion of the spinal cord substance itself, or from local mass effect by tumor. Symptoms may be divided into those arising from compression/involvement of the nerve roots (radiculopathy), spinal cord (myelopathy) or both. Myelopathy can present as subtle to overt motor weakness, proprioceptive difficulties, bowel bladder dysfunction, and/or presence of pathological reflexes. The neurological presentation is often slowly progressive. Muscle weakness may not be detectable on exam early and the adept clinician must be attentive for other signs such as difficulty with manual dexterity, spasticity, imbalance, and/or gait dysfunction.

Pediatric patients can present with unique age-related symptoms/signs of a spinal cord tumor including delayed motor development, progressive scoliosis, or torticollis. In infants or young children subtle neurological deficits may be overlooked due the inability to effectively communicate symptoms. Motor developmental delay may be the first clue in a young child to the presence of a spinal cord tumor [3]. As the young spine develops, scoliosis may become evident, and can be the first presenting sign of a spinal cord tumor [3].

Evaluating patient functional status is important when assessing a patient's overall clinical picture, and as a metric to compare both before and after tumor therapy as well as physical rehabilitation. A commonly used functional assessment tool for use in spinal cord tumor patients, both extramedullary and intramedullary, is the modified McCormick Scale. This is a physician rated scale that is used to determine the preoperative and postoperative global neurological function and walking ability.

(Figure A) Grade of 1 describes a patient with no neurologic dysfunction and a Grade of 5 describes a patient that is para- or quadriplegic and is restricted to a bed or wheelchair [2].

Diagnosis

MRI is the diagnostic modality of choice in a patient with a suspected spinal cord tumor. Both T1 and T2 sequences are useful for narrowing down the possible pathology, defining tumor heterogeneity, and tumor borders, particularly whether there is a potential surgical plane. The location of the tumor relative to the midline or dorsal root entry zone (DREZ), can help the surgeon identify where to enter the substance of the spinal cord if the tumor does not present to a pial surface. Apparent diffusion coefficient (ADC) and gradient echo sequences can be useful in determining the presence of hemorrhage, often seen in patients with intramedullary melanoma, hemangioblastoma, or ependymoma.

It is important to keep in mind various other types of spinal cord pathology in the differential diagnosis, such as demyelinating disease (eg multiple sclerosis (MS), idiopathic transverse myelitis, neuromyelitis optica), infection (abscess), inflammatory disease (sarcoidosis), and vascular (cavernoma, cord infarction from arteriovenous fistula). These may be similar appearance to spinal cord neoplasms and are often suggested by patient history. Cerebrospinal fluid (CSF) markers may be sampled to help rule out the above conditions. For example, elevated IgG index and the presence oF unmatched oligoclonal bands can help diagnose MS, and acetylcholinesterase (ACE) can help determine whether the patient has neurosarcoidosis.

In the absence of specific supporting data, either from history, laboratory, or pathognomonic imaging findings, obtaining tissue is imperative for diagnosis. Tissue from the spinal cord is only safely obtained via an open incisional or excisional tumor resection. In most cases the tumor specimen is obtained during the definitive tumor resection, such as with an ependymoma. If an extensive, diffusely infiltrative astrocytoma is suspected, an open biopsy or subtotal resection can be performed for definitive diagnosis. In most patients, history, laboratory, and/or imaging findings will determine whether to plan for a biopsy or surgical resection of tumor.

Primary Spinal Cord Tumors

Ependymomas

Ependymomas are the most common spinal cord tumors overall and the most common in adults [2, 4]. They account for roughly 2% of all CNS tumors and have a predilection for males though some series suggest no preference [5, 6]. The majority of ependymomas are benign though malignant variants do exist [5]. The average age at diagnosis is between around 30 years of age [4, 5]. Histologically, ependymomas are thought to arise from ependymal glial cells that line CSF spaces. The world health organization places ependymomas into the larger category of ependymal tumors which also includes myxopapillary ependymomas, subependymomas, and anaplastic ependymomas [7]. When it comes to the clinical manifestation and management classical ependymomas and myxopapillary ependymomas are best evaluated in separate categories.

Ependymoma

Roughly half the cases of ependymomas are the traditional variety [4]. These tumors have a predilection for the cervical and thoracic segments of the spinal cord [4]. The WHO further breaks down ependymomas based on their histology into papillary, clear cell, and tanycytic [7].

Most spinal ependymomas present with back pain [2]. Many also have dysesthesias as a result of expansion of the central canal that is believed to impair the spinothalamic tract [2, 5]. Continued progression of the tumor can lead to further pronounced deficits and the involvement of other tracts. It is worth noting that with the prevalence of MRI leading to early diagnosis, weakness and bowel/ bladder dysfunction are less and less common symptoms at time of diagnosis [2].

MRI of the spine with and without gadolinium contrast is the imaging modality of choice. The tumors exhibit hypo-intense or iso-intense signal on T1 images and hyperintense on T2-weighted imaging [8] (Fig. 9.1). In some cases intra-tumoral hemorrhage may produce T1 hyperintensity [8]. They often exhibit a robust enhancement pattern [2, 8]. Some ependymomas may exhibit a "cap sign", which results from hemosiderin deposition from previous hemorrhage and is an area of hypointensity on T2 imaging [8]. A cap sign may be seen approximately 30% of ependymomas, though can be seen in other spinal cord tumors prone to hemorrhage [8]. On tractography, normal fibers tend to be displaced rather than being invaded into [2]. An MRI may further reveal an associated syrinx in up to 60% of cases [6].

The primary treatment for ependymoma is surgical resection. Gross total resection is often feasible because there is often a clear surgical tissue plane between tumor and surrounding parenchyma (Fig. 9.2). Overall progression free survival after surgical resection is approximately 90% at 5 years and 80% at 10 years [9]. Factors that influenced survival included complete versus partial resection and initial histology with myxopapillary ependymomas having poorer outcomes [9]. There have recently been trials of imatinib as a chemotherapeutic agent to treat ependymomas, but the results of these trials have yet to be determined [10]. Adjunctive modalities such as radiotherapy are implemented in cases of partial resection or recurrence, usually employing external beam radiation up to 54 gy [5, 9]. Craniospinal radiation is less well established for spinal cord ependymomas. Overall, for unresectable or partial resections radiation therapy may provide greater progression free survival [5].

Myxopappilary Ependymoma

Myxopapillary ependymomas account for approximately the other 50% of spinal cord ependymomas [4]. This variant has a high predilection for the conus medullaris

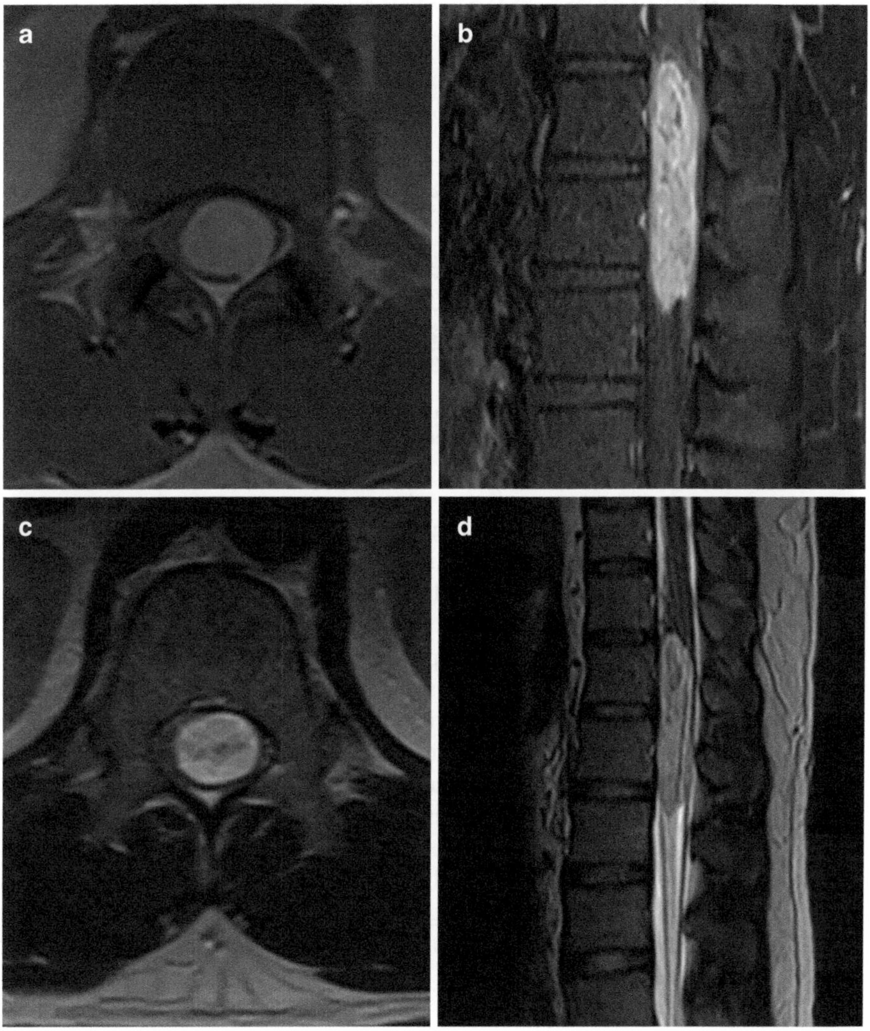

Fig. 9.1 Myxopapillary ependymoma; axial (**a**) T1 pre-contrast and sagittal, (**b**) T1 post-contrast images, axial (**c**) T2 and sagittal (**d**) T2. The tumor is located at the conus medullaris with avid contrast enhancement, strongly suggesting the diagnosis of myxopapillary ependymoma

and the cauda equina [8]. It tends to be more common in males and may have a slightly younger presentation than classical ependymomas (though still more common in adults than pediatric patients) [8]. Patients typically present with low back pain, lumbosacral radiculopathy, and/or bowel and bladder dysfunction [2, 5]. Imaging characteristics on T1 and T2 weighted imaging can be similar to classical ependymomas, and anatomical level can be key distinguishing factors between the two entities [8] (Fig. 9.3).

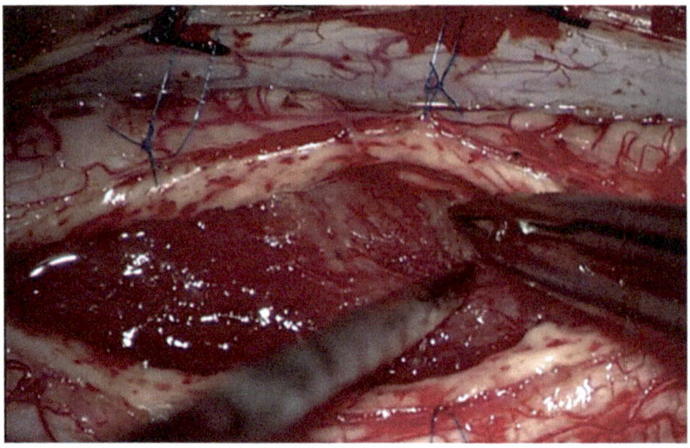

Fig. 9.2 Intraoperative microscope image of a cervical intramedullary ependymoma resection. Note the clearly defined surgical border between tumor and spinal cord. Pial tack up sutures are used to assist with tumor resection

Primary treatment of these tumors is gross total surgical resection, which can be technically difficulty due to tumor friability and adherence to neural elements [11]. In patients where tumor is either partially resected, or there is technical difficulty removing tumor attached to nerve roots, there appears to be a higher incidence of neurological dysfunction, particularly sphincter and gait abnormality [11]. Subtotal resection carries additional risk of seeding the CSF space which can lead to either local recurrence or distant disease in the neuroaxis [11, 12]. Progression free survival after gross total surgical resection is approximately 60–80% at 5 years, though tumors with subtotal resections fare worse [11, 12]. Other prognostic factors include presence of capsule at time of surgery, age and time to diagnosis, as well as tumor histology. Much like classical ependymomas adjunctive radiotherapy is employed in tumors that have a subtotal resection or are unable to resected, with some evidence suggesting improved progression free survival [11, 12]. Whole craniospinal irradiation may be utilized in cases where diffuse dissemination of tumor via CSF is suspected.

Astrocytomas

Astrocytomas are the most common spinal cord tumor in children and second most common in adults [3]. There is no known gender predilection and the median age at diagnosis is around 15 years of age [13]. There are four different WHO grades of astrocytoma: Grade 1= pilocytic, Grade II= diffuse or low grade, Grade III= anaplastic, and Grade IV= glioblastoma (GBM) [7]. The majority of astrocytomas are either grade I or II (up to 80% in some series) [3]. Pilocytic astrocytomas are most commonly found in children, while grade II low grade astrocytomas are most commonly found in adults [14, 15]. GBM is very rarely found in the spinal cord, but when present has a very poor prognosis. The cervicothoracic spine is the most

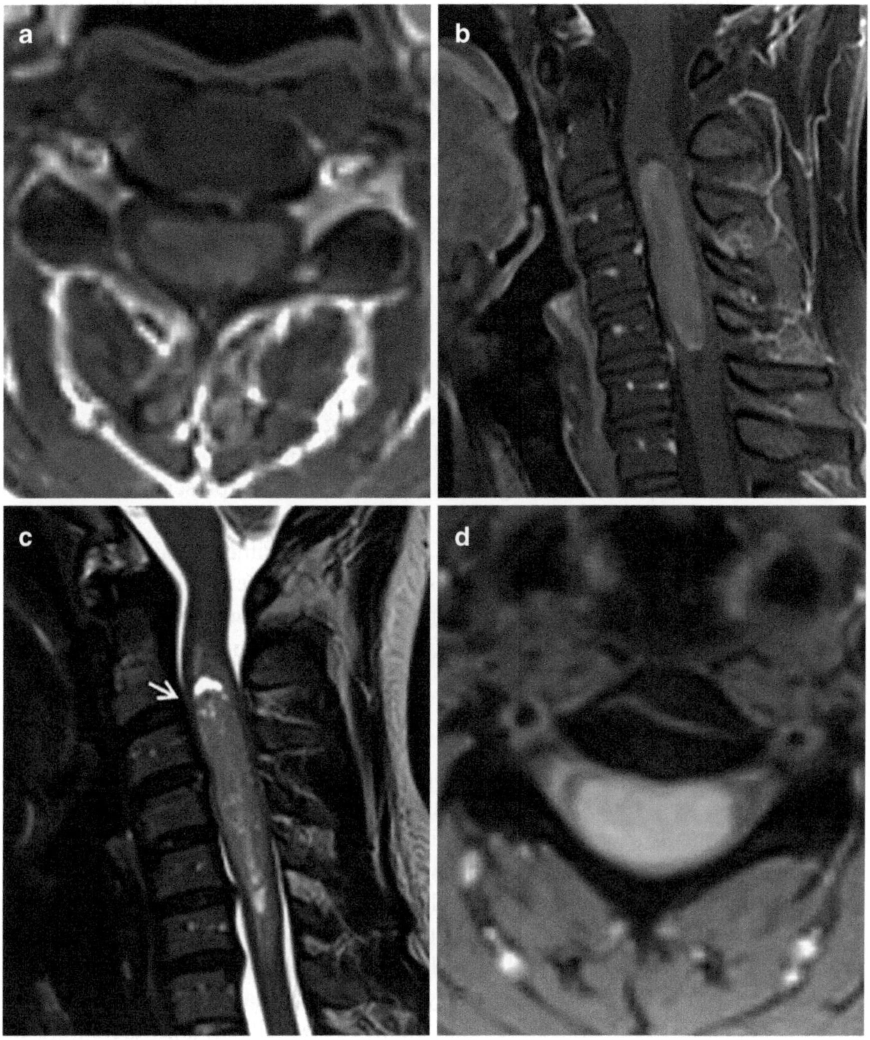

Fig. 9.3 Classical ependymoma; axial (**a**) and sagittal, (**b**) T1 pre-contrast images, axial (**c**) T2 and sagittal (**d**) T2. Pre-contrast T1 imaging is characteristically hypointense where as T2 imaging is more iso to hyperintense. The "cap-sign," a thin hypointense rim of hemosiderin from prior hemorrhage, can be seen at the rostral end of the tumor on T2 imaging (white arrow)

common spinal segment that these tumors are found in, but they can be present anywhere in the spinal cord [8, 16].

Like ependymomas, astrocytomas most commonly present with regional back pain [16]. However, the neurological presentation between the two tumors differs due to the preference of astrocytoma to grow in the periphery of the spinal cord, while ependymoma's tend to be more central in location [2]. Astrocytomas invade fiber tracts rather than displace them as with ependymomas [2]. As such astrocytomas tend to have asymmetric symptoms and are more likely to have weakness on presentation due to corticospinal tract involvement.

MRI shows a hypo-to iso-intense lesion on T1 and hyper-intense lesion on T2 [3]. Most of the astrocytomas enhance with gadolinium though this can be either heterogeneous or homogeneous [2]. Also present on MRI can be necrosis, edema and a cyst with mural nodule. The tumor is usually spread over a greater number of spinal cord segments than ependymomas which can help in distinguishing between the two lesions. In rare cases tumors can span the entire cord and are referred to as holocord tumors [2].

Surgery is the primary treatment modality for astrocytoma. As there are often no clear surgical margins around the tumor, maximum safe resection is the goal [17]. Attempted gross total resection of these tumor can lead to significant morbidity, with up to 40% of patients having decreased neurological function post-operatively [3]. Surgical outcomes vary, with one study reporting approximately 65% of patients had progression of disease at a median follow up of 28 months or a progressive free survival of 35% at 2 years [13]. Higher grade and older age at presentation are associated with worse prognosis [13].

There is a lack of consensus regarding the efficacy of either primary or adjuvant radiotherapy and/or chemotherapy in these tumors [3]. Often these modalities are reserved for patients with unresectable tumor or disease recurrence [3, 10].

Hemangioblastoma

Hemangioblastomas rarely occur in the spinal cord, accounting for approximately 5% of all spinal cord tumors [2]. They can occur either sporadically or as part of a genetic syndrome. If sporadic, the peak incidence of these tumors occurs in adults in the third and fourth decades of life. The majority of spinal hemangioblastomas are diagnosed in patients with von-Hippel-Lindau disease (VHL) [18].

VHL is an autosomal dominant a genetic disorder involving the *VHL* tumor suppressor gene on chromosome 3 [19]. The downregulation of this gene leads to malignancies of the CNS including the eyes (retinal capillary hemangioblastoma), pancreas (cysts and neuroendocrine tumors), kidney (renal cell) and adrenal glands (pheochromocytoma), as well as the epididymis in males (cystadenomas) [19]. Patients who have VHL and are found to have a spinal cord hemangioblastoma tend present earlier than their sporadic counterparts, usually in their second and third decade of life [20]. They often will have tumors found not only in the spinal cord, but also in the cerebellum.

While most spinal cord tumor patients present with gradual onset of neurologic deficits, patients with hemangioblastomas may present with acute symptoms due to tumor hemorrhage. This hemorrhage can be confined solely to the spinal cord parenchyma or extend into the subarachnoid space, which can lead to clinical meningismus [18]. In general, patients with hemangioblastomas tend to have a more rapid progression of symptoms than those of other primary spinal cord tumors due to their inherent vascularity.

The diagnosis of hemangioblastoma requires pathological confirmation but can be strongly suggested by clinical history, particularly VHL patients, as well as pathognomonic imaging findings. Patients with a strong family history or multiple suggestive lesions of the brain and spinal cord on imaging should undergo genetic testing for VHL. Screening for associated malignancies in aforementioned organ systems should also be conducted. Diagnosis of VHL is made clinically but can be confirmed with genetic testing.

Hemangioblastomas originate from embryonic remnant tissues of mesodermal origin, likely undifferentiated mesenchymal cells [2]. They are composed of a dense network of capillary channels which contain endothelial cells, pericytes, and lipid-laden stromal cells. Histology shows reticular pattern of small capillaries and foamy stromal cells.

MRI reveals an iso-intense lesion on T1 weighted imaging and hyperintense lesion on T2 weighted imaging [9, 18]. There is homogeneous enhancement with gadolinium administration. Other distinguishing MRI findings include: presence of flow voids, a homogeneously enhancing hyper vascular nodule with cyst, or syrinx (seen in up to 50% of cases) [9, 18] (Fig. 9.4). Some institutions utilize preoperative angiography, whether CT or DSA, for planning and even preoperative embolization prior to resection though this is not a ubiquitous practice [21–24].

Surgical resection is the primary treatment modality for spinal cord hemangioblastoma [25]. As these tumors are very vascular, piecemeal resection is not recommended. The tumor capsule should be preserved, and gently dissected from the surrounding spinal cord parenchyma. Pre-operative embolization of the tumor can be attempted before surgery to decrease the risk of significant blood loss in the operating room.

Surgical outcomes data is limited as hemangioblastomas are rare. In a large series of 108 predominantly adult patients with VHL associated hemangioblastoma, approximately 70% of patients who underwent surgery had stable neurological exams at 6 months post-surgery [18]. 15% of patients experienced dramatic permanent decline after surgery while fewer, 6%, showed an improvement in their neurological exam [18]. Reported surgical outcomes in patients with sporadic hemangioblastomas suggest that surgical resection results in improved outcomes in most patients [23]. Stereotactic radiosurgery (SRS) is reserved for patients with recurrent or unresectable tumors [26].

Metastases

Metastases to the spinal cord represent 4–8% of CNS metastases and 1–3% of all intramedullary tumors [27, 28]. The majority of patients with spinal cord metastases are adults, typically in the fifth and sixth decades of life [28]. Lung and breast cancer are the most common spinal cord metastases due to the overall incidence of these primary malignancies in the adult population [27, 28]. Other common primaries include renal cell, melanoma, and lymphomas [28].

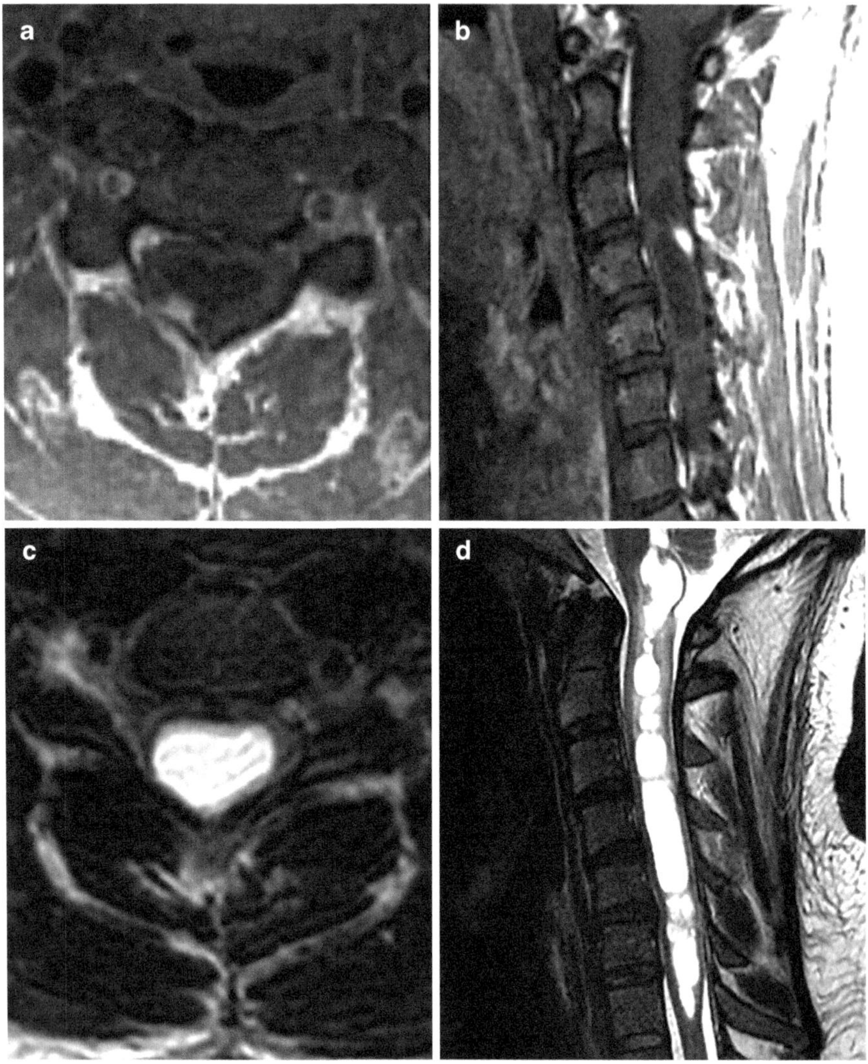

Fig. 9.4 Hemangioblastoma; axial (**a**) and sagittal, (**b**) T1 post-contrast images, axial (**c**) T2 and sagittal (**d**) T2. Note the nodular enhancement on T1 post contrast imaging and presence of cervical syrinx on T2 imaging

Patients with spinal cord metastases primarily present with sensorimotor deficits [27, 28]. Back pain is seen in only seen in 20–30% of patients [28]. Rapid progression of symptoms over days to weeks is more associated with metastases than other primary spinal cord tumors. It is important to note that while the majority of patients have a pre-existing primary malignancy, for some the intramedullary metastasis is the first presenting source of their systemic disease [28].

Imaging findings of spinal cord metastases are generally non-specific. MRI T1 and T2 weighted imaging may have varying levels of intensity. T2 imaging will often reveal peritumoral edema [28]. Most spinal cord metastases demonstrate avid contrast enhancement [28]. In addition to imaging of the affected spinal region, the entire neural axis should be scanned to look for other metastatic foci. CT of the chest, abdomen, and pelvis with and without contrast is recommended to either identify the possible primary source of disease and/or the extant of disease.

The primary treatment for spinal cord metastases is controversial [27, 29]. With advanced microsurgical techniques, surgical resection has been shown to have relatively low morbidity [28, 30]. Factors affecting the decision to proceed with surgery are patient age, degree of neurologic impairment, rapidity of symptom onset, functional performance status, medical comorbidities, tumor radiosensitivity, and presence/absence of leptomeningeal disease [27, 28]. Some surgical series suggest at least some neurological symptomatic improvement or at least preservation of function [28, 31]. In the majority of cases patients with metastases to the spinal cord have mean prognosis of 3–4 months though some studies report rare survival up to 1–2 years or longer [26–29, 31]. A recent case series from MD Andersen has stressed that neurological outcomes and durability of survival is likely tied to the histology of specific metastases and the ability to achieve gross total resection [31]. The authors argue that for radio resistant tumors, in patients with single site involvement and no known leptomeningeal disease, resection results in increased length of neurological preservation, as well as potentially improved overall survival [31].

However many continue to advocate for primary radiation therapy [27]. Stereotactic radiosurgery is increasingly being used and mean survival has ranged from 6–30 months, with mean survival of 17 months [26]. There are no clearly defined guidelines for dosing and fractionation and various strategies have been used such as single doses at 20gy versus 40–50gy given over 10+ fractions [26].

Conclusion

Spinal cord tumors are generally rare entities that typically present with back pain. A high degree of clinical suspicion is necessary to arrive at the appropriate diagnosis, with the utilization of imaging, and ultimately pathology, to confirm the diagnosis. Primary treatment of these tumors consists, for the most part, of maximal safe surgical resection. Radiotherapy is reserved for either partially resected or unresectable tumors.

References

1. Orguc S, Arkun R. Primary tumors of the spine. Semin Musculoskelet Radiol. 2014;18(3):280–99.
2. Mechtler LL, Nandigam K. Spinal cord tumors: new views and future directions. Neurol Clin. 2013;31(1):241–68.

3. Tobin MK, Geraghty JR, Engelhard HH, Linninger AA, Mehta AI. Intramedullary spinal cord tumors: a review of current and future treatment strategies. Neurosurg Focus. 2015;39(2):E14.
4. Chamberlain MC. Ependymomas. Curr Neurol Neurosci Rep. 2003;3(3):193–9.
5. Celano E, Salehani A, Malcolm JG, Reinertsen E, Hadjipanayis CG. Spinal cord ependymoma: a review of the literature and case series of ten patients. J Neuro-Oncol. 2016;128(3):377–86.
6. Klekamp J. Spinal ependymomas. Part 1: intramedullary ependymomas. Neurosurg Focus. 2015;39(2):E6.
7. Louis DN, Perry A, Reifenberger G, von Deimling A, Figarella-Branger D, Cavenee WK, et al. The 2016 World Health Organization classification of tumors of the central nervous system: a summary. Acta Neuropathol. 2016;131(6):803–20.
8. Koeller KK, Rosenblum RS, Morrison AL. Neoplasms of the spinal cord and filum terminale: radiologic-pathologic correlation. Radiographics Rev Publ Radiol Soc North America, Inc. 2000;20(6):1721–49.
9. Bostrom A, von Lehe M, Hartmann W, Pietsch T, Feuss M, Bostrom JP, et al. Surgery for spinal cord ependymomas: outcome and prognostic factors. Neurosurgery. 2011;68(2):302–8. discussion 9
10. Ottenhausen M, Ntoulias G, Bodhinayake I, Ruppert FH, Schreiber S, Forschler A, et al. Intradural spinal tumors in adults-update on management and outcome. Neurosurg Rev. 2018;42(2):371–88.
11. Klekamp J. Spinal ependymomas. Part 2: Ependymomas of the filum terminale. Neurosurg Focus. 2015;39(2):E7.
12. Abdulaziz M, Mallory GW, Bydon M, De la Garza RR, Ellis JA, Laack NN, et al. Outcomes following myxopapillary ependymoma resection: the importance of capsule integrity. Neurosurg Focus. 2015;39(2):E8.
13. Babu R, Karikari IO, Owens TR, Bagley CA. Spinal cord astrocytomas: a modern 20-year experience at a single institution. Spine. 2014;39(7):533–40.
14. Samartzis D, Gillis CC, Shih P, O'Toole JE, Fessler RG. Intramedullary spinal cord tumors: part I-epidemiology, pathophysiology, and diagnosis. Glob Spine J. 2015;5(5):425–35.
15. Gupta A, Dwivedi T. A simplified overview of World Health Organization classification update of central nervous system tumors 2016. J Neurosci Rural Pract. 2017;8(4):629–41.
16. Houten JK, Cooper PR. Spinal cord astrocytomas: presentation, management and outcome. J Neuro-Oncol. 2000;47(3):219–24.
17. Samartzis D, Gillis CC, Shih P, O'Toole JE, Fessler RG. Intramedullary spinal cord tumors: part II-management options and outcomes. Glob Spine J. 2016;6(2):176–85.
18. Mehta GU, Asthagiri AR, Bakhtian KD, Auh S, Oldfield EH, Lonser RR. Functional outcome after resection of spinal cord hemangioblastomas associated with von Hippel-Lindau disease. J Neurosurg Spine. 2010;12(3):233–42.
19. Schmid S, Gillessen S, Binet I, Brandle M, Engeler D, Greiner J, et al. Management of von hippel-lindau disease: an interdisciplinary review. Oncol Res Treat. 2014;37(12):761–71.
20. Hodgson TS, Nielsen SM, Lesniak MS, Lukas RV. Neurological management of Von Hippel-Lindau disease. Neurologist. 2016;21(5):73–8.
21. Bostrom A, Hans FJ, Reinacher PC, Krings T, Burgel U, Gilsbach JM, et al. Intramedullary hemangioblastomas: timing of surgery, microsurgical technique and follow-up in 23 patients. Eur Spine J Off Publ Eur Spine Soc Eur Spin Deform Soc Eur Sect Cervical Spine Res Soc. 2008;17(6):882–6.
22. Snyder LA, Spetzler RF. Resection of sporadic spinal hemangioblastomas. World Neurosurg. 2014;82(5):629–31.
23. Sun HI, Ozduman K, Usseli MI, Ozgen S, Pamir MN. Sporadic spinal hemangioblastomas can be effectively treated by microsurgery alone. World Neurosurg. 2014;82(5):836–47.
24. Deng X, Wang K, Wu L, Yang C, Yang T, Zhao L, et al. Intraspinal hemangioblastomas: analysis of 92 cases in a single institution: clinical article. J Neurosurg Spine. 2014;21(2):260–9.

25. Kothbauer KF. Neurosurgical management of intramedullary spinal cord tumors in children. Pediatr Neurosurg. 2007;43(3):222–35.
26. Hernandez-Duran S, Hanft S, Komotar RJ, Manzano GR. The role of stereotactic radiosurgery in the treatment of intramedullary spinal cord neoplasms: a systematic literature review. Neurosurg Rev. 2016;39(2):175–83. discussion 83
27. Hrabalek L. Intramedullary spinal cord metastases: review of the literature. Biomed Pap Med Fac Univ Palacky Olomouc Czech Repub. 2010;154(2):117–22.
28. Kalayci M, Cagavi F, Gul S, Yenidunya S, Acikgoz B. Intramedullary spinal cord metastases: diagnosis and treatment - an illustrated review. Acta Neurochir. 2004;146(12):1347–54. discussion 54
29. Payer S, Mende KC, Westphal M, Eicker SO. Intramedullary spinal cord metastases: an increasingly common diagnosis. Neurosurg Focus. 2015;39(2):E15.
30. Wilson DA, Fusco DJ, Uschold TD, Spetzler RF, Chang SW. Survival and functional outcome after surgical resection of intramedullary spinal cord metastases. World Neurosurg. 2012;77(2):370–4.
31. Strickland BA, McCutcheon IE, Chakrabarti I, Rhines LD, Weinberg JS. The surgical treatment of metastatic spine tumors within the intramedullary compartment. J Neurosurg Spine. 2018;28(1):79–87.

Hereditary Myelopathy: A Clinical Approach

10

John K. Fink

Contents

Introduction

Hereditary myelopathies are genetic disorders in which major symptoms and neurologic findings arise from impaired function of neurons whose cell bodies or axons are within the spinal cord. In addition to spinal cord localization, hereditary myelopathy syndromes often involve neurologic signs due to pathology outside the spinal cord (e.g. cerebellum or peripheral nerve). Neuronal dysfunction may arise from an abnormality within neurons or from primary extra-neuronal disturbance (e.g. primary glia or blood vessel abnormality) leading to neuron injury.

Why classify extremely diverse disorders, which primarily affect disparate cell types (neurons and glia) by a wide variety of molecular processes simply

J. K. Fink (✉)
Department of Neurology, University of Michigan, Ann Arbor, MI, USA
e-mail: jkfink@umich.edu

B. Greenberg (ed.), *Myelopathy*, https://doi.org/10.1007/978-3-030-99906-3_10

because major (but not all) signs and symptoms localize to spinal cord disturbance? The value of classifying disorders as hereditary myelopathies lies in its clinical utility. These are rare disorders (Table 10.1) with extensive phenotypic variability with which most clinicians have little direct experience. Recognizing

Table 10.1 Syndromic classification of hereditary myelopathies and representative examples

Major syndrome	Representative examples	Diagnostic testing
Spinocerebellar ataxias	SCA 1 through 36	Genetic testing for specific SCA gene mutation; neuroimaging to demonstrate cerebellar atrophy
	Machado-Joseph disease (SCA3)	Genetic testing for specific SCA gene mutation; neuroimaging to demonstrate cerebellar atrophy
	Friedreich ataxia	FRDA gene analysis
	Familial vitamin E deficiency	Serum vitamin E
	Abetalipoproteinemia (Bassen-Kornzweig)	Lipoprotein electrophoresis
	Charlevoix-Saguenay	ARSACS gene analysis
	Partial hexosaminidase deficiency	Leukocyte hexosaminidase assay
Motor neuron disorders	Familial ALS	SOD1 and C9ORF gene analysis Consider gene panels or whole exome sequencing for additional gene analysis
	Spinal muscular atrophy	Survival motor neuron gene analysis Additional gene analysis including BICD2, AR, UBA1, DYNC1H1, and VAPB
	Primary lateral sclerosis (rarely familial)	ALSin gene analysis (for juvenile familial PLS); consider gene panels or whole exome sequencing for additional gene analysis (e.g. C9ORF72, SPG7, DCTN1, PARK2, FIG4)
	Spinobulbar muscular atrophy (Kennedy syndrome)	Androgen receptor gene mutation (CAG repeats)
Leukodystrophies	Subacute combined degeneration (rarely familial)	Serum B_{12}
	5,10 MTHFR deficiency	Plasma homocysteine and methionine, serum folate and vitamin B12
	Multiple sclerosis (occasionally familial)	MRI of brain and spinal cord; CSF analysis; clinical course
	Krabbe disease	Leukocyte β-galactosidase assay
	Metachromatic leukodystrophy	Leukocyte arylsulfatase assay
	Pelizeaus-Merzbacher [1]	Proteolipid protein gene analysis
	Cerebrotendinous xanthomatosis	Serum cholestanol
CNS predominant, motor-sensory axonopathies	Hereditary spastic paraplegia	HSP gene analysis through gene panels or whole exome sequencing
	Adrenoleukodystrophy, Adrenomyeloneuropathy	Serum very long chain fatty acid analysis, ABCD1 gene analysis

Table 10.1 (continued)

Major syndrome	Representative examples	Diagnostic testing
Other disorders	Myelopathy related to Leber optic atrophy and other mitochondrial diosrders	Mitochondrial gene sequencing, analysis of nuclear-encoded mitochondrial genes, lactate, pyruvate muscle biopsy.
	Early-onset Alzheimer disease with spastic paraplegia	Presenilin 1, Presenilin 2, APP gene analysis
	Hypocupremia	Serum copper, serum zinc
	Neurofibromatosis type 2	MRI scan
	Hereditary exostosis with spinal cord compression	CT and MRI scans
	Hereditary hemorrhagic telangiectasia	MRI scan
	Von Hipple Lindau (vHL)	MRI scan and VHL gene analysis
	Tropical spastic paraplegia (due to human T-lymphotropic virus type 1 [HTLV1] infection; may occur in familial clusters)	HTLV1 antibody testing
	Arginase deficiency	Increased plasma arginine, reduced red blood cell arginase
	Biotinidase deficiency	Reduced serum biotinidase
	Syringomyelia (rarely familial)	MRI scan
	Sjögren-Larsson syndrome (SPG54)	DDHD2 gene analysis

their *myelopathic localization* is an important first step to establishing and prioritizing the differential diagnosis.

Note that discussions of hereditary myelopathies do not usually include spinal dysraphisms such as *spina bifida* and other neural tube defects. These disorders have low-hereditability, have been attributed to folic acid deficiency, [2] are occasionally due to chromosome abnormality (e.g. [3], discoverable through karyotype and chromosome microarray analysis), and are usually not due to single-gene mutation [4].

Recognize Hereditary Myelopathy by a Patterns of Motor and Sensory Impairment

The first consideration is whether there are *myelopathic symptoms and signs for which secondary causes have been excluded*. Note that family history of similar disorder is not the first or most critical question during acquisition of a patient's history. For reasons discussed below, family history may be present, absent, unavailable, or ambiguous. Instead, the first question is whether myelopathic localization is "yes/likely" or "no/unlikely" rather than the magnitude of involvement (mild or severe).

Clinical localization to the spinal cord (myelopathy) can be deduced with *highest probability* when one of the following patterns exists: a) "spinal sensory disturbance" (described below); b) length-dependent axonopathy (described below); or c) evidence of anterior horn cell involvement. Although other neurologic signs (e.g. focal, segmental, or hemi-upper motor or sensory deficits certainly *could* result from a spinal cord disturbance (e.g. due to focal or eccentric lesions), their clinical localization to the spinal cord is less certain.

Four patterns of "spinal sensory disturbance". Patterns of spinal sensory disturbance conform to (a) spinal level (all sensory modalities [light touch, vibration and proprioception, pain and temperature] are lost in a relatively uniform pattern below a dermatome (in contrast to a pattern of gradient, distal-greater-than-proximal impairment); (b) central cord sensory impairment ("suspended-dissociated" pattern of band-like loss of spinothalamic sensation [pain and temperature] with preservation of dorsal column function [vibration perception and proprioception]; (c) spinal hemi-section sensory loss ("Brown-Sequard syndrome") in which a hemi-spinal sensory level (all modalities on half the body below a dermatome) occurs with contralateral hemiplegia; (d) isolated dorsal column impairment (reduced vibration and position sensation with preservation of other sensory modalities).

The likelihood of spinal cord localization is greatest when sensory symptoms conform to one of these patterns. Nonetheless, spinal cord localization *cannot be excluded* in subjects with other some sensory disturbances that could be explained by multiple lesions and small, focal, eccentric lesions.

Length-dependent CNS motor axonopathy manifests as corticospinal tract (CST) signs involving upper and lower extremities in a *gradient manner*: Lower extremities are more affected than upper extremities. For example, upper extremities may exhibit asymptomatic, mild hyperreflexia (3+ deep tendon reflexes and Hoffman and Tromner signs) without spasticity or impaired dexterity; while lower extremities exhibit 3+ reflexes at the knees, hamstrings, quadriceps, and adductor spasticity, and sustained ankle clonus (4+ DTRs), with variable lower extremity weakness (particularly in iliopsoas, hamstrings, gluteus medius, and tibialis anterior muscles). With even more mild involvement, upper extremities may be entirely normal, but hyperreflexia is more prominent at the ankles (e.g. 4+) compared to the knees (e.g. 3+).

Clinical Pearl The occurrence of length-dependent CNS motor axonopathy together with length dependent dorsal column impairment (diminished vibration sensation in the toes but not more proximally) is highly suggestive of myelopathy. This pattern is analogous the pattern of distal-greater-than-proximal motor-sensory impairment in subjects with Charcot-Marie-Tooth type II (inherited neuropathy due to primary axon degeneration) in which distal lower extremities are particularly affected.

Anterior horn cell (AHC) involvement is marked by muscle weakness and atrophy with preservation of sensation. Electromyography and nerve conduction studies are valuable in defining anterior horn cell involvement, distinguishing it from peripheral motor neuropathy, and determining whether there is peripheral sensory neuropathy.

Hereditary Myelopathies Often Involve Extra-Spinal Structures Such as the Cerebellum and Peripheral Nerves

In fact, the magnitude of extra-spinal disturbance may equal or exceed myelopathic involvement. Indeed, spinal cord-localized symptoms may represent a phase in an evolving disorder that latter is predominated by extraspinal disturbance (e.g. spastic gait may be a feature of Alzheimer's disease due to presenilin 1 gene mutation (e.g. [5, 6] and sometimes may precede dementia).

As a result, disorders may be classified variably in different schema. For example, inherited cerebellar ataxias with spinal cord involvement (i.e. those with dorsal column or corticospinal tract disturbance) could be classified as "ataxias" (and more specifically as "spino-cerebellar ataxias"; or as myelopathies (more specifically, "myelopathy with cerebellar involvement".

Family History: Consider a Genetic Etiology Even When There Is No Family History of Similar Disorder

While the occurrence of family history of similar disorder suggests both a genetic disorder and potential mode of transmission (dominant, recessive, X-linked, maternal inheritance), the absence of family history does not exclude a genetic disorder. Family history may be absent in X-linked disorders (e.g. adrenomyeloneuropathy), autosomal recessive disorders (e.g. Friedreich's ataxia), mitochondrial disorders with maternal inheritance; subjects with *de novo* mutations for autosomal dominant disorders; and in disorders with incomplete genetic penetrance ("skipping generations"), *forme fruste* manifestations, and variable age-of-symptom onset (including disorders with anticipation in which children may be affected before their parents).

Insidious Onset and Slowly Progressive Course

With several exceptions, hereditary myelopathies have insidious onset (it is not possible to state the month and often not the year when symptoms began) and slow progression (usually over years). Important exceptions are (1) inherited disorders causing hypoxic-ischemic injury or impaired oxygen utilization (vascular disorders and some mitochondrial disorders); (2) inherited disorders associated with focal, space-occupying lesions (e.g. hamartomas, neurofibromas) in which insidious expansion may cross a threshold (often by focal vascular compromise, inflammation, and edema) and cause symptoms to worsen quickly; and (3) disorders associated with seizures, myoclonus, or other paroxysmal event.

Recognize Four Hereditary Myelopathy Paradigms: Spinocerebellar Degeneration, Motor Neuron Disease, Length-Dependent Central Axonopathy, Leukodystrophy

These syndromes arise from variable combinations of deficits involving corticospinal tracts, anterior horn cells, dorsal columns, and spinothalamic tracts. There is overlap between and extreme diversity within these syndromes owing to variation in severity, relative onset, and rate of progression of individual elements and because of variable occurrence of extra-spinal pathology (e.g. peripheral neuropathy, cerebellar ataxia, dementia).

Note that these four patterns do not include presentations for all hereditary myelopathies. Important exceptions are those disorders causing focal or multifocal myelopathy whose presentations may include markedly asymmetric or unilateral spinal motor (upper and/or lower motor neuron deficits) either alone or in combination with spinal sensory impairment. These disorders include familial ALS and disorders mediated through structural abnormalities (e.g. neurofibromatosis), hemangioblastoma (e.g. due to von Hipple-Lindau disease [see [7]]), other vascular malformation, or hypoxia-ischemia including disturbance of oxygen utilization (e.g. some mitochondrial disorders, e.g. [8, 9]).

Spinocerebellar ataxias (SCAs) [10, 11] are recognized by deficits involving (1) cerebellum and (2) corticospinal tracts and/or dorsal columns. Typically, cerebellar midline structures (controlling eye movements, speech, trunk, and legs) are involved more than the cerebellar hemispheres. Corticospinal and dorsal column deficits typically are worse in the legs than the arms. In addition to cerebellar, corticospinal, and/or dorsal column involvement, spinocerebellar degenerations frequently involve motor-sensory peripheral neuropathy (with greatest involvement in the legs). Often, all deficits are not present at the beginning of symptoms but emerge asynchronously as the disorder evolves (for example, lower extremity spasticity and hyperreflexia may be replaced by hypotonia and arreflexia as neuropathy advances). Serial examination, sometimes over two or more years is necessary to appreciate the syndrome and reach a diagnosis.

Gait impairment is typical in spinocerebellar syndromes and usually is wide-based (owing to cerebellar ataxia and various degrees of sensory ataxia from dorsal column impairment and peripheral neuropathy (of variable presence and magnitude). Depending on the degree of corticospinal tract impairment gait disturbance may also have a "spastic gait" pattern (i.e. forward-shifted foot strike, adducted knees, reduced foot dorsiflexion, circumduction, reduced or delayed hip flexion and knee extension).

Case Example (Modified from [12])

A 24 year-old woman presented for evaluation of insidiously progressive gait disturbance that began at ~12 years. There was no family history of similar disorder. The earliest and predominant symptom was balance impairment. Classmates commented that she walked as though intoxicated. There was no dysarthria and no symptoms involving the upper extremities. Slowly, balance impairment became accompanied by paresthesiae in both legs, and subsequently by bilateral foot drop.

Neurologic examination at age 24 revealed normal speech. Saccadic intrusions into smooth pursuit were noted but there was no ocular dysmetria. Upper extremity muscle bulk, tone, and strength and fine motor dexterity were normal. Finger-to-nose testing was normal. There was spasticity in hamstring and quadriceps and weakness in tibialis anterior and iliopsoas muscles. Proprioception was markedly impaired and vibration perception was absent in the toes. In contrast, perception of distally-applied light touch was preserved and pinprick sensation was only minimally impaired. Deep tendon reflexes were normal in upper extremities, hyperactive at the knees, and absent at the ankles. Plantar responses were extensor bilaterally. Gait was wide-based with foot drop bilaterally. Brain magnetic resonance imaging (MRI) was normal. Nerve conduction studies and electromyography were consistent with sensory-motor polyneuropathy.

Neurologic Formulation

The clinical syndrome can be reduced to adolescent-onset, insidiously progressive balance and gait impairment. Neurologic examination identified deficits referable to (a) corticospinal tracts; (b) dorsal columns; (c) peripheral motor-sensory nerves (diminished pinprick sensation and findings and reduced nerve conduction velocities); (d) and subtle deficits involving midline cerebellum (saccadic intrusions into smooth pursuit).

Diagnosis: Friedreich's Ataxia (FA)

Genetic testing demonstrated compound heterozygous frataxin gene mutations: expanded GAA repeat ($[GAA]_{962}$) on one allele and a point mutation on the other allele resulting in amino acid substitution (G130V).

Discussion

FA is the most common form of hereditary ataxia [13, 14]. There is marked variability of age-of-symptom onset (usually in adolescence but may occur later), severity, and degree of peripheral neuropathy, cerebellar involvement, and corticospinal tract involvement. For example, although historically recognized as a form of autosomal recessive ataxia with *areflexia* (the latter owing to a combination of peripheral neuropathy and dorsal root ganglia impairment), it is now recognized that subjects with FA may have retained reflexes and even hyperreflexia and lower extremity spasticity [15]. This underscores the comment that it is the *occurrence* of the neurologic sign (e.g. corticospinal tract impairment) rather than deficit magnitude (mild to severe) that defines a syndrome and helps establish the differential diagnosis. Non-neurologic involvement including diabetes, skeletal abnormalities, and cardiomyopathy may occur [16]. All FA subjects should be evaluated for hypertrophic cardiomyopathy which may be severe (absent in the patient presented).

More than 95% of subjects with FA are homozygous for expanded trinucleotide repeat in a non-coding portion of the frataxin gene. The remaining subjects have either missense mutations or a combination of one missense mutation and one expanded repeat (like subject). Frataxin trinucleotide repeat (GAA) expansions differ from the more common expanded repeats (CAG, encoding polyglutamine) responsible for Huntington chorea, Machado-Joseph disease (spinocerebellar ataxia type 3), and many other spinocerebellar degenerations [17]. Furthermore, frataxin repeat expansions occur in the non-coding portion (intron) are considered to be pathogenic by reducing frataxin mRNA (possibly through locally increased DNA methylation leading to reduced transcription) [49]. Because they occur in introns, pathogenic frataxin mutations may not be reliably detected by whole exome sequencing (which studies transcribed exons) and require specific methods for their detection [13].

Case Example (Modified from [12])

This individual experienced insidious onset, very slowly progressive gait disturbance due to weakness and tightness in his legs and turning-in of his feet. After more than a decade, these symptoms were accompanied by slowly progressive difficulty slurred speech, reduced speech volume, and generalized slowness of all movements. The patient's father, paternal half-brother, and paternal half-sister were similarly affected.

Neurologic examination (age 52, ~14 years after symptom-onset) demonstrated facial bradykinesia, saccadic intrusions into smooth pursuit eye movements, fasciculations in all extremities and the tongue, atrophy of distal upper and lower extremity muscles, and a combination of spasticity (symmetrical) in upper and lower extremities and hyporeflexia in the legs. He was no longer ambulatory after age 55. Re-examination (age 57) showed hypophonia, spastic and hypokinetic dysarthria; lid retraction; saccadic intrusions; sustained end-gaze nystagmus; facial myokymia; and masked facies. There was generalized bradykinesia but no ataxia on finger-to-nose testing. There was atrophy of distal upper and lower extremity muscles and diffuse fasciculations. Weakness of intrinsic hand muscles, and marked lower extremity weakness (worse distally) were also noted. Spasticity, which previously had been a prominent feature, was no longer present. There was a distal-greater-than proximal sensory loss (all modalities) in upper and lower extremities. Deep tendon reflexes were hypoactive in the upper extremities and absent in the lower extremities. Electromyography (at age 52 and 53) revealed chronic, severe, progressive sensorimotor neuropathy primarily of the axonal type. Sural nerve biopsy showed a moderate to severe axonal neuropathy.

Neurologic Localization Deficits were localized to corticospinal tracts (spasticity), peripheral motor-sensory nerves (sensory impairment, hyporeflexia), lower motor neurons (distal atrophy and fasiculations); nigro-striatal pathways (bradykinesia), and a minor degree of midline cerebellar impairment (saccadic intrusions into pursuit eye movements and nystagmus).

The differential diagnosis includes Machado-Joseph disease (MJD, also known as spinocerebellar ataxia type 3, SCA3); other spinocerebellar ataxias associated with peripheral neuropathy (although this would not explain bradykinesia); olivopontocerebellar degeneration (although this would not explain peripheral neuropathy); multisystem atrophy, cerebellar type (although this not explain peripheral neuropathy), mitochondrial encephalomyopathy with peripheral neuropathy; and forms of hereditary spastic paraplegia that also include peripheral neuropathy and cerebellar ataxia (e.g. SPG7, which may have extrapyramidal features).

Diagnosis: Machado-Joseph Disease

Genetic testing demonstrated one expanded SCA3 allele (69 CAG repeats) and one normal SCA3 allele (30 CAG repeats).

Discussion

MJD/SCA3 phenotypes (reviewed in [18]) are highly variable both within and between families. Some phenotype variability (such as age-of-symptom onset and to some extent, symptom severity) correlate with repeat expansion size (earlier onset and more severe symptoms tend to occur in subjects with larger repeat expansions). However, there may also be significant variation in the nature of symptoms. For some subjects, the disorder is predominated by peripheral neuropathy. In contrast, some subjects have less severe neuropathy and the disorder manifests primarily as cerebellar ataxia or spastic paraplegia. Other individuals, such as the one described above, have a complex syndrome including deficits involving corticospinal tracts, peripheral nerve, basal ganglia, and cerebellum.

Clinical Pearl Note that initially prominent spasticity and hyperreflexia gradually resolved and were replaced by areflexia as neuropathy advanced.

Motor Neuron Disorders

Amyotrophic lateral sclerosis (ALS), spinal muscular atrophy (SMA), and primary lateral sclerosis (PLS) are not usually considered myelopathies but typically classified as a "motor neuron disorders". Nonetheless, primary clinical signs in ALS (weakness, atrophy, variable spasticity and hyperreflexia), PLS (weakness, spasticity, hyperreflexia, without atrophy); and SMA (weakness and atrophy without spasticity or hyperreflexia) localize to spinal cord disturbance. Recognizing the myelopathic feature ALS, PLS, and SMA helps expand the differential diagnosis for these syndromes.

Rather than being a single etio-molecular-pathologic entity, the ALSs (plural) are etiologically heterogeneous syndromes in which neuro-degeneration is maximal in spinal and bulbar motor neurons and corticospinal tracts (ALS), involving neurons in the motor cortex and frontotemporal cortex to variable and generally lesser extent. ~10% of ALS subjects have affected first-degree relatives ("familial ALS"). Among these, autosomal dominant inheritance is most common. 25 genes have been implicated in ALS (see review [19]). Among subjects with familial ALS, mutations in C9ORF72 (45%) and SOD1 (20%) are most common [19]. Note that genetic mutations associated with ALS have been identified not only in familial ALS subjects, but sometimes in subjects with no family history of ALS. Identifying a probably pathogenic gene mutation that has been implicated in ALS informs genetic counseling and provides insight into disease mechanisms, but thus far does not impact treatment considerations.

Clinical Pearl Whether identified as an inherited or an "apparently sporadic" disorder, the course and distribution of neurologic signs in ALS are usually quite different than in other inherited myelopathies. As noted above, inherited myelopathies typically begin insidiously, progress slowly, and usually cause relatively symmetric clinical signs. In contrast, particularly early in the disorder, symptoms and signs in ALS may be markedly asymmetric (even localized) and progress relatively faster than other myelopathies. In addition to ALS, inherited disorders causing multifocal myelopathy involving both upper and lower motor neurons and include multiple sclerosis (rarely causes lower motor neuron signs), multifocal structural abnormalities, mitochondrial disorders, and vascular malformations (e.g Von Hipple Lindau disease). Unlike ALS, multifocal spinal cord structural abnormalities would be expected to have sensory deficits which are not present in ALS.

Spinal muscular atrophy (SMA) is an important genetic cause of infant mortality, with pan-ethnic incidence of ~1/10,000 [20]. In spinal muscular atrophy (SMA), neurodegeneration is limited to spinal motor neurons and their peripheral axons. SMA is classified by age-of-symptom onset (infantile, late infantile, juvenile, late onset, types 1 through 4, respectively). Mutations in the survival motor neuron (SMN1) gene are the major cause SMA. These mutations (often deletions) reduce SMN abundance. All subjects have least one (and sometimes more copies) of an SMN pseudogene (SMN2), from which a nearly identical transcript arises and which partially compensates for SMN1 mutation. However, mRNA splicing causes SMN2 transcripts to have markedly reduced stability. Promising therapy is emerging that can correct SMN2 splicing pattern and partially compensate for SMN1 deficiency [21, 22].

Although autosomal recessive SMA due to mutations in survival motor neuron (SMN) gene are the most common cause of the "SMA syndrome", mutations in other genes can also cause similar clinical presentations. Therefore, like ALS, SMA is a genetically heterogeneous syndrome. In addition to SMN, these genes include BICD2, [23] androgen receptor (X-linked spinal bulbar atrophy, [24] also known as Kennedy syndrome), *UBA1* (X-linked), [25] *DYNC1H1*, [26] and *VAPB* [27].

Primary lateral sclerosis (PLS) typically manifests as insidious-onset in adulthood (most commonly in the mid-50's although sometimes earlier), slowly progressive spasticity and weakness in the legs that later involves the arms and hands, speech (spastic dysarthria), and swallowing. In some subjects, symptoms first affect bulbar or upper extremity muscles before lower extremity muscles [28]. Neuropathologic studies demonstrate corticospinal and corticobulbar tract degeneration and to a lesser extent, reduced number of cortical motor neurons [29]. Spinal motor neurons are relatively preserved, there is no (or minimal) atrophy, and EMG is either normal or, late in the course, may show a mild degree of chronic denervation. These features distinguish PLS from ALS. Like ALS, the diagnosis of PLS is based on clinical features and EMG findings, and exclusion of other disorders. PLS diagnostic criteria proposed in 1982 [28] (primarily, an progressive upper motor neuron disorder without lower motor neuron involvement for which other disorders are excluded), are challenged by variable presentations and the occurrence of a mild degree of lower motor neuron involvement [30].

Previously, the occurrence of dorsal column impairment in HSP was considered to distinguish hereditary spastic paraplegia (HSP) from PLS [31]. The observation that some subjects with PLS have impaired vibration sensation, [32] challenges the concept that PLS is exclusively a disorder of corticospinal tracts and corticobulbar axons (and therefore classified as a motor neuron disorder), but instead is actually a length-dependent, motor-sensory central axonopathy (similar to HSP, described below) [33].

In addition to typical, adult-onset PLS, there is a rare childhood-onset, autosomal recessive form of PLS due to ALS2 gene mutation [34]. Depending on the precise location, ALS2 gene mutations either pure upper motor neuron impairment (PLS phenotype); or a combination of upper and lower motor impairment (juvenile-onset, autosomal recessive ALS phenotype). The occurrence of some families with juvenile PLS for whom ALS2 gene mutations are not identified suggests that juvenile PLS is genetically heterogeneous.

PLS is ascertained as an apparently sporadic (non-familial and apparently non-genetic) condition for the vast majority of subjects. Nonetheless, potentially pathogenic mutations in a number of genes (including C9ORF72, SPG7, DCTN1, PARK2, and FIG4) have been identified in "apparently sporadic" PLS subjects [35, 36]. This suggests that PLS, like ALS, is an etiologically heterogeneous *syndrome* and that a number of different genes (and variable molecular abnormalities) can contribute to the disorder even when there is no family history. Furthermore, among gene mutations identified in PLS subjects, note that C9ORF, FIG4, and ALS2 gene mutations also are identified in subjects with ALS; and that SPG7 gene mutation is associated with HSP; and DCTN1 is associated with distal hereditary motor neuropathy and rarely with SMA syndrome. This observation indicates that for some subjects, PLS may be in the same clinico-pathologic spectrum as ALS; in the HSP spectrum for other subjects; and that the cause of PLS for the majority of subjects is not known.

Clinical Pearl Insidiously progressive spastic gait is a common feature of many myelopathies including those that are potentially treatable (e.g. cervical stenosis, B12 deficiency, cerebrotendinous xanthomatosis, 5-methyltetrahydrofolate deficiency) and those that are not yet treatable (e.g. ALS and PLS) [32]. When corticospinal tract deficits (spasticity, weakness, and hyperreflexia) occur in the absence of other signs, it may not be possible to determine on the first evaluation which subjects with insidiously progressive spastic gait a) actually have upper motor neuron predominant ALS and later will develop lower motor neuron findings and be diagnosed with ALS; b) develop family history or evidence of dorsal column impairment, or have an identified HSP gene mutation and be diagnosed as having HSP; c) will develop upper extremity and bulbar muscle involvement and be diagnosed as having PLS; or d) remain as "apparently sporadic" spastic paraplegia [32]. Serial examination including annual electromyography (through the fifth year of symptoms), thorough exclusion of alternate disorders, and caution about prognosis in the early stages prior to definitive diagnosis are recommended.

Case Example

This individual experienced insidious onset of initially subtle gait disturbance in her early 50's. Symptoms progressed very slowly and ~6 years later accompanied by progressive difficulty with fine motor control of her hands and progressively slurred speech. Serial EMGs (performed annually through the fourth year of symptoms) were normal with no evidence of lower motor neuron impairment or peripheral neuropathy. Neuroimaging and laboratory studies (including cerebrospinal fluid examination, syphilis serology, serum B12, folate, very long chain fatty acids) were normal.

Initial neurologic examination (age 56) demonstrated normal speech and cranial nerves; mild iliopsoas and hamstring weakness; spasticity in the hamstrings (mild) and gastrocnemius-soleus (moderate) muscles; and grade 4+ hyperreflexia at the knees and ankles, bilateral extensor plantar responses, and mild spastic gait. Neurologic symptoms continued to worsen slowly. By age 65 she had marked spastic dysarthria, marked lower extremity spasticity, reduced dexterity in the hands, and was minimally ambulatory (required motorized scooter).

Neurologic Localization

Neurologic findings localized to corticospinal tracts serving all extremities (the legs initially and most severely); and corticobulbar tracts serving speech.

Differential Diagnosis and Clinical Diagnosis

The absence of electrophysiologic evidence of peripheral sensory involvement or neuroimaging evidence of white matter disturbance argued against a generalized leukodystrophy; absence of lower motor neuron involvement on serial EMGs argued against ALS. Involvement of upper extremities and speech and the absence of dorsal column involvement argued against a form of hereditary spastic paraplegia.

The exclusion of other disorders and the limitation of neurologic symptoms to corticobulbar and corticospinal tracts is consistent with clinical diagnosis of primary lateral sclerosis.

Case Example (Modified from [12])

Two sisters began having progressive gait impairment at age 2 years, with scissoring and a tendency to drag their toes. Each was the product of uncomplicated full-term gestation, labor, and delivery and each attained developmental milestones normally. Wheelchairs became necessary at ages 10 and 7, respectively. Soon thereafter, each patient began to experience insidiously progressive, upper extremity spasticity, weakness, and decreased dexterity along with dysarthria and dysphagia (which later required gastrostomy tubes). Intelligence was not affected, and using motorized wheelchairs and communicating via typing on keyboards they attended school, ultimately however, upper extremity involvement prevented any functional use of the hands and arms.

Each sister was evaluated for more than 10 years. Examination of the younger (age 20) and older (age 22) sister showed that they were alert, attentive, able to close or move their eyes on command but unable to speak or move their extremities. Each patient had weakness of facial muscles, limited tongue movements, brisk jaw jerk, and drooling. Slowing of downward saccadic eye movements was noted. They had marked spasticity of upper and lower extremities, generalized hyperreflexia, and extensor plantar responses. There was no muscle atrophy or fasciculation. Light touch, pinprick, and vibratory sensations were normal. MRI scans of the brain and spinal cord, EMG, and nerve conduction studies were normal.

Neurologic Localization

Neurologic deficits were referable to corticospinal tracts serving all extremities, corticobulbar tracts serving the face, speech, and swallowing; and to a limited extent, supranuclear control of downward eye movements.

Clinical Diagnosis

Juvenile, familial PLS (also referred to as "infantile ascending spastic paraplegia").

Discussion

These patients, including the occurrence of supranuclear gaze disturbance, are very similar to the juvenile PLS subjects in whom ALS2 mutations were identified [34]. However, genetic evaluation of the patients herein described did not identify homozygous or compound heterozygous mutations in the ALS2 gene. Additional mutations (such as deletions or mutations in non-coding regions) cannot be excluded. Nonetheless, these findings suggest that juvenile-onset, autosomal recessive PLS may be genetically heterogeneous.

Hereditary central motor-sensory axonopathy (CSMA), more commonly known as hereditary spastic paraplegia (HSP), is a group of >80 genetic disorders in which the major, but often not only symptoms are lower extremity spasticity and weakness (occurring in variable proportions and to variable extent) (see reviews [37–39]).

When spasticity and weakness begin in early childhood, symptoms may be non-progressive and resemble spastic diplegic cerebral palsy. When symptoms begin later (e.g after age 5 years) they typically worsen gradually over a period of years, following which the rate of functional decline appears to become slower for many (not all) subjects. "Uncomplicated" syndromes manifest as lower extremity spasticity and weakness frequently accompanied by urinary urgency. "Complicated" syndromes are those in which these symptoms are associated with other systemic or neurologic abnormalities (e.g. peripheral neuropathy, ataxia, intellectual disability, dementia, or muscle wasting). Peripheral neuropathy is a typical or variable feature of ~25% of genetic types of hereditary CSMA/HSP. "Complicated" and "uncomplicated spastic paraplegia syndromes may occur within the same genetic type and sometimes in the same family.

Neurologic examination of subjects with uncomplicated CSMA/HSP demonstrates extremity spasticity, hyperreflexia, and often (not always) weakness in the lower extremities and usually mildly reduced vibration perception in the toes. In uncomplicated spastic paraplegia syndromes, upper extremity strength, tone, and distal dexterity are normal. Nonetheless, it is common to note mild upper extremity hyperreflexia and Hoffman and Tromner signs (correlating with length-dependent axon degeneration, discussed below).

The term "hereditary CMSA" emphasizes neuropathologic findings (reviewed in [38]) shared by a number of different genetic types (e.g. SPG4): distal degeneration of the longest motor and sensory axons in the central nervous system (corticospinal tracts and *fasciculus gracillis* fibers, respectively). Myelin loss is considered secondary to axon degeneration. Whereas relatively shorter corticospinal tracts (those terminating in the cervical region and supplying the upper extremities) are affected to a minor degree (evident as asymptomatic upper extremity hyperreflexia), longer corticospinal tracts (those terminating in the thoracic region and supplying the legs) are more severely affected, causing spasticity and weakness. Sensory disturbance in uncomplicated CSMA/HSP manifests as mildly reduced perception of distally-applied vibration. This correlates with *fasciculus gracilis* axon degeneration that is maxima at their rostral terminals (in the cervicomedullary region). In contrast, there is much less axon degeneration involving relatively shorter *fasciculus cuneatus.*

The length-dependent, motor-sensory axon degeneration in the CMSAs (also known as HSPs) is analogous to length-dependent, motor-sensory axon degeneration occurring in Charcot-Marie-Tooth type 2 (CMT-2) disorders. In fact there is molecular overlap between some types of CMT-2 and CMSA/HSP. For example, mutations in kinesin subunits KIF1A and KIF5A cause CMSA/HSP (SPG30 and SPG10, respectively); mutations in KIF1A also cause hereditary sensory neuropathy; mutations in KIF1B cause CMT2; and mutations in BSCL2 cause hereditary distal motor neuropathy and autosomal dominant HSP associated with distal wasting (SPG17).

Clinical Pearl Reduced distal lower extremity vibration perception in CSMA/HSP is very frequent, *almost always very mild*, and may contribute to balance impairment. Finding marked vibration and proprioception impairment would suggest alternate diagnosis including Friedreich's ataxia, B12 deficiency, folate deficiency, or copper deficiency [40, 41]).

Clinical Pearl For some subjects spasticity (rather than weakness) is the major factor impairing the ability walk. In fact, many subjects are not weak at all. The relative proportions of spasticity and weakness influence symptomatic treatments. Spasticity-reducing medications (such as oral or intrathecal Baclofen) are most helpful when spasticity is the major factor disturbing gait. Conversely, when weakness is the major factor, reducing spasticity may worsen gait.

Case Example

This former college football player experienced insidious onset, progressive gait impairment beginning in his late 20's. There was no family history of similar disorder and no parental consanguinity. Neurologic examination demonstrated normal cranial nerves, normal upper extremity muscle strength, tone, and dexterity; bilaterally symmetric lower extremity spasticity (hamstrings, quadriceps, adductors) without weakness; minimally reduced distal lower extremity vibration sensation with normal light touch perception; lower extremity hyperreflexia; and marked spastic gait. Brain and spinal cord MRI were normal.

Neurologic Localization

Examination showed neurologic deficits referable to corticospinal tracts serving bilateral lower extremities; and to a lesser extent, dorsal column fibers serving bilateral lower extremities.

Diagnosis This individual had adult-onset, apparently sporadic "uncomplicated" spastic paraplegia. Genetic testing identified SPG4/spastin mutation.

Comment

Genetic testing demonstrated potentially pathogenic mutation in the SPG4/spastin gene. This mutation was absent in his parents. This suggests that this individual's adult-onset, "apparently sporadic" spastic paraplegia was due to *de novo* spastin gene mutation. Therefore, as an autosomal dominant disorder, there is a 50% risk of transmitting this mutation to each child. SPG4/spastin-mutation is the single most common form of autosomal dominant CMSA/HSP, responsible for 35–50% of such patients (see reviews[37–39]). Pathogenic SPG4/spastin mutations usually (not always) present as "uncomplicated" progressive spastic paraplegia with onset after childhood. Occasionally, SPG4/spastin mutation-related spastic paraplegia syndromes are complicated, most commonly by peripheral neuropathy or ataxia and rarely other neurologic impairments. Like SPG3/atlastin mutations, onset may occur in infancy and be "non-progressive".

Case Example

The proband had mild, non-progressive, childhood-onset intellectual disability and childhood onset, very slowly progressive spastic gait. Despite cognitive and gait impairment, he was married and worked part-time. Cranial nerves, speech, and upper extremity strength, tone, and dexterity were normal. His son and daughter also had a much greater degree of intellectual disability and more severe lower extremity spasticity than he did. His daughter, who additionally had ataxic dysarthria, late-adolescent onset, upper extremity ataxia, and a degree of upper extremity dystonia, was non-ambulatory.

Neurolocalization

For each subject, neurologic deficits were referable to cerebral hemispheres bilaterally serving cognition; corticospinal tracts serving bilateral lower extremities. In addition, the proband's daughter had deficits referable to midline cerebellum and basal ganglia.

Diagnosis

The syndrome was autosomal dominant spastic paraplegia complicated by cognitive impairment and variable ataxia and dystonia. Genetic testing demonstrated probable pathogenic KIF1A mutation.

Comment

KIF1A mutations cause SPG30 HSP, characterized by cognitive impairment, peripheral sensory neuropathy, and spastic gait. Note that KIF1A mutation-related spastic paraplegia may be transmitted as either autosomal recessive or autosomal dominant disorders [42, 43]. In addition to spastic paraplegia, KIF1A mutations cause autosomal dominant mental retardation (Mendelian Inheritance in man [MIM] phenotype number 614255) and autosomal recessive, hereditary sensory neuropathy type IIC (MIM phenotype number 614213).

Clinical Pearl These patients illustrate features shared by many forms of hereditary CMSA/HSP. First, mutations in a given gene may result in different phenotypes (intellectual disability, spastic gait, sensory neuropathy) that co-exist to variable degrees in each patient.

And second, there is significant variability in the extent of functional disability even within a family. In this family, the father was fully ambulatory without assistance and worked part-time the son ambulated short distances without aids, and the daughter was non-ambulatory.

Case Example

This individual had mild gait disturbance evident in early childhood. Over ~21 years, the gait disturbance began worsening slowly. Neurologic examination at age 47 demonstrated mild ataxic dysarthria, saccadic intrusions into smooth pursuit, mild ocular dysmetria, ataxia on finger-to-nose and heel-to-shin testing. Upper extremity muscle bulk, tone, and strength were normal. There was bilaterally symmetric spasticity in the hamstrings, quadriceps and gastrocnemius-soleus muscles but no lower extremity muscle weakness. Deep tendon reflexes were mildly hyperactive in the upper extremities, markedly hyperactive in the knees and ankles. There was reduced perception of vibration sensation in distal lower extremities. Gait (with a walker) was narrow-based and had forward-shifted heel strike (tending to walk on his toes), and reduced dorsiflexion. His brother was similarly affected.

Neurolocalization

Neurologic deficits were referable to corticospinal tracts serving bilateral lower extremities, cerebellum (midline more than hemispheres), and dorsal columns serving bilateral lower extremities.

Diagnosis

Genetic testing identified heterozygous missense mutation in the SPG7/paraplegin gene.

Comment

SPG7 spastic paraplegia is a relatively common form of spastic paraplegia. SPG7 spastic paraplegia presents with variable phenotypes including uncomplicated spastic paraplegia, spastic ataxia with peripheral neuropathy, optic atrophy, and other neurologic impairments.

Though most commonly identified as an autosomal recessive disorder, there are a number of reports of subjects with single-copy SPG7 gene mutations and pedigrees consistent with autosomal dominant transmission [44]. At least several forms of hereditary CMSA/HSP (e.g. SPG7, SPG11, and SPG30 [described above]) may be transmitted as either autosomal dominant disorders (in which heterozygous mutation is sufficient for disease) or autosomal recessive traits (in which homozygous or compound heterozygous mutations are necessary for disease).

Leukodystrophies are disorders in which the primary abnormality is demyelination or dysmyelination of central nerves (oligodendroglia abnormality) and peripheral nerve (Schwann cell abnormality).

Leukodystrophies are most recognizable when there is both central and peripheral demyelination. They may be harder to recognize and distinguish from hereditary CMSA when peripheral neuropathy is minor or absent. Brain and spinal cord MRI, brainstem and visual evoked potentials, and nerve conduction studies are valuable in evaluating subjects suspected of having leukodystrophy.

Demyelination of corticospinal and corticobulbar tracts, optic, auditory, and peripheral nerves cause spastic gait, spastic dysarthria, reduced distal sensation (n.b.: look for reduced ankle reflexes and distal sensation in subjects with more proximal lower extremity spasticity and hyperreflexia) as well as hearing and vision impairment. Cerebral hemisphere involvement causes intellectual disability, dementia, and seizures (n.b.: seizures are usually late features in leukodystrophies and occur earlier in primary gray matter disorders [poliodystrophies]). Each of these symptoms vary in their intensity and time-of-onset. Therefore, some subjects with leukodystrophies have significant demyelinating peripheral neuropathy, while others have normal peripheral nerve function. Similarly, cognitive impairment may or may not be a major factor early in the disorder.

It is important to note that primary disturbance of myelinating cells (oligodendroglia and Schwann cells) can lead to disturbed function of the axons (axonopathy). Thus, "leukodystrophy" (i.e. primary glial abnormality) may manifest as "motor-sensory axonopathy". An important example is mutation in the proteolipoprotein (PLP) gene. PLP is an oligodendroglia-expressed protein involved in myelin compaction. PLP mutations cause X-linked congenital dysmyelination (Pelizeaus Merzbacher disease). In addition, PLP mutations cause length-dependent axon degeneration manifest as SPG2 HSP/CSMA. Indeed, some mouse models of PLP mutation show axon degeneration instead of demyelination. Other examples of early-onset dysmyelination and later onset length-dependent axonopathy include Connexin 47 (also known as gap Junction protein gamma 2) mutation which causes autosomal recessive hypomyelinating leukodystrophy and autosomal recessive HSP SPG44) [45]. Adrenomyeloneuropathy (AMN) and ALD (adrenoleukodystrophy), X-linked, perioxisomal disorders due to ABCD1 gene mutation were historically considered examples of leukodystrophy (e.g. [12]). The current consensus is that the "default neuropathology" resulting from ABCD1 mutation is length-dependent motor and sensory axon degeneration (AMN phenotype); and that central demyelination (ALD phenotype) occurring in minority of subjects is an inflammatory reaction to axon degeneration [46]. It is not clear why some subjects develop inflammatory demyelination (ALD phenotype) and others (including their identical) develop AMN. Subjects with AMN may not be distinguished by history or examination from other subjects with hereditary CMSA/HSP (noting that peripheral neuropathy, a common feature of AMN, is also a common feature of many forms of CMSA/HSP). This emphasizes the importance of measuring adrenal function and plasma very long chain fatty acids in subjects with progressive spastic paraplegia.

Case Example

This 24-year-old man presented for evaluation of two-years of insidiously progressive gait impairment followed by marked cognitive decline, slurred speech, impaired upper extremity dexterity and three probable seizures. He had mild intellectual disability since early childhood, though completed high school with educational assistance and attended 2 years of community college. A former half-marathon runner, he was now barely ambulatory and required assistance eating: when food was placed on his fork he did not seem to comprehend what to do next. There was no family history of similar disorder.

Neurologic exam demonstrated marked cognitive impairment (for example, he had difficulty reciting the alphabet had difficulty naming objects). He had spastic dysarthria, ptosis, and impaired handwriting. Although he had full muscle strength throughout, there was generalized spasticity and hyperreflexia (mild in the upper extremities and moderate in the legs), extensor plantar responses, reduced vibration perception in his toes, and marked spastic-ataxic gait requiring assistance. Brain MRI revealed advanced cerebral and cerebellar atrophy, and bilaterally symmetric, confluent T2 hyperintensity involving periventricular and deep subcortical regions. Serum vitamin B12 and methylmalonic acid were normal as were plasma very long chain fatty acids, vitamin E, arylsulfatase, galactocerebrosidase, urine organic acids, and serum and urine copper.

Neurolocalization

This individual demonstrated progressive cognitive and gait impairment and had neurologic deficits involving corticospinal tracts and midline cerebellum, and mild deficits affecting dorsal column fibers. Although signs of corticospinal tract impairment were most prominent in the legs, the occurrence of mild spasticity and hyperreflexia in the arms indicated that this was as generalized process. Co-occurrence of dementia suggested a leukodystrophy (confirmed on MRI) primarily involving the CNS (no clinical evidence of peripheral neuropathy). MRI showed cerebral and cerebellar atrophy and confirmed clinical suspicion of leukodystrophy (demonstrating periventricular and confluent deep white matter abnormalities).

Diagnosis and Treatment

Laboratory testing demonstrated markedly elevated plasma homocysteine, homocystinuria, and mildly reduced plasma methionine. Genetic analysis showed homozygous mutations (C677T) in the 5,10-methylene tetrahydrofolate reductase (MTHFR) gene. Testing family members showed that each parent was heterozygous and an as yet asymptomatic younger brother was homozygous for these mutations.

Hyperhomocysteinemia with homocystinuria and hypomethioninemia, in the presence of normal serum folic acid and vitamin B12 suggested 5MTHFR deficiency which was confirmed by genetic testing. Betaine and 5-methyltetrahydrofolate were prescribed. There was marked clinical improvement over the next 12 months. Cognitive abilities returned to baseline and speech and walking markedly improved (spastic gait continued but he was able to ambulate without assistance).

Comment

5,10-Methylenetetrahydrofolate reductase (MTHFR) converts 5,10-methyltenetrahydrofolate to 5-methyltetrahydrofolate, the active form of folate. 5-methyltetrahydrofolate is a necessary co-factor, together with vitamin B12, for conversion of homocysteine to methionine by methionine synthase. Symptoms and signs of B12 deficiency, folate deficiency, and 5MTHFR overlap and include demyelination. 5,10MTHFR deficiency phenotypes are highly variable and include psychomotor developmental delay, epilepsy, thrombo-occlusive disease, and treatable leukodystrophy presenting as adolescent and adult onset spastic paraplegia [47, 48].

Clinical Pearl Treatable leukodystrophies include cerebrotendinous xanthomatosis, B12 deficiency, folate deficiency, 5MTHFR deficiency, and Wilson's disease (leukodystrophy occasionally occurs in Wilson's disease) and mitochondrial disorders (less treatable). For this reason, serum B12, methylmalonic acid, folate, very long chain fatty acids, lactate, pyruvate, serum copper, plasma amino acids (includes homocysteine and methionine), urine amino acids, and serum cholestanol are measured in all subjects with spastic paraplegia and those with leukodystrophy.

Genetic testing has the highest likelihood of yielding unambiguous information when a clinical diagnosis is made and syndrome-specific candidate genes are analyzed. Conversely, it is often difficult to interpret the significance of variations in genes (such as those identified in whole genome or whole exome sequencing) that have little or no known association with the specific syndrome. Importantly, identifying a precise genetic cause of the syndrome does often does not indicate the extent and severity of the individual's symptoms. Each of these syndromes are highly variable. For most conditions, little is known about genotype-phenotype correlation and the contribution of modifying genes and potentially modifying environmental factors. For this reason, a cautious approach to prognosis is advised.

Conclusion

The clinical diversity of hereditary myelopathies limits generalizations about their recognition. Nonetheless, corticospinal tract involvement, ranging from isolated extensor plantar responses or mild hyperreflexia to spastic paraparesis is a common feature of many disorders including it the patients described above (with MJD/SCA3, PLS, HSP, 5MTHFR deficiency, and Friedreich's ataxia). The presence of additional neurologic signs (eg, dorsal column impairment, peripheral neuropathy, ataxia, and muscle atrophy) is essential to clinical recognition of these disorders.

Acknowledgments I am grateful to Dr. Elizabeth Ames (University of Michigan) who assisted with description of the subject with 5MTHFR deficiency; and for the support from the Spastic Paraplegia Foundation and the Paul and Lois Katzman Family without whom our investigations would not be possible.

References

1. Garbern J, Hobson G. Prenatal diagnosis of pelizaeus-merzbacher disease, prenatal diagnosis; 2002;22:1033–35.
2. Garrett GS, Bailey LB. A public health approach for preventing neural tube defects: folic acid fortification and beyond. Ann N Y Acad Sci. 2018;1414(1):47–58.
3. Citraro R, et al. mTOR pathway inhibition as a new therapeutic strategy in epilepsy and epileptogenesis. Pharmacol Res. 2016;107:333–43.
4. Detrait ER, et al. Human neural tube defects: developmental biology, epidemiology, and genetics. Neurotoxicol Teratol. 2005;27(3):515–24.
5. Uttner I, et al. A novel presenilin1 mutation (Q223R) associated with early onset Alzheimer's disease, dysarthria and spastic paraparesis and decreased Abeta levels in CSF. Eur J Neurol. 2010;17(4):631–3.
6. Jimenez Caballero PE, et al. A novel presenilin 1 mutation (V261L) associated with presenile Alzheimer's disease and spastic paraparesis. Eur J Neurol. 2008;15(9):991–4.

7. Lonser RR, et al. Surgical management of spinal cord hemangioblastomas in patients with von Hippel-Lindau disease. J Neurosurg. 2003;98(1):106–16.
8. Lan MY, et al. Leukoencephalopathy with brainstem and spinal cord involvement and lactate elevation (LBSL) with a novel DARS2 mutation and isolated progressive spastic paraparesis. J Neurol Sci. 2017;372:229–31.
9. Tenney JR, et al. Early spinal cord and brainstem involvement in infantile Leigh syndrome possibly caused by a novel variant. J Child Neurol. 2013;28(12):1681–5.
10. Paulson HL. The spinocerebellar ataxias. J Neuroophthalmol. 2009;29(3):227–37.
11. Storey E. Genetic cerebellar ataxias. Semin Neurol. 2014;34(3):280–92.
12. Fink JK. Hereditary myelopathies. Continuum (N.Y.). 2008;14(3):58–74.
13. Xuncla M, et al. Protocol proposal for Friedreich ataxia molecular diagnosis using fluorescent and triplet repeat primed polymerase chain reaction. Transl Res. 2010;156(5):309–14.
14. Bidichandani SI, Delatycki MB. Friedreich ataxia. In: Adam MP, et al., editors. GeneReviews((R)). University of Washington, Seattle University of Washington, Seattle. GeneReviews is a registered trademark of the University of Washington, Seattle. All rights reserved, Seattle, WA; 1993.
15. de Bot ST, et al. Reviewing the genetic causes of spastic-ataxias. Neurology. 2012;79(14):1507–14.
16. Martinez AR, et al. Nonneurological involvement in Late-Onset Friedreich Ataxia (LOFA): exploring the phenotypes. Cerebellum. 2017;16(1):253–6.
17. Paulson H. Repeat expansion diseases. Handb Clin Neurol. 2018;147:105–23.
18. Paulson H. Spinocerebellar ataxia type 3. In: Adam MP, et al., editors. GeneReviews((R)). Seattle, WA: University of Washington; 1993.
19. Brown RH, Al-Chalabi A. Amyotrophic lateral sclerosis. N Engl J Med. 2017;377(2):162–72.
20. Sugarman EA, et al. Pan-ethnic carrier screening and prenatal diagnosis for spinal muscular atrophy: clinical laboratory analysis of >72,400 specimens. Eur J Hum Genet. 2012;20(1):27–32.
21. Parente V, Corti S. Advances in spinal muscular atrophy therapeutics. Ther Adv Neurol Disord. 2018;11:1756285618754501.
22. Meijboom KE, Wood MJA, McClorey G. Splice-switching therapy for spinal muscular atrophy. Genes (Basel). 2017;8(6):161.
23. Yoshioka M, et al. Novel $BICD_2$ mutation in a Japanese family with autosomal dominant lower extremity-predominant spinal muscular atrophy-2. Brain and Development. 2017;40(4):343–7.
24. Grunseich C, Fischbeck KH. Spinal and bulbar muscular atrophy. Neurol Clin. 2015;33(4):847–54.
25. Baumbach-Reardon L, Sacharow SJ, Ahearn ME. Spinal muscular atrophy, X-linked infantile. In: Adam MP, et al., editors. GeneReviews((R)). University of Washington, Seattle University of Washington, Seattle. GeneReviews is a registered trademark of the university of Washington, Seattle. All rights reserved, Seattle, WA; 1993.
26. Das J, et al. A missense mutation in DYNC1H1 gene causing spinal muscular atrophy – lower extremity, dominant. Neurol Neurochir Pol. 2017;52(2):293–7.
27. Nishimura AL, et al. A mutation in the vesicle-trafficking protein VAPB causes late-onset spinal muscular atrophy and amyotrophic lateral sclerosis. Am J Hum Genet. 2004;75(5):822–31.
28. Floeter MK, Mills R. Progression in primary lateral sclerosis: a prospective analysis. Amyotroph Lateral Scler. 2009;10(5–6):339–46.
29. Pringle CE, et al. Primary lateral sclerosis. Clinical features, neuropathology and diagnostic criteria. Brain. 1992;115(Pt 2):495–520.
30. Wais V, et al. The concept and diagnostic criteria of primary lateral sclerosis. Acta Neurol Scand. 2017;136(3):204–11.
31. Fink JK. Progressive spastic paraparesis: hereditary spastic paraplegia and it's relation to primary and amyotrophic lateral sclerosis. Semin Neurol. 2001;21:199–208.
32. Brugman F, et al. Differentiation of hereditary spastic paraparesis from primary lateral sclerosis in sporadic adult-onset upper motor neuron syndromes. Arch Neurol. 2009;66(4):509–14.

33. Fink JK. Upper motor neuron disorders: hereditary spastic paraplegia and primary lateral sclerosis. In: Johnson MV, Adams HP, Fatemi A, editors. Neurobiology of disease. New York: Oxford University Press; 2016.
34. Yang Y, et al. The gene encoding alsin, a protein with three guanine-nucleotide exchange factor domains, is mutated in a form of recessive amyotrophic lateral sclerosis. Nat Genet. 2001;29(2):160–5.
35. Mitsumoto H, et al. Phenotypic and molecular analyses of primary lateral sclerosis. Neurol Genet. 2015;1(1):e3.
36. Chow CY, et al. Deleterious variants of FIG4, a phosphoinositide phosphatase, in patients with ALS. Am J Hum Genet. 2009;84(1):85–8.
37. Fink JK. The hereditary spastic paraplegias. In: Rosenberg R, editor. Molecular and genetic basis of neurologic and psychiatric disease. Lippincott Williams & Wilkins; 2014.
38. Fink JK. Hereditary spastic paraplegia: clinico-pathologic features and emerging molecular mechanisms. Acta Neuropathol. 2013;126(3):307–28.
39. Fink JK (2017). https://rarediseases.org/rare-diseases/hereditary-spastic-paraplegia/
40. Hedera P, et al. Myelopolyneuropathy and pancytopenia due to copper deficiency and high zinc levels of unknown origin II. The denture cream is a primary source of excessive zinc. Neurotoxicology. 2009;30(6):996–9.
41. Jaiser SR, Winston GP. Copper deficiency myelopathy. J Neurol. 2010;257(6):869–81.
42. Cheon CK, et al. Autosomal dominant transmission of complicated hereditary spastic paraplegia due to a dominant negative mutation of KIF1A, SPG30 gene. Sci Rep. 2017;7(1):12527.
43. Roda RH, Schindler AB, Blackstone C. Multigeneration family with dominant SPG30 hereditary spastic paraplegia. Ann Clin Transl Neurol. 2017;4(11):821–4.
44. Sanchez-Ferrero E, et al. SPG7 mutational screening in spastic paraplegia patients supports a dominant effect for some mutations and a pathogenic role for p.A510V. Clin Genet. 2013;83(3):257–62.
45. Orthmann-Murphy JL, et al. Hereditary spastic paraplegia is a novel phenotype for GJA12/GJC2 mutations. Brain. 2009;132(Pt 2):426–38.
46. Ferrer I, Aubourg P, Pujol A. General aspects and neuropathology of X-linked adrenoleukodystrophy. Brain Pathol. 2010;20(4):817–30.
47. Lossos A, et al. Severe methylenetetrahydrofolate reductase deficiency: clinical clues to a potentially treatable cause of adult-onset hereditary spastic paraplegia. JAMA Neurol. 2014;71(7):901–4.
48. Haworth JC, et al. Symptomatic and asymptomatic methylenetetrahydrofolate reductase deficiency in two adult brothers. Am J Med Genet. 1993;45(5):572–6.
49. Greene E, Mahishi L, Entezam A, Kumari D, Usdin K. Repeat-induced epigenetic changes in intron 1 of the frataxin gene and its consequences in Friedreich ataxia. Nucleic Acids Res. 2007;35(10):3383–90.

Activity Based Restorative Therapy (ABRT) in Myelopathies

11

Cristina L. Sadowsky

Contents

The International Classification of Functioning, Disability and Health (ICF) describes functioning at the body, person and societal level; components of functioning and disability are divided into impairments, activity, participation [1] according to the domain it addresses. It is thus helpful to attempt describing a treatment or intervention following this well-defined structure.

Treatment of myelopathies, a vastly inclusive term referring to neurologic changes related to spinal cord dysfunction, require etiology specific and deficit specific interventions as the initial damage to the spinal cord frequently results into long standing neurologic deficits. The etiologies of myelopathies are multiple: degenerative, traumatic, immune, infectious, metabolic, vascular, tumors, etc. and consequences can be grouped into those affecting the central nervous system (CNS), the autonomic nervous system (ANS), the musculo-skeletal system and metabolism.

Over the past 1.5 decades, there has been a paradigm shift in the field of neurorehabilitation, moving the focus from compensation to restoration in order to achieve functional goals. This shift was prompted by accruing evidence that the nervous system is capable of plastic changes and repair and the process is activity dependent [2]. Thus, activity based therapeutic interventions gained more credibility and started flooding the field. From constraint induced movement therapy (CIMT) or forced used therapy, utilized to improve upper limb function following

C. L. Sadowsky (✉)
Kennedy Krieger Institute, International Center for Spinal Cord Injury, Baltimore, MD, USA
e-mail: sadowsky@kennedykrieger.org

B. Greenberg (ed.), *Myelopathy*, https://doi.org/10.1007/978-3-030-99906-3_11

stroke [3] or in children with cerebral palsy [4] to activity based therapy/activity based restorative therapy [5] utilized to improve function in spinal cord related paralysis, activity based programs are becoming more common and mainstream.

The words activity and exercise have been used interchangeably in the past, but they are describing different concepts, with exercise being a subset of physical activity that is "planned, structured and repetitive" and has the objective of maintaining or improving physical fitness [6].

Activity based therapy (ABT) has been described as any therapeutic intervention that is focused on improving muscle function and sensory perception *below* the level of injury [7].These structured interventions attempt to restore function via standardized therapeutic activities based on principles of neuroscience, with the primary premise that the spinal cord, as part of the central nervous system, is plastic and has the ability to recover function [8, 9].

Activity based restorative therapy (ABRT) [10] is defined as a life-long intervention with principles based on activity-dependent neural plasticity, where changes in the nervous and muscular system are driven by repetitive activation of the neuromuscular system *above* and *below* injury level. ABRT intends to deliver repetitive, near-normal amount and quality of activity intended to optimize the function of the neurological system and offset the rapid aging, physical deterioration and secondary complications associated with spinal cord related paralysis.

Key components of ABRT are:

1. Functional Electrical Stimulation (FES)
2. Locomotor Gait Training (LGT)
3. Weight Loading/Bearing
4. Massed Practice
5. Task-Specific Practice

All of the ABRT components have been independently studied in the clinical domain [11–15]; evaluating the combined effect of ABRT on neurologic and day to day function is harder to do, given the individualized application of the different ABRT components during the rehabilitative efforts. Activity can be used to both prime and train the nervous system and the role of each particular instrument varies depending on the timing of intervention [16].

What has consistently been well described on the continuum of impairment, activity limitation and participation is the effect of activity and exercise on the different systems affected by spinal cord disease related paralysis.

As mentioned in the beginning, myelopathies require two domains of intervention and treatment; one related to the cause of the neurologic dysfunction, the other one addressing the consequences. This paper only addresses the latter. It should be noted that few, if any studies looked precisely at the effect of ABRT on the neurologic dysfunction associated with myelopathies in general; most of the interventions have been applied and studied in the traumatic spinal cord injury (SCI) or non-progressive spinal cord disease related paralysis.

The role of activity and exercise at the impairment level can be described throughout the cell-tissue continuum.

A. Cellular basis for role of activity:
   1. New cell birth is activity related in most of the systems affected by the damage characteristic to myelopathies.
      (a) Neurons - Trejo et al. [17] found that exercise induced changes in the adult rat brain, including new neuronal cell birth, is mediated through insulin-like growth factor IGF-I.
      (b) Oligodendrocytes - Krityakiarana et al. [18] demonstrated that 7 days of voluntary exercise increased both nestin-GFP expression and markers for immature oligodendrocytes in the white and gray matter of the intact thoracic cord of a transgenic mice.
      (c) Astrocytes – Chang [19] showed that in a localized model of SCI, exercised rats (given pre-SCI exercise) had significantly higher levels of neuronal and astroglial HSP 72, a lower functional deficit, fewer spinal cord contusions, and fewer apoptotic cells than did non-exercised rats. Also, swimming and a 5 week structured aerobic exercise both decreased neuropathic pain and reversed astrocyte and microglia hyperactivity in the dorsal horn in mice with partial sciatic nerve injury [20].
      (d) Muscle cell – Verdijk et al. [21] found that the type II muscle fiber atrophy associated with normal aging was reversed and the decline in type II muscle fiber satellite cell content was attenuated by a resistance-type exercise training regimen lasting 12 weeks.
      (e) Bone - the integrity and health of the bone depends on a carefully choreographed and balanced osteoblast – osteoclast – osteocyte interplay; exercise and mechanical stimulation play a major role at multiple stages of the bone metabolism: exercise prevents osteocyte death [22]; exercise has been shown to induce mesenchymal cells to differentiate towards osteoblasts [23]; exercise facilitates and conditions osteoblasts to progress toward osteogenic differentiation [24]; 2–4 weeks of exercise in the form of climbing decreases the number of osteoclasts and increases bone mass in mice [25].
   2. Myelination and re-myelination are also activity dependent; Yoon et al. [26] showed that exercise and high fat diet increased the amount of myelin in the lumbo-sacral cord in mice. Low intensity exercise even decreased diabetes related myelin breakdown in the peripheral, sciatic nerve in rats [27].
B. Activity role in tissues/systems affected by myelopathies:
   1. Priming the nervous system:

      It is hard to argue against the fact that exercise improves motor strength and endurance, but exercise also improves motor control; clinical experiments show that exercise can improve motor skills acquisition through a learning, "motor memory" mechanism [28]; in the rehabilitative and sports medicine field, there's ample evidence that exercise improves gait [64, 77, 79]. In the

SCD related population, studies also show that training with exercise therapy, electrical stimulation, or functional electrical stimulation of the upper limb following cervical spinal cord injury leads to improvements in muscle strength, upper limb function and activity of daily living or quality of life [29].

Exercise also affects sensory function and could modulate pain; Sprague-Dawley rats with moderate, unilateral spinal cord contusion at C5 level that exercised exhibited decreased incidence of tactile allodynia [30]; in a peripheral nerve (sciatic) animal injury model, low intensity aerobic exercise regimen suppressed pain-like behaviors, postulated to be mediated by enhancing brainstem 5-HT neurotransmission [31].

Exercise plays a significant role in the modulation of the autonomic nervous system function.

- Cardio-vascular system: there is convincing evidence that some of the protective and therapeutic effects of chronic exercise training are related to its impact on the autonomic nervous system; training induces improvement in vascular function, blood volume expansion, cardiac remodeling, insulin resistance and renal-adrenal function [32]. In one experiment, a single bout of intensive, dynamic arm crank exercise eliminated orthostatic hypotension in 10 individuals with paraplegia [33, 34].
- Genito-urinary system: Ward at al [35] demonstrated in a rat SCI model that repetitive sensory information generated through task-specific stepping and/or loading can improve non-locomotor functions, including bladder function.
- Gastro-intestinal system: physical activity can improve gastric emptying and lower the relative risk of colon cancer in most populations [36] and reciprocal gait orthoses (RGO) driven gait training appeared to improve bowel function in a group of 12 individuals with paraplegia [37].

2. Metabolism: exercise certainly has a well-recognized effect on metabolism, affecting factors like weight, body composition, glucose and lipids processing both in healthy individuals and those with a chronic disease. Specifically, in the SCI population, exercise - like using an indoor hand-bike, appears to be an effective modality to improve body composition, fasting insulin, and insulin resistance levels and fitness [38].
3. Bone mass: there is plenty of evidence that exercise improves bone mass and density in both men and women of different ages: young adult women [39], postmenopausal women [40], adolescent and young men [41] and even middle-aged and older men [42]. In individuals with SCD related paralysis, exercise has not been found to be very effective in preventing bone loss or restoring bone mass [43]; but functional electrical stimulation (ES) using cyclical muscle contraction has been shown to be beneficial to bone mass health [44, 45].
4. Inflammation/immune response: exercise appears to play a role in modulating immune response and inflammation. Dyslipidemia and inflammation are frequently found in some diseases, such as obesity, type 2 diabetes mellitus, and spinal cord related paralysis [46]. Recent literature has identified that

lipids have a pivotal role in the activation of inflammatory pathways, increasing the production of inflammatory cytokines. In one study, aerobic plus resistance training for 1 year showed a protective role in bone mineral content associated with an improvement in adiponectin and leptin concentrations, favoring the control of the inflammatory state related to obesity in 42 adolescents [47]. In addition, exercise-induced modulation of the immune and inflammatory system was described in cancer [48], type 2 diabetes mellitus [49] and SCI [50].

5. Cellular proliferation/tumor formation: exercise appears effective in increasing the birth of various stem cells, their migration and differentiation [51, 52], including neural stem cells [53]. In addition, epidemiological data supports the concept that exercise training can reduce disease risk and mortality for several cancer diagnoses, including breast and colon cancer [54].

Moving to the next ICF domains, those of activity limitation and participation, exercise appears to play a significant role here too. The positive role of exercise on mental health [55, 56], cognitive function [57, 58], quality of life [59, 60] has been vastly documented. Exercise-induced neuroplasticity seems to be the basis of spatial learning and memory improvement, even under neurodegenerative conditions [61].

Now that the role of activity and exercise throughout the impairment-activity-participation continuum has been framed, utilizing ABRT, a well-structured and defined exercise based intervention to implement positive functional changes becomes easier.

In the rehabilitation field, improving function is the ultimate goal. But when dealing with a neurologic etiology for the loss of function, a separation between day to day function and neurologic function needs to be made. Traditionally, rehabilitation only looked at improving the day to day functions, such as feeding, grooming, mobility, transfers, ambulation; the rehabilitative interventions relied heavily on compensatory strategies, utilizing residual neurologic function to improve day to day function. Activity based therapies aim to improve day to day function by restoring neurologic function, taking advantage of the neuro-plastic and neuro-regenerative abilities of the nervous system and guiding the process along. ABRT changes neuro-rehabilitation from a compensatory to a restorative approach.

In 2005, a study was published concluding that in the animal model of ischemic unilateral stroke, behavioral experience with the less-affected forelimb early after unilateral lesions had the potential to increase disuse and dysfunction of the impaired forelimb, consistent with a training-induced exacerbation of learned non-use. These findings were suggestive of competitive processes in experience-dependent neural restructuring after brain damage [62]. In other words, it pointed to the fact that compensatory training has the potential to increase disuse and dysfunction even more.

Another essential difference between traditional, compensatory rehabilitation and the activity based restorative one, is the amount of intervention, in both frequency and length of exposure to the task. In traditional, compensatory rehabilitation, the amount of practice needed to trigger neuroplastic changes is small compared to animal models, thus it is possible that current doses of task-specific practice during rehabilitation are not adequate to drive the neural reorganization [63].

Main features of the compensatory approach/traditional therapy are:

1. Activate nervous system above the level of the lesion
2. Low intensity practice (1 h per day)
3. Non-patterned movements
4. Compensates for loss function
5. Uses compensatory devices

The restorative approach/Activity Based Restorative Therapy features:

1. Activate nervous system above and below the level of the lesion
2. High intensity practice (2–5 h per day)
3. Non-patterned and patterned movements
4. Restores lost function
5. Minimizes or eliminates compensatory devices

ABRT Components

1. Electrical stimulation (estim) involves three types of therapeutic interventions:
   (a) Neuromuscular electrical stimulation (NMES), where electricity is applied across the surface of the skin over the intact peripheral nerve and it evokes an action potential in the nerve fiber which causes an exchange of ions to drive the muscle to contract.
   (b) Functional Electrical Stimulation (FES), where the application of electrical stimulus to a paralyzed nerve or muscle is made with the intention of achieving or restoring a function. FES principle also refers to orthotic substitution (neuroprosthesis).
   (c) Transcutaneous Electrical Nerve Stimulation (TENS), a modality using electricity to modulate pain by exciting the peripheral nerves. Common types of TENS interventions are conventional TENS (sensory), where electrical current activates A beta mechano-receptors; acupuncture like-TENS (motor), where electrical current activates small diameter fibers (A delta or group III) arising from muscles and Intense TENS (noxious), where the electric current activates small A delta cutaneous afferents

   The therapeutic applications of electrical stimulation as it pertains to ABRT in myelopathies are to prevent/reverse disuse atrophy, strengthen the muscle, modulate spasticity and provide orthotic substitution.
2. Locomotor Gait Training (LGT) is an activity-based rehabilitative strategy designed to improve sensory, motor and autonomic function, health and quality of life. It provides sensory cues to re-train neural patterns that will result in effective locomotion and emphasizes recovery of motor function using the intrinsic

mechanisms of the nervous system, rather than compensatory strategies. Proven benefits of locomotor training in SCD related paralysis are increase in walking speed and gait velocity, increase in distance walked and improvements in gait parameters [64].

3. Weight loading, performed by transmitting force across a joint; weight loading is meant to promote joint alignment, bone stress, muscle co-contraction and normalize the afferent input [80, 81].
4. Massed practice is a term used to describe an intervention in which repetitive practice is the primary therapeutic factor. It is meant to promote cortical reorganization; can be motor and sensory driven, or better, combined [13, 14, 65]
5. Task specific practice, also referred to as skill training, has the goal of acquiring new motor skills and induces substantial cortical plastic changes in both the injured and non-injured brain [66–68]

Other therapeutic interventions are added to ABRT's neuro-rehabilitative arsenal as more evidence supporting their effectiveness translate from bench to bedside.

(a) Vibration, specifically whole body vibration is now increasingly used to aid in optimizing bone health [69], improve lower limb blood flow [70, 71], modulate spasticity [72], improve muscle strength and tolerance to upright positioning [73]
(b) Spinal stimulation, transcutaneous or through an implanted device, is able to help achieve full body weight-bearing standing [74] and voluntary movement in individuals with complete cord lesion [75] possibly by enhancing the excitability state of the spinal circuitry [76]
(c) Aquatherapy, where weightlessness and buoyancy are added to the LGT, massed practice and task specific training [78], has been found to improve function in individuals with SCD related paralysis, but is underutilized.

ABRT and Technology

ABRT is heavily reliant on technology. Indeed, technology can be used for several reasons in individuals with neurologic paralysis:

(a) To achieve movement/motor function:
   - External device: FES orthosis for foot drop, robotics/exoskeletons for gait training and community ambulation, Brain Machine Interface (BMI) for sailing, virtual reality for motor training/skill acquisition
   - Internal implant: FES bowel/bladder system to insure continence, BMI for eating, epidural implant to achieve standing/walking [2]

(b) To insure accessibility: mobility devices/wheelchairs, robots to help Instrumental Activities of Daily Living ("The Butler"); voice activation for environmental control

(c) To allow for sustained exercise and physical activity [77]:
   - Information and communication technology for knowledge dissemination, to improve accessibility and compliance
   - Interactive technology for engagement, training and compliance
   - Electronic gauges for monitoring performance
   - FES driven exercise systems for motor training and endurance building

Finally, ABRT aims to facilitate integration in normal living, participation in sports, recreation and leisure activities, thus addressing both the ICF's participation component and the restorative mission included in its' title.

Much remains to be studied in the application and benefits of utilizing an activity based restorative rehabilitation program when addressing consequences related to neurologic insults like those induced by myelopathies: the specific interventions, the exact dosing, the best methods to evaluate its' effectiveness, the cost in effort and currency. And to have a pragmatic view of why using a restorative approach is better than compensating for the deficit is helpful. Lastly, specific research on the effectiveness of ABRT in myelopathies needs to be done; addressing each etiology in well-designed clinical trials might be too large of a task, but utilizing pooled, well collected mega-data and analyzing clinical effectiveness is in the realm of doable.

References

1. World Health Organisation (WHO). International classification of functioning, disability and health: ICF. Geneva: WHO; 2001.
2. Fakhoury M. Spinal cord injury: overview of experimental approaches used to restore locomotor activity. Rev Neurosci. 2015;26(4):397–405.
3. Kwakkel G, Veerbeek JM, van Wegen EE, Wolf SL. Constraint induced movement therapy after stroke. Lancet Neurol. 2015;14(2):224–34. Intensive training of motor function and functional skills among young children with cerebral palsy: a systematic review and meta-analysis. BMC Pediatr. 2014; 14: 292. 0.1186/s12887-014-0292-5
4. Jones ML, Evans N, Tefertiller C, Backus D, Sweatman M, Tansey K, Morrison S. Activity-based therapy for recovery of walking in individuals with chronic spinal cord injury: results from a randomized clinical trial. Arch Phys Med Rehabil. 2014;95(12):2239-46.e2. https://doi.org/10.1016/j.apmr.2014.07.400. Epub 2014 Aug 4
5. Caspersen CJ, Powell KE, Christenson GM. Physical activity, exercise, and physical fitness: definitions and distinctions for health-related research. Public Health Rep. 1985;100(2):126–31. PMCID: PMC1424733
6. Backus D, Apple D, Hudson L, Acevedo R. Systematic review of activity-based interventions to improve neurological outcomes after SCI January 1998-March 2009; 2017. Available at: www.bu.edu/drrk/research-syntheses/spinal-cord-injuries/activity-based-interventions. Accessed 10 Nov 2017
7. Dromerick AW, Lum PS, Hidler J. Activity-based therapies. NeuroRx. 2006;3(4):428–38.
8. Sadowsky CL, McDonald JW. Activity-based restorative therapies: concepts and applications in spinal cord injury-related neurorehabilitation. Dev Disabil Res Rev. 2009;15(2):112–6. https://doi.org/10.1002/ddrr.61. Review. PMID: 19489091
9. Dolbow DR, Gorgey AS, Recio AC, Stiens SA, Curry AC, Sadowsky CL, Gater DR, Martin R, McDonald JW. Activity-based restorative therapies after spinal cord injury: inter-institutional

conceptions and perceptions. Aging Dis. 2015;6(4):254–61. https://doi.org/10.14336/AD.2014.1105. eCollection 2015 Aug 1. Review
10. Martin R, Sadowsky C, Obst K, Meyer B, McDonald J. Functional electrical stimulation in spinal cord injury: from theory to practice. Top Spinal Cord Inj Rehabil. 2012;18(1):28–33. https://doi.org/10.1310/sci1801-28. PMCID: PMC3584753
11. Hubli M, Dietz VJ. The physiological basis of neurorehabilitation – locomotor training after spinal cord injury. Neuroeng Rehabil. 2013;10:5. https://doi.org/10.1186/1743-0003-10-5. Published online 2013 Jan 21. PMCID: PMC3584845
12. Beekhuizen KS, Field-Fote EC. Massed practice versus massed practice with stimulation: effects on upper extremity function and cortical plasticity in individuals with incomplete cervical spinal cord injury. Neurorehabil Neural Repair. 2005 Mar;19(1):33–45.
13. Hoffman LR, Field-Fote EC. Functional and corticomotor changes in individuals with tetraplegia following unimanual or bimanual massed practice training with somatosensory stimulation: a pilot study. J Neurol Phys Ther. 2010 Dec;34(4):193–201. https://doi.org/10.1097/NPT.0b013e3181fbe692.
14. Spooren AI, Janssen-Potten YJ, Kerckhofs E, Bongers HM, Seelen HA. ToCUEST: a task-oriented client-centered training module to improve upper extremity skilled performance in cervical spinal cord-injured persons. Spinal Cord. 2011;49(10):1049–54. https://doi.org/10.1038/sc.2011.54. Epub 2011 Jun 7
15. Morreale M, Marchione P, Pili A, Lauta A, Castiglia SF, Spallone A, Pierelli F, Giacomini P. Early versus delayed rehabilitation treatment in hemiplegic patients with ischemic stroke: proprioceptive or cognitive approach? Eur J Phys Rehabil Med. 2016;52(1):81–9. Epub 2015 Jul 27.E
16. Trejo JL, Carro E, Torres-Alemán I. Circulating insulin-like growth factor I mediates exercise-induced increases in the number of new neurons in the adult hippocampus. J Neurosci. 2001;21(5):1628–34.
17. Krityakiarana W, Espinosa-Jeffrey A, Ghiani CA, Zhao PM, Topaldjikian N, Gomez-Pinilla F, Yamaguchi M, Kotchabhakdi N, de Vellis J. Voluntary exercise increases oligodendrogenesis in spinal cord. Int J Neurosci. 2010 Apr;120(4):280–90. https://doi.org/10.3109/00207450903222741.
18. Chang CK, Chou W, Lin HJ, Huang YC, Tang LY, Lin MT, Chang CP. Exercise preconditioning protects against spinal cord injury in rats by upregulating neuronal and astroglial heat shock protein 72. Int J Mol Sci. 2014 Oct 20;15(10):19018–36. https://doi.org/10.3390/ijms151019018.
19. Almeida C, DeMaman A, Kusuda R, Cadetti F, Ravanelli MI, Queiroz AL, Sousa TA, Zanon S, Silveira LR, Lucas G. Exercise therapy normalizes BDNF upregulation and glial hyperactivity in a mouse model of neuropathic pain. Pain. 2014;156(3):504–13. https://doi.org/10.1016/j.pain.0000000000000065. PMID: 25633251 [Epub ahead of print]
20. Verdijk LB, Snijders T, Drost M, Delhaas T, Kadi F, van Loon LJ. Satellite cells in human skeletal muscle; from birth to old age. Age (Dordr). 2014 Apr;36(2):545–7.
21. Fonseca H, Moreira-Gonçalves D, Esteves JL, Viriato N, Vaz M, Mota MP, Duarte JA. Voluntary exercise has long-term in vivo protective effects on osteocyte viability and bone strength following ovariectomy. Calcif Tissue Int. 2011;88(6):443–54. https://doi.org/10.1007/s00223-011-9476-2. Epub 2011 Mar 18
22. Maredziak M, Smieszek A, Chrzastek K, Basinska K, Marycz K. Physical activity increases the total number of bone-marrow-derived mesenchymal stem cells, enhances their osteogenic potential, and inhibits their adipogenic properties. Stem Cells Int. 2015;2015:379093.
23. Menuki K, Mori T, Sakai A, Sakuma M, Okimoto N, Shimizu Y, Kunugita N, Nakamura T. Climbing exercise enhances osteoblast differentiation and inhibits adipogenic differentiation with high expression of PTH/PTHrP receptor in bone marrow cells. Bone. 2008;43:613–20.
24. Mori T, Okimoto N, Sakai A, Okazaki Y, Nakura N, Notomi T, Nakamura T. Climbing exercise increases bone mass and trabecular bone turnover through transient regulation of marrow osteogenic and osteoclastogenic potentials in mice. J Bone Miner Res. 2003 Nov;18(11):2002–9.

25. Yoon H, Kleven A, Paulsen A, Kleppe L, Wu J, Ying Z, Gomez-Pinilla F, Scarisbrick IA. Interplay between exercise and dietary fat modulates myelinogenesis in the central nervous system. Biochim Biophys Acta. 2016;1862(4):545–55. https://doi.org/10.1016/j.bbadis.2016.01.019. Epub 2016 Jan 26
26. Gulsen I, Demiroglu M, Aycan A, Ucler R, Alaca I, Orhon ZN, Kanter M. Effects of low-intensity treadmill exercise on sciatic nerve in experimental diabetic neuropathy. Anal Quant Cytopathol Histpathol. 2016 Apr;38(2):95–102.
27. Skriver K, Roig M, Lundbye-Jensen J, Pingel J, Helge JW, Kiens B, Nielsen JB. Acute exercise improves motor memory: exploring potential biomarkers. Neurobiol Learn Mem. 2014;116:46–58. https://doi.org/10.1016/j.nlm.2014.08.004. Epub 2014 Aug 14
28. Lu X, Battistuzzo CR, Zoghi M, Galea MP. Effects of training on upper limb function after cervical spinal cord injury: a systematic review. Clin Rehabil. 2015;29(1):3–13. https://doi.org/10.1177/0269215514536411. Epub 2014 Jun 4
29. Detloff MR, Smith EJ, Quiros Molina D, Ganzer PD, Houlé JD. Acute exercise prevents the development of neuropathic pain and the sprouting of non-peptidergic (GDNF- and artemin-responsive) c-fibers after spinal cord injury. Exp Neurol. 2014;255:38–48. https://doi.org/10.1016/j.expneurol.2014.02.013. Epub 2014 Feb 19
30. Bobinski F, Ferreira TAA, Córdova MM, Dombrowski PA, da Cunha C, Santo CCDE, Poli A, Pires RGW, Martins-Silva C, Sluka KA, Santos ARS. Role of brainstem serotonin in analgesia produced by low-intensity exercise on neuropathic pain after sciatic nerve injury in mice. Pain. 2015 Dec;156(12):2595–606. https://doi.org/10.1097/j.pain.0000000000000372.
31. Fu Q, Levine BD. Exercise and the autonomic nervous system. Handb Clin Neurol. 2013;117:147–60. https://doi.org/10.1016/B978-0-444-53491-0.00013-4.
32. Engelke KA, Shea JD, Doerr DF, Convertino VA. Enhanced carotid-cardiac baroreflex response and elimination of orthostatic hypotension 24 hours after acute exercise in paraplegics. Paraplegia. 1992 Dec;30(12):872–9.
33. Engelke KA, Shea JD, Doerr DF, Convertino VA. Autonomic functions and orthostatic responses 24 h after acute intense exercise in paraplegic subjects. Am J Physiol. 1994;266(4 Pt 2):R1189–96. Erratum in Am J Physiol. 2007 Oct;293(4):R1771
34. Ward PJ, Herrity AN, Smith RR, Willhite A, Harrison BJ, Petruska JC, Harkema SJ, Hubscher CH. J Neurotrauma. 2014;31:819–33.
35. Bi L, Triadafilopoulos G. Exercise and gastrointestinal function and disease: an evidence-based review of risks and benefits. Clin Gastroenterol Hepatol. 2003 Sep;1(5):345–55.
36. Sun JL, Zhong SZ, Ouyang YT, Tang D, Xian QL. Beneficial effects of reciprocating gait orthosis on bladder and bowel functions in paraplegia patients. Nan Fang Yi Ke Da Xue Xue Bao. 2008 Jun;28(6):1019–21.
37. Kim DI, Lee H, Lee BS, Kim J, Jeon JY. Effects of a 6-week indoor hand-bike exercise program on health and fitness levels in people with spinal cord injury: a randomized controlled trial study. Arch Phys Med Rehabil. 2015;96(11):2033-40.e1. https://doi.org/10.1016/j.apmr.2015.07.010. Epub 2015 Aug 5
38. Mosti MP, Carlsen T, Aas E, Hoff J, Stunes AK, Syversen U. Maximal strength training improves bone mineral density and neuromuscular performance in young adult women. J Strength Cond Res. 2014;28(10):2935–45. https://doi.org/10.1519/JSC.0000000000000493. PMID: 24736773
39. Howe TE, Shea B, Dawson LJ, Downie F, Murray A, Ross C, Harbour RT, Caldwell LM, Creed G. Exercise for preventing and treating osteoporosis in postmenopausal women. Cochrane Database Syst Rev. 2011 Jul 6;7:CD000333. https://doi.org/10.1002/14651858.CD000333.pub2.
40. Strope MA, Nigh P, Carter MI, Lin N, Jiang J, Hinton PS. Physical activity-associated bone loading during adolescence and young adulthood is positively associated with adult bone mineral density in men. Am J Mens Health. 2015;9(6):442–50. https://doi.org/10.1177/1557988314549749. Epub 2014 Sep 18

41. Bolam KA, van Uffelen JG, Taaffe DR. The effect of physical exercise on bone density in middle-aged and older men: a systematic review. Osteoporos Int. 2013;24(11):2749–62. https://doi.org/10.1007/s00198-013-2346-1. Epub 2013 Apr 4
42. Biering-Sørensen F, Hansen B, Lee BS. Non-pharmacological treatment and prevention of bone loss after spinal cord injury: a systematic review. Spinal Cord. 2009;47(7):508–18. https://doi.org/10.1038/sc.2008.177. Epub 2009 Jan 27
43. Dudley-Javoroski S, Shields RK. Asymmetric bone adaptations to soleus mechanical loading after spinal cord injury. J Musculoskelet Neuronal Interact. 2008;8:227–38.
44. Frotzler A, Coupaud S, Perret C, et al. High-volume FES-cycling partially reverses bone loss in people with chronic spinal cord injury. Bone. 2008;43:169–76.
45. Lira FS, Rosa Neto JC, Antunes BM, Fernandes RA. The relationship between inflammation, dyslipidemia and physical exercise: from the epidemiological to molecular approach. Curr Diabetes Rev. 2014;10(6):391–6.
46. Campos RM, de Mello MT, Tock L, Silva PL, Masquio DC, de Piano A, Sanches PL, Carnier J, Corgosinho FC, Foschini D, Tufik S, Dâmaso AR. Aerobic plus resistance training improves bone metabolism and inflammation in adolescents who are obese. J Strength Cond Res. 2014 Mar;28(3):758–66. https://doi.org/10.1519/JSC.0b013e3182a996df.
47. Koelwyn GJ, Wennerberg E, Demaria S, Jones LW. Exercise in regulation of inflammation-immune Axis function in cancer initiation and progression. Oncology (Williston Park). 2015 Dec;29(12):908–20.
48. Karstoft K, Pedersen BK. Exercise and type 2 diabetes: focus on metabolism and inflammation. Immunol Cell Biol. 2016;94(2):146–50. https://doi.org/10.1038/icb.2015.101. Epub 2015 Nov 16
49. Neefkes-Zonneveld CR, Bakkum AJ, Bishop NC, van Tulder MW, Janssen TW. Effect of long-term physical activity and acute exercise on markers of systemic inflammation in persons with chronic spinal cord injury: a systematic review. Arch Phys Med Rehabil. 2015;96(1):30–42. https://doi.org/10.1016/j.apmr.2014.07.006. Epub 2014 Jul 24
50. Shi XC, Cai MX, Tian ZJ. Research advance on cardiomyocyte proliferation induced by aerobic exercise and stem cell mobilization. Sheng Li Ke Xue Jin Zhan. 2014 Aug;45(4):276–81.
51. Skovgaard D, Bayer ML, Mackey AL, Madsen J, Kjaer M, Kjaer A. Increased cellular proliferation in rat skeletal muscle and tendon in response to exercise: use of FLT and PET/CT. Mol Imaging Biol. 2010 Dec;12(6):626–34. https://doi.org/10.1007/s11307-010-0316-y.
52. Luo J, Hu X, Zhang L, Li L, Zheng H, Li M, Zhang Q. Physical exercise regulates neural stem cells proliferation and migration via SDF-1α/CXCR4 pathway in rats after ischemic stroke. Neurosci Lett. 2014;578:203–8. https://doi.org/10.1016/j.neulet.2014.06.059. Epub 2014 Jul 7
53. Pedersen L, Christensen JF, Hojman P. Effects of exercise on tumor physiology and metabolism. Cancer J. 2015 Mar-Apr;21(2):111–6. https://doi.org/10.1097/PPO.0000000000000096.
54. Biddle SJ, Asare M. Physical activity and mental health in children and adolescents: a review of reviews. Br J Sports Med. 2011;45(11):886–95. https://doi.org/10.1136/bjsports-2011-090185. Epub 2011 Aug 1
55. Matta Mello Portugal E, Cevada T, Sobral Monteiro-Junior R, Teixeira Guimarães T, da Cruz RE, Lattari E, Blois C, Camaz Deslandes A. Neuroscience of exercise: from neurobiology mechanisms to mental health. Neuropsychobiology. 2013;68(1):1–14. https://doi.org/10.1159/000350946. Epub 2013 Jun 15
56. Hötting K, Röder B. Beneficial effects of physical exercise on neuroplasticity and cognition. Neurosci Biobehav Rev. 2013;37(9 Pt B):2243–57. https://doi.org/10.1016/j.neubiorev.2013.04.005. Epub 2013 Apr 25
57. Bherer L. Cognitive plasticity in older adults: effects of cognitive training and physical exercise. Ann N Y Acad Sci. 2015 Mar;1337:1–6. https://doi.org/10.1111/nyas.12682.
58. Park SH, Han KS, Kang CB. Effects of exercise programs on depressive symptoms, quality of life, and self-esteem in older people: a systematic review of randomized controlled trials. Appl Nurs Res. 2014;27(4):219–26. https://doi.org/10.1016/j.apnr.2014.01.004. Epub 2014 Jan 30
59. Latimer-Cheung AE, Pilutti LA, Hicks AL, Martin Ginis KA, Fenuta AM, MacKibbon KA, Motl RW. Effects of exercise training on fitness, mobility, fatigue, and health-related

quality of life among adults with multiple sclerosis: a systematic review to inform guideline development. Arch Phys Med Rehabil. 2013;94(9):1800-1828.e3. https://doi.org/10.1016/j.apmr.2013.04.020. Epub 2013 May 10
60. Cassilhas RC, Tufik S, de Mello MT. Physical exercise, neuroplasticity, spatial learning and memory. Cell Mol Life Sci. 2016;73(5):975–83. https://doi.org/10.1007/s00018-015-2102-0. Epub 2015 Dec 8
61. Allred RP, Maldonado MA, Hsu And JE, Jones TA. Training the "less-affected" forelimb after unilateral cortical infarcts interferes with functional recovery of the impaired forelimb in rats. Restor Neurol Neurosci. 2005;23(5–6):297–302. PMID: 16477091
62. Lang CE, Macdonald JR, Reisman DS, Boyd L, Jacobson Kimberley T, Schindler-Ivens SM, Hornby TG, Ross SA, Scheets PL. Observation of amounts of movement practice provided during stroke rehabilitation. Arch Phys Med Rehabil. 2009 Oct;90(10):1692–8. https://doi.org/10.1016/j.apmr.2009.04.005.
63. Morawietz C, Moffat F. Effects of locomotor training after incomplete spinal cord injury: a systematic review. Arch Phys Med Rehabil. 2013;94(11):2297–308.
64. Kattenstroth JC, Kalisch T, Peters S, Tegenthoff M, Dinse HR. Long-term sensory stimulation therapy improves hand function and restores cortical responsiveness in patients with chronic cerebral lesions. Three single case studies. Front Hum Neurosci. 2012 Aug 25;6:244. https://doi.org/10.3389/fnhum.2012.00244.
65. Adkins DL, Boychuk J, Remple MS, Kleim JA. Motor training induces experience-specific patterns of plasticity across motor cortex and spinal cord. J Appl Physiol. 2006;101:1776–82. https://doi.org/10.3389/fnhum.2012.00244. eCollection 2012
66. Pascual-Leone A, Nguyet D, Cohen LG, Brasil-Neto JP, Cammarota A, Hallett M. Modulation of muscle responses evoked by transcranial magnetic stimulation during the acquisition of new fine motor skills. J Neuro-Oncol. 1995;74:1037–45.
67. Butler AJ, Page SJ. Mental practice with motor imagery: evidence for motor recovery and cortical reorganization after stroke. Arch Phys Med Rehabil. 2006;87(12 Suppl 2):S2–11. PMID: 17140874
68. Davis R, Sanborn C, Nichols D, Bazett-Jones DM, Dugan EL. The effects of whole body vibration on bone mineral density for a person with a spinal cord injury: a case study. Adapt Phys Activity Q. 2010;27(1):60–72.
69. Herrero AJ, Menéndez H, Gil L, Martín J, Martín T, García-López D, et al. Effects of whole-body vibration on blood flow and neuromuscular activity in spinal cord injury. Spinal Cord. 2011;49(4):554–9.
70. Menéndez H, Ferrero C, Martín-Hernández J, Figueroa A, Marín PJ, Herrero AJ. Acute effects of simultaneous electromyostimulation and vibration on leg blood flow in spinal cord injury. Spinal Cord. 2016;54(5):383–9.
71. Ness LL, Field-Fote EC. Effect of whole-body vibration on quadriceps spasticity in individuals with spastic hypertonia due to spinal cord injury. Restor Neurol Neurosci. 2009;27(6):621–31.
72. Felter C. Curr Phys Med Rehabil Rep. 2017;5:99. https://doi.org/10.1007/s40141-017-0155-8.
73. Rejc E, Angeli C, Harkema S. Effects of lumbosacral spinal cord epidural stimulation for standing after chronic complete paralysis in humans. PLoS One. 2015;10(7):e0133998. https://doi.org/10.1371/journal.pone.0133998. eCollection 2015
74. Angeli CI, Edgerton VR, Gerasimenko YP, Harkema SJ. Altering spinal cord excitability enables voluntary movements after chronic complete paralysis in humans. Brain. 2014;137(Pt 5):1394–409. https://doi.org/10.1093/brain/awu038. Epub 2014 Apr 8
75. Minassian K, Hofstoetter US. Spinal cord stimulation and augmentative control strategies for leg movement after spinal paralysis in humans. CNS Neurosci Ther. 2016;22:262–70. https://doi.org/10.1111/cns.12530.
76. Lai B, Young HJ, Bickel CS, Motl RW, Rimmer JH. Current trends in exercise intervention research, technology, and behavioral change strategies for people with disabilities: a scoping review. Am J Phys Med Rehabil. 2017 Oct;96(10):748–61. https://doi.org/10.1097/PHM.0000000000000743.

77. Hortobágyi T, Lesinski M, Gäbler M, VanSwearingen JM, Malatesta D, Granacher U. Effects of three types of exercise interventions on healthy old adults' gait speed: a systematic review and meta-analysis. Sports Med. 2015 Dec;45(12):1627–43. https://doi.org/10.1007/s40279-015-0371-2.
78. Recio AC, Stiens SA, Kubrova E. Curr Phys Med Rehabil Rep. 2017;5:108. https://doi.org/10.1007/s40141-017-0158-5.
79. Bonini-Rocha AC, Andrade ALS, Moraes AM, Gomide Matheus LB, Diniz LR, Martins WR. Effectiveness of circuit-based exercises on gait speed, balance and functional mobility in people affected by stroke: a meta-analysis. PM R. 2017;pii:S1934-1482(17)31386-2. https://doi.org/10.1016/j.pmrj.2017.09.014. [Epub ahead of print]
80. Tatara AM, Lipner JH, Das R, Kim HM, Patel N, Ntouvali E, Silva MJ, Thomopoulos S. The role of muscle loading on bone (re)modeling at the developing enthesis. PLoS One. 2014;9(5):e97375. https://doi.org/10.1371/journal.pone.0097375. eCollection 2014
81. Fineberg DB, Asselin P, Harel NY, Agranova-Breyter I, Kornfeld SD, Bauman WA, Spungen AM. Vertical ground reaction force-based analysis of powered exoskeleton-assisted walking in persons with motor-complete paraplegia. J Spinal Cord Med. 2013 Jul;36(4):313–21. https://doi.org/10.1179/2045772313Y.0000000126.

Index

B. Greenberg (ed.), *Myelopathy*, https://doi.org/10.1007/978-3-030-99906-3

GPSR Compliance

The European Union's (EU) General Product Safety Regulation (GPSR) is a set of rules that requires consumer products to be safe and our obligations to ensure this.

If you have any concerns about our products, you can contact us on ProductSafety@springernature.com

In case Publisher is established outside the EU, the EU authorized representative is:

Springer Nature Customer Service Center GmbH
Europaplatz 3
69115 Heidelberg, Germany

Batch number: 10732090

Printed by Printforce, the Netherlands